UNDERSTANDING EMERGING EPIDEMICS: SOCIAL AND POLITICAL APPROACHES

ADVANCES IN MEDICAL SOCIOLOGY

Series Editor: Barbara Katz Rothman

Series Editor for Volumes 5–6: Gary L. Albrecht

Series Editor for Volumes 7–8: Judith A. Levy

Recent Volumes:

ADVANCES IN MEDICAL SOCIOLOGY   VOLUME 11

UNDERSTANDING EMERGING EPIDEMICS: SOCIAL AND POLITICAL APPROACHES

EDITED BY

ANANYA MUKHERJEA

City University of New York

United Kingdom – North America – Japan
India – Malaysia – China

Emerald Group Publishing Limited
Howard House, Wagon Lane, Bingley BD16 1WA, UK

First edition 2010

British Library Cataloguing in Publication Data
A catalogue record for this book is available from the British Library

ISBN: 978-1-84855-080-3
ISSN: 1057-6290 (Series)

Awarded in recognition of
Emerald's production
department's adherence to
quality systems and processes
when preparing scholarly
journals for print

INVESTOR IN PEOPLE

CONTENTS

v

LIST OF CONTRIBUTORS

Frederick Attenborough	Department of Geography, Loughborough University, Loughborough, UK
Kathryn Burrows	Department of Sociology, Rutgers University, New Brunswick, NJ, USA
William D. Cabin	Richard Stockton College of New Jersey, Pomona, NJ, USA
Fernando Dias de Avila-Pires	Tropical Medicine Department, Oswaldo Cruz Institut, Rio de Janeiro; Human Ecology and Health Group, Federal University of Santa Catarina, Florianópolis, Brasil
Shari L. Dworkin	Department of Social and Behavioral Sciences, University of California, San Francisco, CA, USA
Maya K. Gislason	Department of Sociology, School of Law, Politics & Sociology, University of Sussex, Brighton, UK
Márcia Grisotti	Sociology and Political Science Department/Human Ecology and Health Group, Federal University of Santa Catarina, Florianópolis, Brasil
Hanna Grol-Prokopczyk	Department of Sociology, University of Wisconsin-Madison, Madison, WI, USA
Alana J. Hermiston	Department of Sociology, Trent University, Ontario, Canada
Mike Jolley	Department of Sociology, CUNY Graduate Center, New York, NY, USA

Sara Kuppin	Independent Scholar, New York, NY, USA
Antonio Maturo	Università di Bologna, Bologna, Italy
Ananya Mukherjea	Sociology and Women's, Gender, and Sexuality Studies, CUNY College of Staten Island, Staten Island, NY, USA
Tinaz Pavri	Department of Political Science, Spelman College, Atlanta, GA, USA
Victor W. Perez	Department of Sociology and Criminal Justice, University of Delaware, Newark, DE, USA
Thomas Rotnem	Political Science and International Studies, Southern Polytechnic State University, Marietta, GA, USA
Danae Roumis	Independent Scholar, Boston, MA, USA
Jeffrey Shantz	Criminology, Kwantlen Polytechnic University, British Columbia, Canada
Daniel Skinner	Political Science, Ramapo College of New Jersey, Mahwah, NJ, USA
Deborah A. Sullivan	School of Social and Family Dynamics, Arizona State University, AZ, USA
Manuel Vallée	Sociology Department, University of California, Berkeley, CA, USA

ACKNOWLEDGMENTS

I would like to acknowledge all the efforts of Series Editor Barbara Katz Rothman and of Zoe Sanders and the other staff at Emerald who have worked on this volume and facilitated its production. I am also grateful for the generous feedback and support for this project that I received from Arunava Mukherjea and Jeffrey Bussolini.

INTRODUCTION

The concept of the emerging epidemic can evoke many different responses, but it is a major topic of our time, garnering attention in scholarship across the sciences, social sciences, and humanities, in the mass media, and in popular fiction and films. There is a designated journal and multiple study centers devoted to understanding, monitoring, and ultimately defeating emerging epidemics. Regardless of the venue, however, emerging epidemics create a great deal of popular fear, and they symbolize the continuing (and new) vulnerabilities of our late modern age. The contributors to this volume attempt to put this significance in context, offering critical, historical, structural, social constructionist, ecological, and political economic perspectives on the concept altogether or on specific epidemics. These authors deeply consider the knowledge we make of emerging epidemics and the meaning that knowledge has in our lives. Throughout this volume, social and economic justice and the representation of the needs of politically marginalized groups are matters of particular concern.

The first part of the volume comprises three chapters that examine epidemics in local context. Shantz and Roumis focus on *relatively* small areas that serve diverse functions – Toronto during the SARS crisis, and the response to malaria in the Ngorongoro Conservation Area, Tanzania – while Pavri and Rotnem provide an international comparison of the HIV/AIDS epidemics in India and Russia – large, multicultural, and dynamic nations that share some patterns of political change and economic growth.

Next Grisotti and Dias de Avila-Pires unpack the history and the definition of the term "emerging epidemics," using case studies from Costa Rica and Brazil to illustrate their discussion. Gislason, Dworkin, and Mukherjea offer political and historical accounts of three longstanding epidemics that, in "emerging," have created social or moral panic. Gislason shows that the information presented about West Nile Virus on the Public Health Agency of Canada's Web site is produced through a series of negotiations of power, knowledge-making processes, and disciplinary techniques reflected in Canadian society and elsewhere. Dworkin's chapter uses Vietnam's response to its HIV/AIDS epidemic as a case study to illuminate how several governments have responded to the emerging and concentrated phases of their own HIV/AIDS epidemics and to underscore important questions to be addressed in policy making. Mukherjea locates pandemic influenza within the history of the 20th and young 21st centuries and questions what insights this history might offer as to how preventative public health and disaster preparedness programs can, or ideally should, work and complement each other.

In the third part, Skinner, Cabin, Attenborough, and Perez take on the thorny questions of rhetoric, categorization, and epistemology. They apply these questions to the medicalization of male circumcision in the United States (Skinner), to the growing issue of developing home care policy in response to what appears to be an emerging Alzheimer's epidemic (Cabin), to the wily scientific history of the 2003 SARS epidemic (Attenborough), and to the political processes behind the determination that there is such a thing as a new autism epidemic (Perez).

Part IV considers the limits (and their breaching) of the uses of an "emerging epidemic" model, specifically with respect to psychiatric disorders and social control. Maturo and Burrows offer two different social constructionist critiques of understanding bipolar disorder as an epidemic condition. While the two authors are largely in agreement, Maturo focuses on the increasing medicalization of mood overall while Burrows addresses the difficulty of accurately counting cases and their increase. Both authors examine the nebulous and shifting process of diagnosing bipolar disorder. Kuppin and Vallée apply these same questions to depression and attention deficit disorder and ask, as well, what the repercussions are when these conditions are considered growing epidemics. Jolley looks at the epidemic as metaphor and as a reified category in his chapter on the history of youth deviance being pointed out as a particularly troubling and growing phenomenon, as linked to the nature of being young itself, and as "diseased" and "contagious."

The book is completed by a part devoted to obesity as a case study of different ways of understanding the uses of "epidemic" as a concept loaded with multiple meanings. Deborah A. Sullivan, Hanna Grol-Prokopczyk, and Alana Hermiston look at this issue from three perspectives. Sullivan considers what structural, economic, and behavioral trends and patterns are contributing to the obesity epidemic, how these factors intersect with other modes of social power (such as class and race), and what constitutes an effective, or ineffective, response. Grol-Prokopczyk examines, historically and politically, how obesity came to be termed an epidemic at all and calls into question the uses and abuses of medicalizing overweight and obesity. Hermiston's social constructionist essay focuses on the conceptual elision in the developing medical understanding of obesity as a disease itself, especially as one seen to be "contagious."

Because obesity is widely and institutionally referred to as an epidemic and because this is a relatively recent designation and, further, because obesity differs in its nature from the infectious, psychiatric, or cognitive disorders discussed thus far in the volume, it offers a rich test case for the many questions of method, definition, power, knowledge, and public health put forth in the book overall. We hope these questions can shed light on the social significance of emerging epidemics and their effects on our lived experiences. That level of lived experience, of the welfare of individuals and communities, is where I would like to focus the reading and application of the chapters and ideas in this volume.

Ananya Mukherjea
Editor

PART I
POLITICAL ECONOMIC AND ECOLOGICAL MATTERS: GAGING THE IMPACT OF AN EPIDEMIC

CAPITALISM IS MAKING US SICK: POVERTY, ILLNESS AND THE SARS CRISIS IN TORONTO

Jeffrey Shantz

ABSTRACT

Purpose – *For much of the first half of 2003 world attention was captured by news of a mysterious but deadly virus that was claiming lives in places as distant as Toronto and Beijing. In a matter of months there were around 8,000 infections and over 689 deaths related to severe acute respiratory syndrome (SARS). In my hometown, Toronto, 43 people died of SARS during the outbreaks of 2003.*

Approach – *This chapter examines issues of class and poverty in emergence of SARS. The chapter begins with a discussion of the political economy of the emergence of SARS, and its relation to the spread of the virus. It then discusses issues of public policy, and particularly neo-liberal cuts to social services and public spending, that set the stage for the SARS outbreak, influenced its impact and contributed to the failures of response in Ontario.*

Findings – *Through analysis of the lack of social resources available to working people in the province and the prioritizing of corporate, particularly tourism industry, concerns, the chapter illustrates how issues of class underpinned public responses to SARS, exacerbating problems.*

Understanding Emerging Epidemics: Social and Political Approaches
Advances in Medical Sociology, Volume 11, 3–18
Copyright © 2010 by Emerald Group Publishing Limited
All rights of reproduction in any form reserved
ISSN: 1057-6290/doi:10.1108/S1057-6290(2010)0000011005

The chapter concludes by giving attention to the need for social solidarity and community mutual aid.

Contributions to the field – *The chapter shows the extent to which neo-liberal governments prioritize business security above the health and social security of workers and reveals some of the ways in which the pressures of capitalist social relations make people ill.*

INTRODUCTION

For much of the first half of 2003 world attention from Hong Kong to Geneva was captured by news of a mysterious but deadly virus, similar to pneumonia, that was claiming lives in places as distant as Toronto and Beijing. As accounts of the virus' growing toll became regular occurrences by February, severe acute respiratory syndrome (SARS) became part of the global lexicon. In a matter of months there were around 8,000 infections and over 689 deaths related to SARS. In my hometown, Toronto, 43 people died of SARS during the outbreaks of 2003.

The recent outbreaks of SARS in Toronto shone a harsh light on the inadequacies and outright failures of neo-liberal public health policies and practices. They also showed clearly the extent to which neo-liberal governments prioritize business security above the health and social security of workers. Even more than this, however, the SARS crises revealed some of the ways in which the pressures of capitalist social relations make people ill.

Public health officials first received warnings of SARS in early February and a full-blown crisis was emerging by March. By late April Ontario's Conservative (Tory) Premier of the day, Ernie Eves, had not even recalled the legislature, which had been on hiatus since Christmas, to devise a plan for dealing with the various aspects of the crisis. For weeks the Conservative plan appeared to consist of little more than suggestions to 'wash your hands' or 'continue to eat in Chinatown'. Governments only responded, and even then largely in terms of public relations, after the embarrassment of the late-April World Heath Organization (WHO) travel advisory and the threat of losses for tourist industry owners.

Even worse, the provincial government's rush to assure tourists that the crisis was over following the WTO advisory seems to have played a major part in a renewed outbreak during the end of May. The nurses' unions reported publicly that prior to the second outbreak their warnings to the government that it was too soon to let up on SARS went unheeded

(Boyle & Mallan, 2003; Diebel, 2003). Clearly public relations, rather than public health, were at the forefront of Conservative concerns.

This chapter examines issues of class and poverty in emergence of SARS. These issues are also examined in relation to the public response to SARS in Toronto. Issues of poverty and illness are crucial in addressing emerging epidemics, especially in the global age in which diseases can travel the globe in hours rather than years. The chapter begins with a discussion of the political economy of the emergence of SARS, and its relation to the spread of the virus. It then discusses issues of public policy, and particularly neo-liberal cuts to social services and public spending, that set the stage for the SARS outbreak, influenced its impact and contributed to the failures of response in Ontario. Through analysis of the lack of social resources available to working people in the province and the prioritizing of corporate, particularly tourism industry, concerns, the chapter examines how issues of class underpinned public responses to SARS, exacerbating problems. The chapter concludes by giving attention to the need for social solidarity and community mutual aid in a context of emerging epidemics within capitalist globalization and questions why diseases and illnesses impacting poor people have received less attention and fewer resources than those largely impacting members of the global tourist classes.

SARS, ECOLOGY AND CAPITALIST POVERTY

In May 2003, researchers with the WHO traced the emergence of SARS to the Dongyuan market cages where various animal species, including threatened and endangered species, are regularly sold for human consumption. The SARS virus was found in six masked palm civets, a type of ferret that is served as food, as well as in a raccoon dog and a badger. Tens of thousands of civets are sold to restaurants in Guangdong each year.

Because of the poverty of market vendors, the markets are lacking proper facilities to maintain hygienic conditions. This along with the cramped quarters puts the animals under great stress, a condition that can activate coronaviruses. Such conditions also mean that it becomes more likely that viruses are passed to each other and to humans. These conditions make the markets susceptible to transfers of previously hidden viruses from animals to humans.

While experts went on to blame 'outdated farming practices' and over-population for the outbreaks of viral strains in China, the root cause is more likely poverty and the conditions of work that go along with poverty. Unfortunately analysts have not looked more closely at this crucial factor.

Of course SARS is only one example of viral outbreaks related to environmental destruction and the intersection of ecological damage and poverty. Many viruses that already exist in nature are beginning to emerge and turn up in humans as a result of deteriorating ecological conditions, especially deforestation. Ebola in Africa and the Nepa virus in Malaysia are only two examples. As humans come to occupy newly opened natural areas or expand into wilder areas, they come into contact with previously inaccessible pathogens or their natural hosts.

MAKING ONTARIO SUSCEPTIBLE: IMPACTS OF NEO-LIBERAL RESTRUCTURING

Health care in Canada operates in a complex space where federal and provincial mandates intersect. Health care is considered a provincial responsibility but the majority of funding is provided by the federal government through the national Medicare program. The federal Liberal government has instituted, over three consecutive majority terms beginning in 1993, a massive reduction of funding transfers to the provinces. Beginning in 1995 the federal government removed regulations covering health care transfers that had previously ensured the funding went directly to health care. This move meant that monies that had previously been earmarked specifically for health care could now be spent on any other area the provincial government deemed necessary. This left Ontario's governments free to apply $987 million in federal health transfer money to such areas as hydro cost overruns (Diebel, 2003, p. A8). Previously such moves would have been met with a financial penalty and a future loss of funds. This situation was compounded when former finance minister and former Prime Minister, Paul Martin, cut $6 billion from health care transfers to Ontario over four years between 1995 and 1999.

Most of the harm to Ontario's health care system has been inflicted by the provincial Progressive Conservative (Tory) government. SARS, like the Walkerton tragedy before it, which saw several people die and hundreds become sick after privatization and cuts to water inspection contributed to *E. coli* contamination of the town's drinking water, revealed the extent of the damage done to the health care system in Ontario by the Tories. When the Tories assumed power in 1995 under the leadership of Eve's predecessor

Mike Harris, they pursued a stated policy of creating a crisis in public services in order to encourage privatization and cutbacks. Harris withdrew $1.3 billion from hospitals to underwrite a policy of tax cuts for the wealthy and corporations (Diebel, 2003, p. A1). With regard to health care, Harris maintained that Ontario employed too many nurses and worked to reduce staffing levels by laying off thousands of nurses. Between 1995 and 1999, 25,000 hospital positions were cut in Ontario (Diebel, 2003, p. A8). In addition, much of nursing in the province was casualized with 50% of nurses working part-time, often holding down two or three jobs at separate hospitals. Only 18 months prior to the SARS outbreak the government fired five leading laboratory scientists who worked with a Toronto reference laboratory unit that monitored coming infections and new disease threats. 'Hospitals and public health units across Ontario relied on their work' (Toronto Star, 2003b, p. A9).

Under-funded and under-staffed infection surveillance and control in hospitals played a part in the spread of SARS. Contaminated medical equipment and improper hygiene, which have been identified as emerging problems in Ontario's hospitals, contributed to the progress of SARS (Nikiforuk, 2003, p. A23). The source of these problems resides partly in the privatization of such services in Ontario's hospitals since 1995. 'The evangelical search to save money in hospitals has also assisted and fortified microbes' (Nikiforuk, 2003, p. A23).

The provincial government also downloaded public health costs onto already cash-strapped municipalities in 1998. At the time of the SARS outbreak, less than 83% of what is required in public health services according to provincial standards is actually being delivered in Ontario (Diebel, 2003, p. A8). Despite the concerns raised by SARS, the funding level is still below necessary amounts. Much of the responsibility has been passed onto municipalities that lack the resources to cope properly. In Toronto, the public health department requires $5 million to reach a full complement of staff (Toronto Star, 2003a, p. F6). Due to budget constraints resulting from chronic under-funding by the provincial government, the department was short 65 workers around the time preceding, during and following the SARS outbreak. During the crisis people were pulled off of other programs to assist with SARS and health workers had to be brought to Toronto from other areas of the province.

The Tories' privatization of front-line health services played a major part in the province's inability to keep up with the SARS outbreak. Likewise cuts to health care put systems under greater strain and left fewer resources to pick up the extra work (resulting in delays for people requiring other services). Not only does Ontario's health care system have little or no room for 'surge capacity', the insurance against unexpected outbreaks or emergencies, but it also lacks adequate capacity to meet ongoing needs, a problem that persists to the present day. SARS was a relatively narrowly confined illness, affecting primarily health care workers and family members of SARS patients, which should have been quickly and easily contained. Unfortunately few Ontario hospitals have the necessary number of infection-control nurses, as outlined by provincial recommendations. The diminished state of Ontario's health care system, with inadequate facilities and staff levels for proper infection control, means that 'the spread of infections such as SARS is inevitable' according to the former chief of infectious diseases at Toronto's Hospital for Sick Children (quoted in Diebel, 2003, p. A8). This already untenable situation was exacerbated by the response to the outbreak which saw the closing of hospitals to all but the most serious cases and the cancellation of hundreds of operations. Several otherwise avoidable deaths during the crisis were attributed to delayed or canceled operations (Diebel, 2003). Clearly public health care in Ontario requires a substantial increase in resources.

RESTRICTED RESPONSES

During the SARS outbreak in Toronto, provincial health authorities attempted to control the outbreak by declaring a health emergency and implemented widespread restrictions on the non-urgent use of hospital-based procedures at each of the Greater Toronto Area's (GTA) 32 hospitals. Using a retrospective analysis of hospital admission data from the GTA prior to, during and after the SARS outbreak, two sets of investigators (Schull et al., 2007; Schabas, 2007) concluded that hospital restrictions resulted in only a modest decrease in the rate of admissions. Worse, hospital restrictions may have inhibited potentially seriously ill patients from seeking medical attention. Many people with serious conditions had surgeries canceled because hospitals were considered contaminated areas, and some of those people died. At three hospitals of the University Health Network, 1,050 surgical procedures were canceled as a result of SARS, including transplants, cancer and heart surgeries, hip and knee replacements and lens implants (Singer, 2007). As well, radiation, chemotherapy, dialysis physiotherapy and other treatments were canceled (Singer, 2007). Singer (2007) concludes that there may have been as many people who died from other illnesses who could not access hospitals as died from SARS.

In Toronto, thousands of people were placed in quarantine. Richard Schabas, Chief Medical Officer of Health for Hastings and Prince Edward Counties, argues that the use of quarantine during the SARS outbreak was ultimately ineffective as it is, counter to popular wisdom, in most infectious disease outbreaks. According to Schabas (2007) the practice not only wasted resources, but it also served to substantially heighten public anxiety and intolerance. Schabas concludes that SARS was not controlled through the use of quarantine but through the effective isolation of cases within the hospitals. Schabas (2007) argues that the experience of SARS makes clear that quarantine should have a very limited role in contemporary public health.

Singer (2007) suggests that restrictions of liberty, in the face of serious and imminent harm, must be relevant, legitimate and necessary, using the least restrictive methods reasonably available. It would appear that in the case of SARS in Toronto, these conditions were not met. Indeed they were not even approached. Singer (2007) also argues that society has a duty to ensure that those quarantined receive adequate care, are not kept in quarantine for unduly long periods and are not abandoned or psychosocially isolated. Again the experiences of quarantine in Toronto under SARS raise questions about the degree to which these obligations were fulfilled. While Singer (2007) also raises the need to eliminate economic barriers, such as income loss, that would prevent someone from following a quarantine order, it is quite clear that such economic supports were largely absent. Furthermore, restrictions were enacted against the informed analysis of front-line health workers.

These recent reports suggest strongly that dramatic measures used to address the outbreak, particularly quarantine, travel restrictions and the limiting of non-urgent use of hospital-based procedures, were largely ineffective, and more, even counter-productive. In fact, hospital restrictions may have inhibited patients who were ill with potentially serious illnesses from seeking medical attention. Schull et al. (2007) found that decreases in the admissions for serious acute conditions, such as gastrointestinal bleeding, heart attacks and pulmonary embolisms, were greater in the Toronto area, suggesting that people may have been inhibited from accessing specialized care.

Despite these conclusions, however, following the SARS outbreak, the Government of Canada passed the Quarantine Act of 2006 which strengthened the ability of health authorities to detain people believed to have been exposed to a communicable disease. In the view of government officials the legislation, and the imposition of travel restrictions, represents a major step forward in developing preparedness in the event of a widely anticipated influenza pandemic. Critics such as Dr. Schabas counter that both the SARS experience and the particular biology of influenza should raise significant warning signs about the use of quarantine and travel restrictions during an influenza pandemic. In his view, not only would the costs of trying to establish quarantine be enormous, but also a system seeking to restrict travel and quarantine air passengers would be threatened with a descent into chaos (Schabas, 2007). Schabas argues that national borders are not, and indeed, never have been, important lines of defense against infectious diseases. Yet it might be noted that the focus on detention and restrictions on mobility fit well with the broader emphasis on border controls and detention that have characterized Canadian social policy, particularly with regard to immigrant populations, since the terrorist attacks of 11 September 2001.

Rather, for Schabas, the proper defense is found in sanitation and hygiene, overall health and proper general medical care. Other factors, such as the ready availability of immunization, antibiotics and antiviral drugs, also play important parts. Yet it is precisely areas of sanitation, hygiene and access to regular and suitable medical care that have been weakened by almost two decades of neo-liberal governance in Ontario. Indeed, cuts to social spending for the poor and unemployed leaving thousands of families without proper diets and nutrition, declines in adequate social housing stocks, reduced health care expenditures and the shortage of family doctors in the province, as well as the lack of public coverage for pharmaceuticals all contribute to a context in Ontario in which the population is left more susceptible to broad health problems.

SARS AND WORK

The problems caused by the lack of public health resources were compounded by the failure of any level of government to compensate workers who had to go under quarantine and the failure to compensate anyone who was not quarantined but thought they had symptoms and should stay home from work. That this failure played a part in the spread of SARS in Toronto, and in the spread of panic over SARS, was highlighted when an infected nurse from Mount Sinai hospital took the inter-city commuter 'GO Train' and Toronto Transit Commission (TTC), urban rapid transit, to work on 14 and 15 April because she could not afford to miss.

By mid-June, the province had still failed to increase hospital resources and staff. At St. Michael's hospital 30 extra health care workers were required for SARS duty during the second outbreak. Even double-time wages were not enough to entice many workers to put themselves at risk given the inadequacies of resources that remained. A Ministry of Labour investigation during the outbreak found St. Michael's, as well as North York General, to be in violation of the Workplace Health and Safety Act for having provided inadequate equipment and training to nurses, including SARS masks that did not fit. The hospitals responded by threatening mandatory work to deal with the SARS cases. Finally, during the second outbreak, after weeks of serving stress-filled overtime shifts and suffering some of the city's highest infection rates, nurses, through their union, put forward a demand for 'danger pay'. No amount of danger pay could make up for the tragic fact that SARS left two nurses dead while making dozens more ill.

Incredibly, other hospitals responded by laying off nurses. Lakeridge Health Corporation laid off 15 registered practical nurses, including 11 who were in quarantine at the time. Premier Eves responded to criticisms about the firings by claiming it was part of the province's attempt to build a 'flexible system' that 'would be able to move resources as we need them within the health-care system' (quoted in Boyle & Mallan, 2003, p. A6). Indeed further layoffs were proposed as hospitals scrambled to make up a deficit of approximately $400 million. Of course the flexibilization of health care, a key aspect of Tory policy, had already placed the system in an extremely vulnerable position.

Singer (2007) suggests that under SARS Toronto health care workers were, for the first time in a generation, forced to weigh their obligations to care for the sick against serious and imminent health risks to themselves and their families. With dozens of medical workers, primarily nurses, contracting SARS, difficult choices confronted health care workers across the city in a context in which hospital administrations and the government only heightened the stress that those workers faced. Putting their lives at risk to help others, health care workers feared contagion for themselves and their families and being shunned by others who viewed them as potentially infectious (Singer, 2007). Many struggled with reduced human contact with sick and dying patients and the burdens imposed by cumbersome and uncomfortable equipment they were required to wear to protect themselves (Singer, 2007). Loss of work and disrupted work routines, without proper compensation or support, added to stress. Many more lost work as their hospitals restricted admissions.

Singer (2007) argues that, as health care workers have a duty to care, society and its institutions have a reciprocal duty to assist health workers. Policies in health care institutions should not penalize workers either financially, socially or emotionally. Workers must be compensated for loss of work on a dollar-for-dollar basis. As well information and support must be made available to workers, both so that they understand the risks they are facing and to ensure that their safety is regarded and protected as much as possible. None of these circumstances was adequately present during the SARS outbreak. Furthermore, health care workers' duty to care must be met by a mutual respect for their need to care for themselves, both as a human right and in order to ensure that they can properly carry out their work.

Institutions have an obligation to present clear guidelines so that workers know what is expected of them and what support and assistance they can expect (Singer, 2007). Workers must also be rewarded or penalized for following sensible practices such as staying home when they are sick. Singer (2007) suggests that rather than sending workers home when fewer staff are needed, better use of people's time and desire to help might be made in communicating with patients and their families by phone to help overcome the isolation and alienation felt when people are quarantined and loved ones have restricted access to each other.

Governments were also absent in offering assistance to workers suffering layoffs and reduced hours in industries, especially hospitality and tourism, negatively affected by SARS. As late as 27 May, Hotel Employees, Restaurant Employees (HERE) Local 75 was still requesting, unsuccessfully, meetings with federal Industry Minister Allan Rock and Human Resources Minister Jane Stewart. Local 75 president Paul Clifford noted: 'There has been no additional funds from senior levels of government directed towards hospitality workers. No EI [employment insurance] funds, no waiving of the two-week waiting period for EI, no relaxing of EI regulations and many workers and their families are going under' (quoted in McGran, 2003b, p. A6).

During the second outbreak more than 7,000 people were quarantined. Incredibly, compensation packages were still not made available. More than two months into the outbreak the federal Liberal government finally waived the two-week waiting period for claims. Unfortunately they did nothing to relax eligibility regulations, a factor which was particularly relevant given that many hospitality and restaurant workers are part-time and therefore not eligible to receive EI payments under the normally tight EI restrictions. As well it should be pointed out that EI payments do not cover full wages, even for the already lowly paid workers in hotel and restaurant industries. Similarly, nothing was forthcoming to assist tenants facing evictions or people unable to make utilities payments due to SARS layoffs or work cutbacks (Goosen, Pay, & Go, 2003).

SARS AND CIRCUSES: TOURISM AND TORONTO'S ECONOMIC AILMENTS

That each level of government was more concerned with helping tourist industry bosses rather than workers was clear in who received compensation or subsidy packages. Provincial money has come as subsidies to capital, especially those involved in entertainment industries such as Mirvish Entertainment (producers of such theatre spectacles as *The Lion King* and *Mama Mia*) and Rogers Communications (owners of the Toronto Blue Jays baseball team and notorious for not paying their cable installers). Exclusive restaurants and hotels also received subsidies.

For the most part the federal Liberal government, which precipitated the crises in health care by gutting health transfers to Ontario by $6 billion, offered such 'symbolic support' as holding a cabinet meeting at an exclusive Toronto hotel, to and from which they were chauffeured with great haste. Other responses were little more than gimmicks, including the proposal to pay the Rolling Stones $10 million in public money to put on a 'free' concert. Ironically this was the same amount as the total federal relief package to compensate laid-off and quarantined workers and affected small businesses.

Tourism in Toronto had been ill for some time before the SARS outbreak. A spokesperson for the TTC, which runs the city's subway and buses, noted that the TTC had experienced a general city-wide falloff in ridership prior to any word of SARS. This echoed independent research into TTC ridership declines and budget cuts (Munro, 2002).

Like the entertainment industry giants, however, the TTC was not about to lose an opportunity. Promoting downtown events among Torontonians, the Transit Commission urged residents to 'find out what it's like to be a tourist in your own town'. The TTC public address system broadcast messages from prominent Torontonians encouraging its 800,000 riders to 'wine, dine, entertain and shop in Toronto'. Suggestions for being a hometown tourist included, in a familiar vein, going to the theatre, trying a new restaurant and, incredibly, staying in a hotel. These 20-s messages were broadcast every 15 min in 69 subway stations. So again capital's cure for whatever ails you is 'go shopping'. This was, of course, reminiscent of George W. Bush's plea for Americans to go shopping after 9–11.

SARS simply provided a fortuitous cover for governments at all levels to obscure the relation of government policies, and the whims of investors and speculators, to economic troubles in Ontario. In fact, manufacturing and retail are vastly more significant aspects of Toronto's economy that have suffered from changes in global economies and government bungling.

Two key factors behind recent economic concerns have received almost no mention: the Canadian dollar and rising electricity costs. The dollar's increase in value has played a far greater part in the tourism drop-off than SARS and has also affected demand in the United States, which takes 85% of Canadian exports. The dollar surged from a record low of 62.1 cents (US) in January to a six-year high of 74 cents (US) in May. The Tory deregulation of utilities has resulted in a doubling of electricity costs for many companies, raising costs to twice the levels in Quebec.

SOME SURGERY REQUIRED

Anger over the Tories' part in mishandling the outbreak, as part of their larger mismanagement of services, played a part in the provincial elections at the end of 2003. The Tories suffered a devastating loss as the provincial Liberals captured one of the largest majorities in Ontario's history. Tellingly, Premier Eves (now former Premier) canceled two prior election announcements, including one that had been planned for the week in which the second outbreak occurred, lest the election become a referendum on Tory health care policies. Anger over the Tory bungling of the SARS crisis was still running high, extending into their support base among suburban consumers in the regions surrounding Toronto, at the time of October's election and likely contributed to the loss of several key Tory ridings in the city's suburbs. Notably, health minister Clement, a major figure in the party, was among the casualties.

Now into a second term, the provincial Liberal government has failed to maintain its election commitment to restore funding and resources to Ontario's health care system. This is probably not too surprising given the actions of the federal Liberals to undermine medical care in Canada over the last decade. Indeed the provincial Liberals, upon taking office, broke their promise to end a private–public hospital venture.

SOLIDARITY AND HEALTH: AN ALTERNATIVE GLOBALIZATION

Infectious diseases can now travel the globe quickly, in a matter of hours rather than years. In a globalized world the need for solidarity becomes crucial (Singer, 2007). This has long been a central theme of the alternative globalization movements that have emerged to mobilize for a globalization of social justice, fairness and equality rather than a globalization of 'free trade', markets and economic exploitation. Solidarity means working on the basis of mutual aid and support with others who are less powerful, wealthy or healthy (Singer, 2007). A key challenge of the global era is to understand and address the complex interconnections between globalization and health and to develop ways to overcome global health inequalities in different regions (Singer, 2007). Some of the instability and indeed trauma of globalization might be lessened through the nurturing of a global health ethic of solidarity. Health impacts are felt far more severely and do greater damage in poor, rural areas, but diseases can spread to wealthier, urban areas, as SARS showed, so those in wealthier centers have a self-interested, rather than purely compassionate, reason for developing an ethic of solidarity in dealing with health issues. Health, in privileged nations, is linked with health, or the lack of health, in poorer nations, especially as distinctions between domestic and foreign policy become blurred in the global age (Singer, 2007). Addressing this will, of course, require significant socio-political shifts.

As Singer (2007) suggests, along with solidarity we need transparency, honesty and good communication over health issues at global levels. Information sharing becomes a crucial part of ensuring the public good globally. This may involve the development of new governance mechanisms, and should, as alternative globalization advocates have argued, be carried out as part of a democratization process that includes greater citizen involvement in national as well as global governance. One example might include citizen fora and community panels, and transnational community organizations which bring together grassroots community members to share information and resources. This would involve the participation of health care workers but also unionists and workers in relevant industries such as food production, bringing people together across borders to share ideas and material resources that might allow for a restructuring of work and subsistence such that the causal conditions behind major outbreaks are avoided or lessened. It is not coincidental that SARS and, more recently,

H1N1 have roots in farming practices within conditions of poverty and insufficient resources. Other example would include the inclusion of health care workers and their union representatives within community policy panels.

Health must be viewed as a global public good, despite being treated nationally, regionally or locally (Singer, 2007). Local action and global action must be connected and coordinated. National governments cannot hide health information that might serve to protect others (Singer, 2007). Neo-liberal governance and the increased marketization of health care and food production, within multinational corporate contexts, have served to privatize health care and environmental regulations precisely at a time when private issues have globally public consequences. At the same time the neo-liberal emphasis on individualized health care and decreases to public welfare leave growing numbers of people susceptible to harm, without adequate resources to care for themselves and their communities.

Solidarity will mean addressing infrastructural needs globally. This will include the development of suitable public health laboratories, information systems, health communication capabilities, data gathering, storage and analysis capacities and epidemiological capacities (Singer, 2007). There is also a need to develop response capacities to deal with outbreaks, especially within poorer countries. This includes training in public health and an influx of resources to ensure health workers are properly deployed (Singer, 2007).

BEYOND SARS: THE HIDDEN ILLNESSES OF CLASS

The frantic, if inadequate, attention given to SARS, by both media and governments, highlights other class-related issues in Canadian health care. Other recent outbreaks in Toronto, such as tuberculosis, Norwalk virus and Hepatitis A, have received less attention because there is a sense among governments that these diseases are confined to poor and homeless populations and not likely to spread to the population at large. SARS had such impact because it affected suburbanites, consumers and, potentially, tourists.

Street nurses, those trained nurses who devote themselves to assisting homeless and street-involved individuals and tending to their many health issues, Crowe and Hardill (2003) note that the TB outbreak in Toronto shelters in 2001 was predicted by front-line health workers as early as 1994; yet the city and province did nothing to change the conditions – overcrowding and poor shelter conditions, lack of affordable housing and community-based programs such as drop-in centers and unsatisfactory nutrition – that allow for the spread of such illnesses. Horribly, three homeless people died of consumption in Canada's richest city in 2001 (Crowe & Hardill, 2003). Almost 40% of shelter residents have been exposed to TB (Crowe & Hardill, 2003).

The conditions that underlie the spread of TB are really the same as those that underlie the spread of SARS: the insecurity of capitalist economics which forces people to spend much of their lives working for wages lest they face the consequences of homelessness and hunger. Many workers know that they are a paycheck away from being homeless and too many of us are faced with the decision to pay the rent or feed the kids. Lack of access to and control over the necessities of life, which are owned and controlled by various profit-seeking bosses, and the forced compulsion to work to survive undermine the capacities of individuals and communities to make their health a priority.

As Crowe and Hardill (2003) affirm, 'food, income, safety and housing protect people's health. Simply stated, housing is protection from disease'. A guaranteed income might provide the same protection. Clearly a broad-based program for community health would include not only increased funding for public health departments, but also more affordable housing, improved conditions in shelters, nutrition programs, a minimum wage increase to a living wage level and increased welfare rates (or better a guaranteed income).

SARS, and the social response to it, brought together many of these crucial issues. It showed fundamentally and often starkly that emerging epidemics are about political economy as much as anything. SARS brought to the fore relations of inequality, power, poverty, democracy and governance and the distribution of resources within capitalist societies such as Canada in the global period. It showed that relations of power and inequality are central in giving rise to epidemics but also in inhibiting the capacities of people, such as health care workers, to respond adequately, despite their often heroic efforts. Even advanced health care systems are imperiled by persistent disparities in wealth and access to resources and decision-making processes. These are lessons that must still be learned and acted upon in light of ongoing threats of emerging epidemics in the current period. As more people are negatively impacted through economic crisis, and as economic 'recovery' programs retrench neo-liberal policies and re-distribute public resources to private capital, the lessons of SARS, and its social underpinnings, press even more forcefully upon us.

REFERENCES

Boyle, T., & Mallan, C. (2003). Quarantined nurses laid off by hospitals. *Toronto Star*, June 12, pp. AI, A6.
Crowe, C., & Hardill, K. (2003). What would nightingale say? *Toronto Star*, April 24.
Diebel, L. (2003). 10 questions for a SARS inquiry. *Toronto Star*, June 8, pp. A1, A8.
Goosen, T., Pay, C., & Go, A. (2003). Healing the scars in post-SARS Toronto. *Toronto Star*, May 19.
McGran, K. (2003). Toronto's economic worries flood back. *Toronto Star*, May 27, p. A6.
Munro, S. (2002). *Transit's lost decade: How paying more for less is killing public transit.* Toronto: Toronto Environmental Alliance.
Nikiforuk, A. (2003). Why hospitals can be bad for your health. *Toronto Star*, May 6, p. A23.
Schabas, R. (2007). Is the quarantine act relevant? *Canadian Medical Association Journal*, *176*(13), 1840–1842.
Schull, M. J., Stukel, T. A., Vermeulen, M. J., Zwarenstein, M., Alter, D. A., Manual, D. G., Guttmen, A., Laupacis, A., & Schwartz, B. (2007). Effect of widespread restrictions on the use of hospital services during and outbreak of severe acute respiratory syndrome. *Canadian Medical Association Journal*, *176*(13), 1827–1832.
Singer, P. (2007). *Ethics and SARS: Learning from the Toronto experience.* Toronto: Joint Centre for Bioethics, University of Toronto.
Toronto Star. (2003a). Lessons from SARS (3): Time to reinvest in public health. *Toronto Star*, June 28, p. F6.
Toronto Star. (2003b). Ill-planned cuts hurt SARS fight. *Toronto Star*, May 9, p. A9.

FALSE PERCEPTIONS AND *FALCIPARUM*: A POLITICAL ECOLOGY OF MALARIA IN THE NGORONGORO CONSERVATION AREA IN TANZANIA

Danae Roumis

ABSTRACT

Purpose – *This chapter aims to provide a cross-section of some social, political, cultural, and economic factors that contribute to the conditions of illness, specifically malaria, in an area of Tanzania where both land and population have been marginalized to varying degrees over time. It also suggests the relevance of such considerations in the planning and implementation of public health interventions in the region.*

Methodology/approach – *This chapter elaborates upon a case study conducted by the author in the Ngorongoro District in Tanzania in 2006. A political ecology framework is used to guide the discussion.*

Findings – *Malaria in the Ngorongoro Maasai community can be more fully understood by incorporating critical social science perspectives into health-related analyses, by allowing for a greater appreciation of the complex history behind current configurations of infrastructure and*

Understanding Emerging Epidemics: Social and Political Approaches
Advances in Medical Sociology, Volume 11, 19–41
Copyright © 2010 by Emerald Group Publishing Limited
All rights of reproduction in any form reserved
ISSN: 1057-6290/doi:10.1108/S1057-6290(2010)0000011006

sociopolitical interactions in the region. Assuming that equity is of concern, this appreciation can contribute to ensuring that all populations in the country have the opportunity to benefit from the public health momentum in Tanzania.

Contribution to the field – *Much attention is justifiably directed toward the social and economic consequences of infectious diseases in developing countries. Tanzania alone accounts for a large proportion of malaria cases and deaths worldwide. This chapter recognizes that malaria is one of the many elements in an ecological system continually integrating cues from nature and society, and uses that framework to demonstrate the importance of qualitative analysis in view of the copious international funding and assistance for control measures.*

INTRODUCTION

In recent years Tanzania has multiplied its efforts against endemic malaria, as one of the five countries that account for 50 percent of global malaria deaths and 47 percent of all malaria cases (RBM, 2008), and where 100 percent of the population is at risk (WHO, 2008). The dominant species in Tanzania, *Plasmodium falciparum*, is also the most deadly of the four human types. Much attention is thus rightfully directed toward the social and economic consequences of infectious diseases in such developing countries. For example, it has been estimated that Africa loses about US$ 12 billion annually in direct and indirect costs due to malaria and that malaria constrains economic growth by an average of 1.3 percent annually (RBM, 2007). However, the socioeconomic and political determinants of such diseases are often overlooked, underestimated, or misunderstood. Malaria is not the result of a linear or static process, but is one of the many elements in an ecological system continually integrating cues from nature and society. As such, critical perspectives on intervention must accompany efforts to prevent, control, and eradicate it. This chapter discusses the sociopolitical preconditions of illness, specifically malaria, in an area of Tanzania where both land and population have been marginalized in different ways over time, and suggests the relevance of such considerations in the design and implementation of current public health interventions in the region.

The specific situation of malaria in the Ngorongoro Conservation Area (NCA) in northern Tanzania sheds light on a discrepancy between policy goals and reality – namely the inadequate services or opportunities provided to the human population in order to meet basic needs. This contradiction premises an inquiry into the contextual backdrop of the formulation and implementation of those policy goals. This chapter is not meant as a comprehensive review of the malaria prevention and control strategies or indicators in Tanzania, nor is it an ethnographic account of health and illness in this Maasai community. Rather, it is a case study of some characteristics of an epidemic among a particular population, which draws links to the environment and the country more broadly. It begins with an overview of malaria in Ngorongoro and a background of the ecological relationship between Maasai pastoralism and the Ngorongoro lands. It then continues with a historical account of the ideological paradigms, and actions taken thereof, that have shaped land use and management objectives over the past several decades in the Ngorongoro District. This section is guided by a few key points, including the ways that ideological paradigms have fed into policy formulation, misrepresentating of socioeconomic and ecological realities "on the ground" in the NCA, and some effects on Maasai self-sufficiency and the increased burden of malaria of successive interventions built upon these paradigms. The current management configuration is then discussed, detailing heavy influence by international as well as domestic interests in conservation and tourism. The present and somewhat paradoxical reliance of conservation activity on the tourist industry, as well as the social and economic space that tourism occupies in the NCA, are highlighted as important factors in this discrepancy. While malaria, in times past, had not posed as serious a burden on the Maasai community due to their extensive mobility and the climatic characteristics of the Ngorongoro highlands, the present conditions under which the Maasai must negotiate socially, culturally, economically, and politically combined with a warming climate and continued encroachment of tourism and conservation infra-structure have contributed to an upsurge of malaria, as well as other diseases, among the Maasai community in the past few years.

MALARIA IN NGORONGO

The pages of the Endulen Hospital record books are brimming with malaria diagnoses, and compel the observer to wonder why, in a time of vast knowledge and constant innovation, the burden of a preventable and treatable disease has been intensifying for the Maasai in the NCA. The answer to this question transcends the epidemiological present, and involves an exploration of historically rooted management issues, their perceptual milieu, and their ecological consequences. Since the early 1900s, policies shaping the management of the Ngorongoro lands, including conservation policies, have had several adverse effects on the economic and social well-being of the Maasai who live there. Despite the fact that their well-being is listed as a core objective in the NCA mission statement, the Maasai residents face myriad hardships that include an escalating burden of disease. In order to initiate proper reparations, it is therefore necessary to explore the question of health outcomes as corollaries of mismanagement.

A case study of malaria prevention in the NCA was undertaken by the author in 2006 during five weeks of field research and observation, semi-structured interviews, and data collection at the Endulen Hospital, as well as semi-structured interviews in the villages in the Ngorongoro District. The Endulen Hospital is the only full hospital inside the conservation area, supplemented by a government clinic at the entrance gates, and comprises a catchment spread over approximately 830 ha of land area. In community interviews, malaria was identified as a prime concern with regard to accessing and affording adequate measures of prevention and treatment in light of a perceived escalating burden. According to the Maasai, their communities previously experienced a lesser burden of malaria due to climate in the chillier highlands, and a mobile lifestyle. However, as more pastoralists are forced to be sedentary in a warming highland climate, the burden of malaria has increased.

In the Ngorongoro setting, the Endulen Hospital records indicate an increasing burden of malaria but even then it is understated because numerous cases do not present to the hospital for reasons related to the difficulties of transportation and cost, home misdiagnosis, or other factors. For example, many of the distant villages rely on the hospital's outreach services for care, and episodes often occur between scheduled visits. Implementing an effective treatment policy at the Endulen Hospital also poses financial sustainability concerns. Coartem®, the artemisinin-based combination therapy (ACT) drug artemether–lumefantrine, is currently the first-line recommendation for Tanzania. But it costs about 10,000 Tanzanian shillings (about US$ 8[1]), which can amount to about 20 times more than a dose of Fansidar® (sulfadoxine/pyrimethamine), a second-line drug (Endulen Hospital Physician,[2] personal communication to author, 2006).[3] Second-line drugs become necessary only when treatment failure of first-line drugs is confirmed parasitologically by blood slide within 14 days of a patient initiating ACT (after 14 days first-line drugs may in most cases be tried again), or when active drug resistance is encountered (WHO, 2006). Hospital staff fear that a cost increase to patients would discourage purchase and/or adherence.

The recent World Malaria Report (WHO, 2008) reports on at-risk countries' malaria burden, vector and parasite profiles, stratification of risk, and control programs. These figures are crucial for assessing the type of health infrastructure, financing schemes, and breadth of resources needed to alleviate the disease burden in a given locality. However, the present study aims to illustrate that such measures do not always speak to the role of malaria in time and space with regards to the structural – that is, social, political, and economic – facilitators of the parasite's proliferation. In other words, alleviating the disease burden does not necessarily address its determinants, and calculations of resource requirements often fail to accurately identify barriers in implementation. Of course, one assumes that a population or community would be better off with a reduced malaria burden, but in order for such changes to truly last, the conditions under which the disease was facilitated (i.e., under which the parasite and vector's survival was accommodated) must also be mitigated. A sustainable control strategy calls for matched cogency toward the determinants of the disease and the nuances of intervention. Furthermore, tackling the determinants of a disease that disproportionately affects vulnerable populations targets the very conditions of vulnerability, namely the socioeconomic and political conditions related to poverty.[4]

The eradication of malaria in many parts of the developed world continues to serve as a great success story in the public health arena. Still, malaria has remained an unfortunate fact of life in places where structural prerequisites for successful control programs, including those that would target the aversion of drug resistance, are weak or missing. In this way, it is justified to focus on the most immediately effective forms of malaria control in areas where it is consistently causing illness, lower productivity, and other significant impacts. However, the focus on managing an epidemic by troubleshooting it should not overshadow the need to ensure durable social, economic, and political structures for sustaining favorable conditions for health and well-being. Furthermore, scientific knowledge about the parasite has been growing exponentially. Advancements in genomic research have been ongoing for years, while malaria vaccine trials in their second and third phases are already under way in many African countries including Tanzania. But public health indicators will not reflect such developments without structures in place to implement the technology properly and equitably.

Currently, owing to the limited capacity of the Endulen Hospital and the conservation regulations in the area, conditions relevant to subsistence and health for the Maasai residents are often insecure. Positioning the problems related to malaria control in the NCA in a sphere of ecological, historical, and socioeconomic perspectives imparts a view of the area as a space within which shifting interests in the lands and human population have fostered vulnerability – a predicament which is too often overshadowed by the geographical grandeur and romanticism ascribed to the NCA. The intention of such inquiry is to "direct attention away from the body to a wider range of external facts" where health is considered in terms of "its setting, and its conditions and constraints" (Lewis, 1993, p. 88). The infusion of critical perspectives does not undermine the role of biomedical interventions. Rather it embraces their potential and offers guidance about whether, when, and how they might be used appropriately by considering pressing needs in terms of longstanding contextual challenges.

POLITICAL ECOLOGY: A FRAMEWORK FOR LOOKING PAST THE SYMPTOMS

One must look deeper than the clinical symptoms that indicate an epidemic to delineate the interactions, activities, and conditions involved in everyday life that affect an individual's or a community's ability to maintain physical and social well-being. I use the definition put forth by anthropologist Arturo Escobar et al. (1999, p. 4) to introduce the political ecology framework that characterizes the following discussion:

> Defined as the articulation of biology and history, political ecology examines the manifold practices through which the biophysical has been incorporated into history – more accurately, in which the biophysical and the historical are implicated with each other .... Each articulation has its history and specificity and is related to modes of perception and experience, determined by social, political, economic, and knowledge relations, and characterized by modes of use of space, ecological conditions, and the like. It will be the task of political ecology to outline and characterize these processes of articulation and its goal to suggest potential articulations realizable today and conducive to more just and sustainable social and ecological relations.

This method of inquiry is particularly useful for investigating the way that history has influenced the current malaria situation in Ngorongoro as well as the available channels of remediation through which the Maasai must navigate. These channels at minimum comprise both local and national political structures as well as physical and environmental circumstances. In turn, these factors have the ability to either promote or imperil the security of both human and natural life.

At the same time, the influence of history must be recognized as a collective of human actions and interactions mediated and motivated by philosophies, ideologies, interests, objectives, and intentions. Particularly in this context, perception as a mediator plays a major role. In this study, the term denotes the conceptual construction of a subject, in contrast with a perspective informed by empirical observation, and implies an inconsistency between the two. Although tracing the influence of perception invariably involves a degree of subjectivity, this factor must not be ignored when it is of real, practical import. The permeation of perceptions into policy often facilitates their reproduction on the ground level, rendering policy-making a practice that can inaccurately define behavior instead of reasonably regulating it. For instance, colonial officials in the 1920s noted that Maasai were engaged in small-scale cultivation but dismissed it as strange and anomalous, as they firmly believed that pastoralists do not cultivate (Hodgson, 2001), rather than recognizing this as a last resort survival strategy in a time of herd fragility and food shortage. Subsequent bans on cultivation by regulatory authorities combined with other barriers to the acquisition of grain caused major subsistence problems for the Maasai. In these and other ways explicated below, perceptions have steadily worked within ideological paradigms to mask the ecological and socio-economic realities in the NCA. The political ecology framework allows the integration of a wide range of contextual factors that interact with the population in question and ultimately play a part in the persistence of the disease.

MAASAI PASTORALISM AND HEALTH IN ECOLOGICAL PERSPECTIVE

The NCA is made up of its landmark caldera, the largest intact in the world, along with mountainous highlands, forests and woodlands, depressions, swamps, streams and soda lakes, grassy pastures, and several volcanic peaks. Seasonal rainfall results in alternating periods of drought and heavy rain (Homewood & Rodgers, 1991). The NCA is also of archaeological significance due to its proximity to some of the most important remains of ancient humans, flora, and fauna. The diverse climate and topography make for an aesthetically unique and marvelous landscape, but also present a variety of challenges for its approximately 60,000 Maasai residents (UNESCO, 2007 estimate of Ngorongoro Maasai population).

Transhumant pastoralism is the primary productive system of the Maasai and as such is socially coded and culturally integrated into daily life (see

Galaty, 1977; Århem, 1985; Spear & Waller, 1993; Hodgson, 2001 for more ethnographic accounts of the Maasai). Transhumance is characterized by intervallic movement and settlement according to seasonal conditions. In the Ngorongoro lands, climatic fluctuations result in marked dry and wet seasons that correspond to Maasai patterns of movement across land as well as altitude. Altitudinal transhumance is perhaps the crux of successful pastoralism in this particular ecosystem. For the Maasai, the lowland plains make up the traditional home base and wet-season grazing lands while the highlands serve as dry-season and drought-period reserves. The transhumant resource allocation system allows pastures to recover properly from grazing pressures. The Maasai traditionally partition their communities by territorial sections and localities that determine grazing rights and parameters, a system conducive to moving large groups in search of water and grazing, while livestock signify food and economic security, confer wealth and status, serve as a medium of exchange, and represent social relationships (Århem, 1986). In this way economy and society are bound by their joint role in maintaining the ecological balance between humans, livestock, and the natural environment (Århem, 1981).

Furthermore, mobility confers protection to both humans and livestock against disease. The highlands are dry-season grazing grounds, but the Maasai prefer to live on the plains where "cattle thrive better and fatten quicker ... [and] Humans are less liable to bronchial trouble than in the damp, misty highlands, and because the waters are temporary, malaria usually presents little problems [sic]" (Ndaskoi, 2006, p. 10). Periodic movements avert parasite accumulation within homesteads (Homewood & Rodgers, 1991) and protect cattle from diseases such as malignant catarrhal fever (MCF), easily contractible from wildebeest. Where mobility is the central tenet of transhumant pastoralism and risk aversion, restrictions as are currently in place against habitation and grazing in the lowland Serengeti plains and designated areas in the NCA are fundamentally at odds with the extensive nature of pastoralism, and undermine its integrity as both a function of and contributor to a healthy environment.

Adaptation to the Ngorongoro environment also intermittently involves controlled burning of pasture as well as small-scale cultivation. Burning, typically carried out at the end of a season, confers additional assurance that grazing lands will recover for the next period of use by releasing nutrients in the soil to stimulate new growth. This practice also kills ticks and parasites (Århem, 1981) and reduces the habitat of the tsetse fly, the vector for trypanosomiasis (Homewood & Rodgers, 1991), which can affect both humans and livestock. Without controlled burning, the carrying capacity of the land can be reduced (Johnsen, 2000) by allowing wildfires and inedible grasses to spread. Although it has since been officially accepted as a way to monitor invasive species (UNESCO, 2007), the previous longstanding ban by conservation authorities on burning serves as an additional example of a policy driven by dogmatic perceptions, such as that burning is always destructive.

Maasai have intermittently engaged in small-scale cultivation in order to survive severe dry-climate conditions, and reconstitute their herds. Waller (1999) points out that cultivation can be an indicator of processes related to the struggle for resources and survival, especially in consideration of the population and their motivations. The climatic cycles of the Tanzanian highlands precipitate malaria transmission at particular points of the year (Jones et al., 2007). If cultivation is banned at the points when pastoralist production is already reduced, the results of food shortage can be dramatic. Droughts and famine followed by heavy rains, combined with economic hardship and difficulty accessing grain, are particular harbingers of an impending epidemic (Packard, 1984). In addition to posing general health risks, malnutrition increases susceptibility to the malaria parasite, and exacerbates the severity of infection, especially in vulnerable groups such as pregnant women and children under the age of five years. Therefore, the resilience of the Maasai both economically and against disease largely depends on the plasticity of subsistence activities in times of need. A systematic disregard of such coping strategies by restrictive conservation policies, which have already limited first-resort mobility practices, threatens to short-circuit the balance of Maasai pastoralism and the maintenance of health and well-being. It was recently reported that over 34,000 households in the Ngorongoro District faced a critical food shortage, with district officials calling for emergency food aid. This shortage follows a period of drought claimed as the worst in recent history impacting pastoralists in the area particularly, due to lack of pasture and water for their livestock (IPP Media, 2009). Drought not only affects food supply, but can also devastate herd size, forcing some families to become more sedentary and potentially less economically viable in a livestock-based economy.

MANAGING THE MAASAI AND DEFINING THE NGORONGORO CONSERVATION AREA

Historically, management of the NCA has been misinformed by an inaccurate assessment of the relationship between the land and its inhabitants. This exemplifies the importance of recognizing how knowledge and information is produced and used, especially in the context of devising strategies for disease prevention and control. As anthropologist Dorothy Hodgson (1999, p. 221) explains, "Part of the problem is the formulation of the problem itself, especially the image of pastoralists that shape how scholars, policy-makers and development practitioners understand the problems of pastoralists, and then design and implement development interventions to solve them." Several phases of management including colonial, post-independence, and modern periods illustrate this point.

Colonial authority obstructed proper transhumance by instituting boundaries and restrictions that were politically and economically expedient and neither ecologically nor socially sound. After arriving in the Ngorongoro lands in the 1890s, the Germans appropriated preferential land for European settlers, compacting the Maasai and their herds into a Reserve. When the British inherited the mainland called Tanganyika in the 1920s, they resumed these coercive approaches with multiplied vigor. Despite having undermined the sound resource allocation system by asserting indirect rule, the British proceeded to evaluate Maasai pastoralism without due regard to their interventions. For instance, they concluded that pastoralism caused land degradation by using as evidence the activity of livestock within the compact Reserve. The fusion of this opinion with strapping moral judgments gave way to a series of paternalistic management prescriptions: the 1925 Arusha District Annual Report, which had been written for reporting to central colonial authorities, states, "It is a commonly accepted dictum that the pastoralist is a stage behind the Agriculturalist in the process of evolution and development" (cited in Hodgson, 2001, p. 73), and that, "A nomadic pastoralist without any bounds governing his wandering and the wanderings of his herds will be a menace to active progress and can only induce chaos and lack of administrative control" (cited in Hodgson, 2001, p. 48). Ndaskoi (2006, p. 11) observes that the British "had wandered all the way from little England," highlighting the one-sided perception in the above assessment. Moreover, the perception of wandering diluted the strategy, methodology, and utility of transhumance – indeed it may have neglected to acknowledge any system at all. The Maasai were forced to acquire grazing and cattle-movement permits, to pay a development tax for which they seldom, if ever, received compensatory benefits, and to purchase access to water resources from European settlers. Colonial policies thus weakened the productive capacity of the pastoral system, and coerced a dependence on external administrative structures.

Then in 1951, the Serengeti National Park (SNP) was established, originally encompassing the expanse of the Ngorongoro lands. Perception shifted from a view of the land as an underutilized resource to one requiring rigorous, proactive protection, partly due to extensive hunting by colonialists. Since the notion of the national park was developed in the United States based on the Yellowstone model, some of its tenets were immaterial to the realities of the NCA. "The separation of nature and culture lied at the heart of Western concepts of environmental preservation. It was accepted that for wildlife to be preserved, special areas free from human habitation must be created" (McCabe, 2002, p. 66). Although regulations undermined traditional systems of environmental management and adaptive behavior, they were seen as part and parcel of a new mandate for conservation. The shift from Maasai Reserve to national park also signified the appropriation of land by the public administration, rendering any activity on the land either compliant or in violation of laws with misguided ecological foundation. Indeed there is much to be said for stringent environmental protections, especially in light of climate change and globalization. However, the Maasai were disturbed by the idea that conservation, as defined by Westerners, could only be carried out in the absence of human co-existence, and anti-conservation sentiments materialized.

Tensions and conflicts over the next few years led to the split of SNP into the plains section, which retained the name, and the remaining portion, the NCA. The NCA Ordinance of 1959 formally introduced the concept of multiple land use: "The Serengeti Committee of Enquiry, 1957, recommended that Ngorongoro Crater Highlands be made a special conservation unit, administered by the government, with the object of conserving water supplies, forest and pasture – primarily in the interests of man, but with due regard for the preservation of wild animal life" (Parliament of Tanganyika, 1959). Unfortunately, ensuing conservation policies, such as bans on controlled burning, effectively regarded neither the well-being of man nor the environment. The Maasai were subject to a process of marginalization that, in words, claimed to prioritize their interests. They were cloaked by a rhetoric that misrepresented their needs and afforded them narrow channels through which to communicate their concerns, or participate in healthy debate on conservation. For example, some Maasai claim that their system "conserves because it is a natural duty, it is conservation for its own sake" while outside conservationists do so because of its economic utility (Olenasha, Ole Seki, & Kaisoe, 2001). Also, the Maasai harbor a societal taboo against the consumption of wild meat, and hunt only occasionally, mostly against dangerous animals in defense of their herds. Likewise, the act of felling trees is laden with social meaning dictating reasonable limits for only direct and necessary use of the resources.

IMAGE, IDENTITY, AND INTERVENTION IN THE NGORONGORO CONSERVATION AREA

In 1961, Tanganyika became an independent nation, and in 1964 joined with the islands of Zanzibar to become the United Republic of Tanzania. In a modernizing Tanzania, anything that symbolized the past came under scrutiny and often under harsh pressure to transform. Julius Nyerere, Tanzania's first president, is credited with instituting what is often referred to as an African brand of socialism, which served as the foundation for subsequent countrywide interventions such as Ujamaa villagization. *Ujamaa*, meaning brotherhood, lent its name to the formal resettlement effort instituting cooperative villages meant to bring the nation's more than 120 ethnic groups into a common Tanzanian identity. Even under well-meaning intentions of unity and solidarity, villagization was not always implemented rationally:

> First, the boundaries of the Conservation Area are wholly arbitrary and meaningless in the context of pastoral land use. They cut right through social units and areas utilized for dry and wet season grazing by pastoralists living both inside and outside the conservation area ... Secondly, the village is an arbitrarily defined unit in the context of pastoral resource use. In actual practice, villages are grouped together in larger and loosely defined socio-economic units characterized by joint utilization of grazing land and salt licks. (Århem, 1981, p. 16)

Even by the time that the 1975 Village Act made villagization compulsory, many Maasai had registered for villages without actually moving, in order to benefit from the stock dipping stations. State perceptions of the fundamental inability of Maasai to reform were reinforced by their reaction to ecologically and socially inappropriate interventions. In the 1960s, tensions ran high and conflict – sometimes violent and on occasion resulting in the arrest of Maasai – ensued between Maasai communities and conservation area authorities.

At the same time, a government-commissioned campaign in the late 1960s, called Operation Dress-up, began to pressure the Maasai to abandon their traditional dress for modern clothing and participate in the development of the Tanzanian state in the name of "the eradication of ignorance, disease and poverty" (Schneider, 2006, p. 107). Maasai women were often denied medical treatment if they were dressed in traditional garments. This mindset relegated them as symbols of an obsolete past:

> The African elite who took power embraced the modernist narrative with its agenda of progress. For them, the Maasai represented all they had tried to leave behind, and persisted as icons of the primitive, the savage, the past. Thus, although Maasai people had undergone significant changes in their pastoralist production system during the colonial period, their image as pastoralists and its associations with traditionalism and primitivism obscured their changing realities. (Hodgson, 1999, p. 225)

The interventions of this period perpetuated images of the Maasai as exceptions – both the land they lived on and their way of life were peripheral in the overall scheme of the Tanzanian state, and were made to appear as if some quality of innate conservatism justified their destitution. Indeed it reflects political scientist James Scott's (1998, p. 3) European model of statecraft in which "... social simplifications ... permitted a more finely tuned system of taxation and conscription [and] made possible quite discriminating interventions of every kind, such as public-health measures, political surveillance, and relief for the poor."

Also in the same period, the US Agency for International Development (USAID) initiated a US$ 23 million project, the Maasai Livestock and Range Development Project (MLRDP), in the attempt to improve the quality of livestock for the purpose of increasing yields in beef production. The underlying objective was to bring the Maasai into a productive system and economic scheme that was an assumed improvement upon their existing methods with little regard for the fact that beef production was not the bottom line of Maasai pastoralism. The Maasai, interested in the prospect of increased access to resources, concentrated around dams and water developments to defend these resources from migrant farmers, causing rapid degradation around the stations and counteracting the multiple land-use principles on which the NCA was based as well as the fundamental practices of transhumance. In 1979, the MLRDP was halted at the behest of President Nyerere, who feared that it was threatening the success of Ujamaa, while the overall failure of the MLRDP project was attributed to the Maasai.

The Maasai were labeled as inefficient and primitive when the colonizers were first appropriating land, and then were later deemed a threat to the conservation goals of the SNP. Once the NCA was established, their interests were defined disproportionately by non-Maasai charged with the management of the park. When Tanzania became independent, the pressure to modernize stressed a participatory nationalism whereby the Maasai, cast as resistant to change, continued to be viewed as emblems of the past.

In fact, it was mostly during the post-independence and modernization period that political representation of the Maasai in the Conservation Authority was formally done away with (Olenasha et al., 2001). While the details of colonial, post-independence, and conservation-based management schemes may at first seem removed from the analysis of malaria prevention and control, it is important to consider the exact reasons for physical barriers to accessible health and welfare services as well as the competing economic interests that influence Maasai pastoralism and coping mechanisms. In the above examples, defining the identity and needs of a population or community was done explicitly but without reliable follow-through. In the following years, a new economic plan came about, touting even more promise and thus responsibility to the local environment and population.

TOURISM AND CONSERVATION: HARMONIOUS INTERACTION?

During the mid to late 1970s, the augmented international interest in the NCA drew attention to tourism as an economic strategy benefiting objectives of both the state and conservation bodies. Current management is most heavily influenced by the ideological paradigm uniting conservation and tourism. A 1975 government act vested authority of the NCA in the newly structured Ministry of Natural Resources and Tourism. In 1979, UNESCO and the World Conservation Union (IUCN) deemed the NCA a World Heritage Site. In 1981, the Ngorongoro Crater Highlands and its contiguous ecosystems were recognized as the Ngorongoro–Serengeti Biosphere Reserve, a positive recognition in light of the fact that the NCA is under a different administrative authority than Tanzania National Parks Administration (TANAPA) which oversees the SNP. The 1982 NCA management plan echoed UNESCO's recognition of the "longstanding harmonious interaction" between man and environment (Homewood & Rodgers, 1991). But these designations were spread opaquely over a history of management that consistently undermined this harmony, and the blanket recognition of the importance of pastoralism in the Ngorongoro lands veiled its increasingly apparent disrepair. Changes in the way the land was conceived, managed, and shared still have direct effects on the Maasai, especially in terms of the infrastructure and services needed to address health concerns and other basic needs. "[B]y changing economic perceptions of the value of NCA to the nation, tourism can change policies of land use which themselves radically affect pastoralist futures" (Homewood & Rodgers, 1991, p. 6).

When Ali Hassan Mwinyi assumed the Tanzanian presidency in 1985, Nyerere's socialist agenda was redirected into a capitalist scheme emphasizing privatization and foreign investment where free market ideals replaced those of brotherhood and unity. Mwinyi believed that tourism was the most promising way of improving Tanzania's economic status (Neumann, 1995). Between 1985 and 1990, tourist visitation increased by about 600 percent (Neumann, 1995), and then by 200 percent between 1990 and 2000 (UNESCO, 2007). Between 2002 and 2006, visitor numbers in the NCA jumped from about 126,000 to 359,000 (de Groot & Ramakrishnan, 2005) in this continually increasing pattern. The annual income from tourism can generate up to 60 percent of the total NCA budget (UNEPWCMC, 2008). Between 2006 and 2007, the total income amounted to about 27 billion Tanzanian shillings plus 12 billion from other sources (approximately US$ 21 million and 9 million, respectively) such as fines, concession fees, service provision to lodges such as water and electricity, and foreign investment (UNESCO, 2007). According to UNESCO (2007), Tanzania has introduced a strategy to reach 1 million tourist visits annually by 2010.

International interest and tourist marketing has nurtured the same aspects of Maasai culture that had come under scrutiny in the preceding decades and has recycled them for use as a necessary part of the experience of nature and authenticity in the NCA. "Indeed, tourism is a safe place for practices that are contested in other spheres, for in tourism they function in a privileged representational economy" (Bruner & Kirshenblatt-Gimblett, 1994, p. 448). Through the joint venture of conservation and tourism, images of the Maasai as part of a living past borne out of reforms such as Operation Dress-up are put to use for the benefit of the state via the "re-representation of 'traditions' as something valuable, and not inherently bad" (Talle, 1999, p. 123). Tourist literature markets the NCA as an Eden, and the Maasai as charmingly antediluvian. "The 'tourist gaze' ... influences everything from destination images projected, to tour content and attraction design, to community members' identities, to local environmental management needs and concerns" (Meletis & Campbell, 2007). In other words, the neo-liberalization of the state propagated "re-regulation" whereby "previously untradeable things" became valuable commodities (Igoe & Brockington, 2007).

The official website of the NCA claims that "cultural tourism ... encourages residents to share their values with the outside world and provides them with direct financial benefits" (Ngorongoro Conservation Area, n.d.). Of these financial benefits, the sale of handicrafts and photographic opportunities are most frequently cited. But in order for tourism to benefit the local population, its profits must be allocated fairly and adequately in ways that improve the quality of life of the Maasai. Having their pictures taken and selling wares for minimal prices does little if anything to this end – in fact, it only furthers their reliance on the external cash economy. Further, it casts the Maasai as part of the attraction and the landscape, painting a portrait of deliberate perceptions rather than fostering interaction with reality. Historically, Maasai were treated as if their pastoral system was damaging to the environment. In contrast, foreigners traverse the NCA in vehicles that damage the land and pollute the air, and are accommodated in lodge facilities that use clean water daily while the Maasai often travel long distances daily on foot to fetch water from outdoor, unclean sources. Yet, so long as the experience of visiting the NCA is framed partly in terms of stereotypes, the acquisition of essential goods and services that determine health and well-being might continue to somehow be seen as anomalous.

Modification of tourism policies and activities, however, might improve the situation by fostering greater participation of the Maasai in manage- ment decision-making processes, scaling down the amount of tourist consumption and impact to a sustainable level, while considering the local population, and adjusting some of the restrictions and regulations on the Maasai that have been inherited from previous management regimes. This would address the conflicts regarding material resource allocation in the NCA and would represent a move toward management philosophy better aligned with the realities of the NCA lands and population. It is important to acknowledge that international bodies of conservation such as UNESCO, UNEP, IUCN, and the Man and Biosphere (MAB) program now openly recognize and promulgate a view of development and conservation in the NCA that involves integration of pastoralism with conservation-oriented management. According to IUCN World Heritage criteria, the NCA is a Managed Resource Protected Area, where priority is given to long-term protection of biological diversity as well as "a sustainable flow of natural products and services to meet community needs" (UNEP-WCMC, 1994). While an important foundation, considering potential influences on the tourist gaze, concrete and cooperative actions need to reflect these views.

Present initiatives of the IUCN aim to "build recognition of the many ways in which human lives and livelihoods, especially of the poor, depend on the sustainable management of natural resources" (IUCN, 2008). But there is value in recognizing the ways in which the livelihoods of natural resources also depend on the sustainable management of human lives. A greater degree of Maasai participation in management can alter the way that its objectives are achieved. This is not a novel concept, especially to the Maasai. Homewood and Rodgers (1991, p. 239) point out a paradox of conservation-justified tourism: "Fifty zebra-striped tourist buses a day in the Crater are acceptable: one Maasai grain truck a week, bound for Nainokanoka, is not." This exemplifies the existence of usable infrastructure, that is, that there are enough roads and vehicles to deliver grain. Tourism infrastructure developments over the years have further encroached upon traditional grazing lands, contributing to the reduction in transhumant pastoralist capabilities without remediation. While the famed environment and natural splendor of the area may be touted, in the end the enterprise has been just income-generating, consumptive tourism that happens to take place in a conservation area. In fact, in 2009 the UNESCO World Heritage Committee threatened to remove the NCA from its list of World Heritage Sites because of ecological damage done by human activity, citing the extreme consumption of tourism as well as, perhaps without enough consideration, pastoralist activities (eTN, 2009). It is thus perhaps a matter of enacting a regular process of equitable distribution and creative cooperation toward sustainable management in line with the original objectives of multiple land use.

In the past decade, a few non-governmental organizations have been formed by the Maasai, aimed at disseminating their message to a wider audience and fostering an organized community effort for improved living conditions (Neumann, 1995; Honey, 1999). A Pastoral Council comprised of Maasai liaisons to the NCAA has existed since the early 1990s. Another group offers services such as veterinary care for maintaining herd health and integrity. The organization called ERETO theoretically functions as a cooperative between the Maasai and the NCAA. However, only a marginal portion of the NCAA profits benefit these groups – only 1.2 billion Tanzanian shillings (approximately US$ 920,000) were allocated to the Pastoral Council for the fiscal year 2006–2007 (UNESCO, 2007) – and the Maasai continue to express overall dissatisfaction with the management (Coffin, 2007). Therefore, the body of regulations that determine what, when, and how any health interventions can be introduced into the system will be successful only when bargaining parties are considered colleagues, not competitors.

The malaria situation is essentially an issue of access to resources, including natural, political, social, and material resources, and such access has often been obstructed by interventions mediated by inaccurate perceptions about the activities and ecological role of the Maasai. Disease occupies a social and political space as a problem faced by societies on several scales, and dealt with via adaptive strategies and behaviors. Management policy, which includes tourism guidelines, must be seen as a potential whose capacity and form is molded by the method of evaluating a situation. Community perspectives reflect this notion, noting that the NCA has the means to work with the Maasai system, but that practical improvements need to be made (Coffin, 2007).

Malaria existed before the onset of its present scope, and Maasai pastoralism was not a static entity before the advent of colonialism. But when a preventable and curable disease becomes a major and increasing burden on a population whose interests are supposed to be part of the governing legislation, especially in such a localized context and in the face of the compounding effects of sedentarization and land tenure insecurity, that burden becomes an indicator of management process gone awry. In his studies of forced migration among the Maasai of southern Kenya, historian Lotte Hughes (2006, p. 130) asserts that with respect to subsistence and disease, "confinement in reserves had put an end to traditional Maasai coping mechanisms." The Maasai system is adept at coping with hardship based on environmental unpredictability, but has been injured severely by the type of hardship that has undermined the mechanisms used to deal with it. In addition, perceptions about the compatibility between tourism and conservation that are not implemented with careful deliberation about the environment and community at hand are at least partly responsible for the effects of such enterprise on Maasai well-being and health.

CONCLUSIONS: LOOKING FORWARD AFTER LOOKING BACK

Addressing the malaria situation in Ngorongoro thus means addressing its historically rooted foundations. Historical anthropologist Nicholas Thomas (1996, p. 9) explains that "historical processes and their effects are internal to social systems and ... attempts to analyze societies without reference to history are likely to embody both theoretical errors and substantive misinterpretations." Failing to take history into account in such cases can lead to a view of the malaria situation as one of stationary endemicity, whereby administrative authority is seen to play a negligible part in the upsurge of the disease. It also carries the potential of blaming the cultural and social practices of the Maasai for their own burden of disease without taking into account their ongoing dialectical interface with management policy. Mutual trust is paramount in this context and it represents an area of immense potential for the improvement of NCA–Maasai relations. Without calibrating perspective by an accurate understanding of the situation, connections between disease burden and population become skewed by the very perceptions that led to its proliferation in the first place. "Improvements in community health and education have to start from the conditions given by the pastoral environment and the transhumant mode of life" (Århem, 1985, p. 108). The ability of the Maasai to deal with poverty conditions and illness has been compromised by the factors detailed above.

Ultimately, the capacity of Endulen Hospital to improve upon its quality of care delivery and acceptability in the community will come into question. This is especially in consideration of the fact that malaria is not the only illness that burdens the population here, as is the case in many resource-poor settings. The Maasai of Ngorongoro are also burdened by widespread tuberculosis, an AIDS epidemic evermore closing in on this population, as well as other communicable and zoonotic diseases. The most recent Millennium Ecosystem Assessment emphasizes the need for "a reconciliation between ecology, economics, and ethics" (de Groot & Ramakrishnan, 2005, p. 460). There are several ways that the community and conservation authorities can come together, however, toward more socially just service delivery. One prospect for change that can be made within the system involves the rise of human rights documentation as a legislative stencil. Guided by principles of availability, access, acceptability, and quality, human rights-based approaches would serve both the environment and the people and might bring income-generating activities to a more justifiable place in the NCA. The inclusion of these principles into the NCA policies might also serve to specify a definition of Maasai well-being that they can use to defend the resources necessary for their survival, and facilitate accountability. By engendering ongoing conservations, these mediating principles might also clarify perceptions from the Maasai point of view regarding foreign intervention and management intentions. "Both public health and human rights recognize the ultimate responsibility of governments to create enabling conditions necessary for people to make and effectuate choices, cope with changing patterns of vulnerability, and keep themselves and their families healthy" (Brundtland, 2005, p. 61).

Perhaps cooperation can lead to a system whereby entrance fees directly support a certain set of expenses borne by the Endulen Hospital. Another suggestion, based on the abundance of evidence that nutritional well-being is of the utmost importance in the context of malaria, might be to use the tourism infrastructure already in place, such as roads and vehicles, to increase transport of grain and nutritional supplements, as well as the actual lodge facilities to store them, of course contingent on agreements with the Maasai. A combination of veterinary and human health services might also be considered in remote villages. Of course, improved transparency and good governance on the part of the NCA Authority underscores any progress at all.

In the NCA in Tanzania, Maasai residents report a crescendo in malaria incidence, coinciding with changes in seasonal climate patterns and the continuation of environmental management policies driven by both international conservation agendas and the economic promise of the tourist industry. They have also specifically voiced wishes for more outposts or dispensaries in those villages farther from Endulen Hospital. This paper has elucidated a variety of ways in which such policies have been misinformed, and several principles that must find legitimate space in the NCA's management in order to initiate an effective dialog on malaria and other health matters among stakeholders. Laying out the context of poverty and disease in the area can serve as a useful prelude to such discussions.

As Tanzania was listed as one of the best provisioned countries with antimalarials and ACTs in 2006 (WHO, 2008), it should be ensured that populations marginalized and at risk have the opportunity to benefit equally from these circumstances. With small bits of several things – awareness of perception, understanding of ecological relationships, and initiative toward an inclusive management approach – malaria can be practically and effectively addressed. Malaria is one of many issues in the NCA, and is, itself, a symptom of other, deeper issues. But progress must start someplace, and the record books of the Endulen Hospital are no worse than any other.

NOTES

1. All currency conversions as of August 2009.
2. Name is not given to protect the confidentiality of hospital staff.
3. These prices reflect the costs to Endulen Hospital. Currency conversions are recent, but the amount they reflect in shillings was reported to the author in 2006. This involves a degree of uncertainty, and there may also be variability in the price of ACT drugs depending on the source and the process of delivering the drugs to health facilities. However, it is widely known that although highly effective, ACT drugs cost a considerable and often restrictive amount more than second-line drugs.
4. For more on vulnerability, risk, and human rights see Gruskin, Grodin, Annas, and Marks (2005).

ACKNOWLEDGMENTS

Ashe naleng/Asante sana to the Maasai community of Ngorongoro and the Endulen Hospital staff for their generous hospitality and great insight. Many thanks also to the Ngorongoro Conservation Area Authority, the University of Dar es Salaam, and the Associated Colleges of the Midwest. Special thanks for valuable input extended to Nai Oloorubat, John and Robin Greenler, Charles Saanane, Audax Mabulla, Endulen camp staff and students, Florian Schneider, Russell Tuttle, Mark Lycett, and Greg Beckett.

REFERENCES

Århem, K. (1981). *Maasai pastoralism in the Ngorongoro Conservation Area: Sociological and ecological issues.* BRALUP Research Paper no. 69. Bureau of Resource Assessment and Land Use Planning, University of Dar es Salaam, Dar es Salaam.

Århem, K. (1985). *Pastoral man in the Garden of Eden: The Maasai of the Ngorongoro conservation area, Tanzania.* Uppsala, Sweden: University of Uppsala, Department of Cultural Anthropology in cooperation with The Scandinavian Institute of African Studies.

Århem, K. (1986). Pastoralism under pressure: The Ngorongoro Maasai. In: J. Boesen, K. J. Havnevik, J. Koponen & R. Odgaard (Eds), *Tanzania: Crisis and struggle for survival* (pp. 239–251). Uppsala, Sweden: Scandinavian Institute of African Studies.

Brundtland, G. H. (2005). The UDHR: Fifty years of synergy between health and human rights. In: G. Sofia, M. Grodin, G. Annas & S. Marks (Eds), *Perspectives on health and human rights* (pp. 59–62). New York: Taylor and Francis Group, LLC.

Bruner, E. M., & Kirshenblatt-Gimblett, B. (1994). Maasai on the lawn: Tourist realism in East Africa. *Cultural Anthropology, 9*(4), 435–470.

Coffin, J. (2007). *Wildlife–livestock disease interface and potential climatic effects, a case study: Understanding dynamics in the Ngorongoro Conservation Area.* Unpublished B.A. thesis, Macalester College.

de Groot, R., & Ramakrishnan, P. S. (2005). Cultural and amenity services. In: R. Hassan & N. Ash (Eds), *Ecosystems and human well-being: Current state and trends, volume 1. Findings of the condition and trends working group of the millennium ecosystem assessment* (pp. 455–476). Washington: Island Press.

Escobar, A., Berglund, E., Brosius, P., Cleveland, D. A., Hill, J. D., Hodgson, D. L., Leff, E., Milton, K., Rocheleau, D. E., & Stonich, S. C. (1999). After nature: Steps toward an antiessentialist political ecology. *Current Anthropology, 40*(1), 1–30.

eTN (eTurboNews). (2009). Africa's UNESCO Ngorongoro Conservation Area faces significant ecological threats. Available at http://www.eturbonews.com/9119/africas-unesco-ngorongoro-conservation-area-faces-significant-eco (accessed August 2009).

Galaty, J. G. (1977). *In the pastoral image: The dialectic of Maasai identity.* Ph.D. thesis, University of Chicago.

Gruskin, S., Grodin, M., Annas, G., & Marks, S. (Eds). (2005). *Perspectives on health and human rights.* New York: Taylor and Francis Group, LLC.

Hodgson, D. L. (1999). Images & interventions: The problems of pastoralist development. In: D. Anderson & V. Broch-Due (Eds), *The poor are not us: Poverty & pastoralism in Eastern Africa* (pp. 221–239). Oxford: Ohio University Press.

Hodgson, D. L. (2001). *Once intrepid warriors: Gender, ethnicity, and the cultural politics of Maasai development.* Bloomington: Indiana University Press.

Homewood, K., & Rodgers, W. A. (1991). *Maasailand ecology: Pastoralist development and wildlife conservation in Ngorongoro, Tanzania.* Cambridge, UK: Cambridge University Press.

Honey, M. (1999). *Ecotourism and sustainable development: Who owns paradise?* Washington, DC: Island Press.

Hughes, L. (2006). *Moving the Maasai: A colonial misadventure.* Basingstoke: Palgrave Macmillan in association with St. Antony's College.

Igoe, J., & Brockington, D. (2007). Neoliberal conservation: A brief introduction. *Conservation and Society, 5*(4), 432–449.

IPP Media. (2009). Starving Ngorongoro sends out food SOS. Available at http://ip-216-69-164-44.ip.secureserver.net/ipp/guardian/2009/03/26/134082.html (accessed 30 March 2009).

IUCN (International Union for the Conservation of Nature). (2008). About IUCN. Available at http://cms.iucn.org/about/ (accessed 10 March 2008).

Johnsen, N. (2000). Placemaking, pastoralism, and poverty in the Ngorongoro conservation area, Tanzania. In: V. Broch-Due & R. A. Schroeder (Eds), *Producing nature and poverty in Africa* (pp. 148–172). Uppsala: Nordiska Afrikainstitutet.

Jones, A. E., Uddenfeldt Wort, U., Morse, A. P., Hastings, I. M., & Gagnon, A. S. (2007). Climate prediction of El Nino malaria epidemics in north-west Tanzania. *Malaria Journal, 6*(162), 1–15.

Lewis, G. (1993). Some studies of social causes of and cultural response to disease. In: C. G. N. Mascie-Taylor (Ed.), *The anthropology of disease* (pp. 73–124). Oxford: Oxford University Press.

McCabe, J. T. (2002). Giving conservation a human face? Lessons from forty years of combining conservation and development in the Ngorongoro conservation area, Tanzania. In: D. Chatty & M. Colchester (Eds), *Conservation and mobile indigenous peoples: Displacement, forced settlement, and sustainable development* (pp. 61–76). New York: Berghahn Books.

Meletis, Z. A., & Campbell, L. M. (2007). Call it consumption! Re-conceptualizing ecotourism as consumption and consumptive. *Geography Compass, 1*(4), 850–870.

Ndaskoi, N. (2006). Root causes of the Maasai predicament. *Fourth World Journal, 7*(1), 28–61.

Neumann, R. P. (1995). Local challenges to global agendas: Conservation, economic liberalization and the pastoralists' rights movement in Tanzania. *Antipode, 27*(4), 363–382.

Ngorongoro Conservation Area. (n.d.). Ngorongoro Conservation Area. Available at http://www.ngorongoro-crater-africa.org/home.html (accessed 25 February 2008).

Olenasha, W., Ole Seki, W., & Kaisoe, M. (2001). Case study 4: Tanzania: The conflict between conventional conservation strategies and indigenous conservation system: The case study of Ngorogoro Conservation Area. Available at http://www.forestpeoples.org/documents/africa/tanzania_eng.pdf (accessed August 2009).

Packard, R. M. (1984). Maize, cattle and mosquitoes: The political economy of malaria epidemics in colonial Swaziland. *Journal of African History, 25*(2), 189–212.

Parliament of Tanganyika. (1959). *Ngorongoro Conservation Area, principal legislation 1959* (Chapter 413 of the Laws, Suppl. 59). Dar es Salaam: Government of Tanganyika.

RBM (Roll Back Malaria). (2007). Technical design, affordable medicines facility-malaria (AMFm) Available at http://rbm.who.int/partnership/tf/globalsubsidy/AMFmTechProposal.pdf (accessed July 2009).

RBM (Roll Back Malaria). (2008). Global Malaria Action Plan. Available at http:// www.rollbackmalaria.org/gmap/ (accessed October 2008).

Schneider, L. (2006). The Maasai's new clothes: A developmentalist modernity and its exclusions. *Africa Today, 53*(1), 101–129.

Scott, J. C. (1998). *Seeing like a state: How certain schemes to improve the human condition have failed.* New Haven: Yale University Press.

Spear, T. T., & Waller, R. (1993). *Being Maasai: Ethnicity and identity in East Africa.* London: Ohio University Press.

Talle, A. (1999). Pastoralists at the border: Maasai poverty & the development discourse in Tanzania. In: D. Anderson & V. Broch-Due (Eds), *The poor are not us: Poverty & pastoralism in Eastern Africa* (pp. 106–124). Oxford: Ohio University Press.

Thomas, N. (1996). *Out of time: History and evolution in anthropological discourse* (2nd ed.). Ann Arbor: University of Michigan Press.

UNEP, World Conservation Monitoring Centre. (1994). World database on protected areas. Available at http://www.unep-wcmc.org/wdpa/index.htm (accessed 6 February 2008).

UNEP, World Conservation Monitoring Centre. (2008). Ngorongoro Conservation Area, Tanzania. Available at: http://www.unep-wcmc.org/sites/wh/pdf/Ngorongoro.pdf (accessed July 2009).

UNESCO. (2007). *Ngorongoro Conservation Area, United Republic of Tanzania: Report of the reactive monitoring mission,* 29 April–5 May. World Heritage Committee, Thirty-first Session. Paris: UNESCO.

Waller, R. (1999). Pastoral poverty in historical perspective. In: D. Anderson & V. Broch-Due (Eds), *The poor are not us: Poverty & pastoralism in Eastern Africa* (pp. 20–49). Oxford: Ohio University Press.

WHO. (2006). Guidelines for the treatment of malaria. Available at http://www.who.int/ malaria/docs/TreatmentGuidelines2006.pdf (accessed 18 September 2008).

WHO. (2008). World malaria report. Available at http://www.who.int/malaria/wmr2008/ malaria2008.pdf (accessed 18 September 2008).

POLICY, POLITY, AND THE HIV CRISIS IN EMERGING ECONOMIES: INDIA AND RUSSIA COMPARED

Tinaz Pavri and Thomas Rotnem

ABSTRACT

Purpose – *In this chapter, we compare the cases of India and Russia as they address the spread of HIV-AIDS in their respective countries. The countries, former Cold War allies, have embarked upon a path toward economic liberalization in the past decade and a half. In Russia's case, this came with political upheaval. In India's case, liberalization started with tentative steps and reached more full-blown economic and social liberalization in recent times. Both have also had to deal with the rapid spread of HIV-AIDS within their societies which brings with it the threat of derailing recent economic progress.*

Methodology – *A comparative case-study method is used to make comparisons between these countries which are facing similar challenges but whose approaches to them differ.*

Findings – *The chapter looks at how the government and a tradition-bound society in both cases have addressed the crisis. While both governments are recently becoming more serious about sustainable responses to the spread of the disease, in India's case this response has been buttressed by social liberalization unleashed by recent economic success.*

Understanding Emerging Epidemics: Social and Political Approaches
Advances in Medical Sociology, Volume 11, 43–57
Copyright © 2010 by Emerald Group Publishing Limited
All rights of reproduction in any form reserved
ISSN: 1057-6290/doi:10.1108/S1057-6290(2010)0000011007

Contributions to the field – *We argue that social liberalization, as in the case of India, has made an impact in terms of the spread and acceptance of prevention education. This has positive implications for those countries where liberalization has changed traditional societies and where these changes are being used to battle the HIV-AIDS crisis.*

INTRODUCTION

In the past decade and a half, India and Russia have both embarked upon their own revolutions, the former a consolidated democracy, opening up its markets to foreign investment as never before and starting down the road to economic liberalization, the latter echoing in some measure India's economic liberalization path but within the context of a political transition that has taken on recent authoritarian overtones. As the following pages will show, the two countries warrant comparison on a number of issues: both were late and reluctant entrants into the HIV policy-making community, the crisis facing both is grave, and in both cases it has implications for the continuation of the economic growth that has included them in the Bric (Brazil, Russia, India and China) bloc. In addition, the former Cold War allies have faced the challenges of largely traditional societies that have limited the range of governmental and societal responses to addressing the disease's spread.

Although the first cases of HIV infection were reported in the 1980s in both India and what was then still the Soviet Union, both countries did not really start grappling with the crisis until the 1990s. Further strides have only been made, particularly in India's case, in the new millennium. The potential consequences of the advance of this epidemic in both cases are grave, threatening to cause large-scale demographic change, particularly in Russia where the population is rapidly graying and has already declined by some 6 million since 1991 (The Economist, 2006) and economic disturbances as funds are diverted from economic development and infrastructure improvement to treatment and hospitalization of those affected with HIV/AIDS. At the micro-level, the costs of doing business will be driven upwards, as benefits and pension systems become swiftly under-financed and rehiring and retraining expenses increase precipitously (Gunther, 2004). Furthermore, productivity among the workforce would suffer, and at the individual level, private savings rates would unavoidably fall, decreasing capital formation.

World Bank forecast estimates of the economic consequences of a moderate to severe HIV/AIDS crisis on Russia's investment and growth trajectories demonstrate that the *annual* percentage change in investment growth may vary from -2.54 to -14.50 by 2020, while the *annual* percentage change in gross domestic product (GDP) growth may vary from -4.68 to as much as -25.44 by 2020 (Ruehl, Pokorovsky, & Vinogradov, 2002). A more recent analysis argues that the economic impact of HIV points to a -4.15 drop in Russian GDP by 2010 (Twigg, 2007). In India, UNAIDS predicts a 1% per year cut in economic growth over the next decade which would lead to a decline in per capita income also (Zaheer, 2006).

This chapter looks comparatively at the cases of India and Russia, former allies during the Cold War, both weathering the challenges and reaping the fruits of the new, global economy as they liberalize their markets, and both operating within the context of traditional societies that struggled to acknowledge first the existence and then the rapid spread of the disease in their countries. The governments in both countries also hesitated early on in the crisis in searching for policy solutions. More recently, however, it appears that the Indian government and NGOs have become more forceful in playing a greater and more visible role in spearheading efforts addressing the pandemic. We analyze this phenomenon as we compare the two countries, the development of the crises in both, and the present-day efforts to address its spread. We aver that economic liberalization (and its concomitant social liberalization) has had a significant impact on the way that the disease is viewed and addressed in India but that in Russia the response has been largely governmental, perhaps due to the stifled state of civil society in the post-communist country. The chapter first examines the Indian case and then the Russian case. It then offers a comparative analysis of the two before concluding.

INDIA

In India, the first AIDS case came to light in 1986 in the southern city of Chennai. The initial spread of the disease appeared concentrated in those segments of the population that were consistent with reported patterns in other developing world countries including Russia, sex workers, their clients, and intravenous drug users (IDUs). From this core population, it spread rapidly to other population sub-groups including heterosexual and homosexual males. The disease initially appeared to concentrate in the more urbanized states such as Karnataka, Tamil Nadu, and Maharashtra, but it has since spread to all states.

In 2006, India became the country that had the largest number of AIDS cases at more than 5 million (Goodspeed, 2006); in percentage terms it is currently 0.3% of the population. UNAIDS predicts 1.9% of the population being affected by 2019 (Pembry, 2005). However, other agencies including the WHO predict that AIDS has reached its peak and appeared to be stabilizing (Misra, 2005). Other agencies caution that this might be misleading, since stabilization appears to be greatest in the large cities where the greatest prevention awareness has taken place and that in more remote or rural areas, the rates might still be increasing but might not be effectively recorded.

In the time since the identification of the first case, India has experienced dramatic change on the economic front, with the fruits of its economic liberalization policy which began in 1990 under the Congress party government of P.V. Narasimha Rao beginning to come to light on many levels. Although the country is still grappling with critical problems on many levels including pervasive poverty, the high rates of growth – between 6% and 9% GDP annually – have swelled the ranks of the middle class (today understood to represent those Indians earning between $2,000 and 20,000 a year, even while the average per capita income is only $800), attracted unprecedented foreign investment, created new markets for consumer goods and services, and led to a social liberalization that globalization brought in its wake in the form of television shows, films, cultural exchanges, cutting-edge creativity in the arts and fashion industries, etc. In turn, this has revolutionized India's social climate, particularly in urban areas, with greater openness, dialog, and experimentation with hitherto taboo ideas and subjects including sexuality.

The early days of the disease, however, were quite different. India in the 1980s was still relatively much more tradition-bound and this Indian tradition dictated that a disease that was linked to sexual activity could not be freely discussed in the public domain. Consequently, prevention messages linked to condom use or safe sex were also deemed hardly acceptable in the public arena. The impact of recent globalization had not yet been felt, television shows and films from other countries were not freely viewed, and far fewer Indians had the means to travel. Hence, existent cultural and social norms against discussing sexuality mitigated against the spread of prevention programs. Those who were infected suffered the brunt of society's disapproval. Bureaucratic agencies routinely disputed international estimates of the spread of AIDS in India and argued that their data showed a much slower growth of the disease. In fact, a government agency to address the pandemic, the National AIDS Control Organization (NACO), was set up as late as 1992, six years after the first HIV case was discovered (Pembry, 2005).

From the late 1990s and into the new millennium, there has been a sea change in India's economic sphere and, to a great extent as a result, we argue, in its social fabric. Much has been written about India's new economy and the many changes that have come about after liberalization and most of these authors have been optimistic and positive about this new growth.[1] Less has been written linking economic liberalization to social liberalization, but we are arguing that this has in fact been the case. A plethora of films, radio, television shows, and literature by new Indian authors addressing cutting-edge social issues that would have been inconceivable a decade and more ago are today the norm. At least in urban India, women have acquired greater societal freedoms, families have shaken the yoke of the joint-family generational burden and struck out on their own, and greater individualism including for women is becoming more the norm. India's celebrity culture fuelled by the premier spot Bollywood holds is setting the trend for these greater freedoms with Bollywood actors and actresses routinely flouting societal norms and inspiring the younger generation to do the same. When India's greatest pre-occupation, Bollywood actors and actresses, engage in openly non-traditional sexual behavior patterns, the masses take their cues from them.

India's AIDS policies and prevention programs in recent times appear to have been "liberalized," to some extent by the changes that have become evident in the economic and social spheres. In 2002, BBC World Service Trust coordinated an integrated campaign that involved All India Radio and Doordarshan, India's first TV channel. Bollywood celebrities are joining forces to lend their tremendous appeal to the tackling of the disease along with the non-governmental sector. The first mainstream AIDS movie, *Phir Milenge* (We Will Meet Again), was released in 2004 (Bollywood, 2006). Bollywood actors Hrithik Roshan and Farhan Akhtar attended the 26th International AIDS Candlelight Memorial in Mumbai and have pledged to increase awareness (Mumbai's AIDS, 2009) and cricketer Dhoni has become actively involved in different awareness campaigns (Dhoni Creates, 2008).

Avahan, the NGO funded by the Bill and Melinda Gates foundation, has been at the forefront of innovative programs that have brought the plight of AIDS to Indian society and raised awareness, while still continuing the daily work of funding numerous programs all across the country that address prevention and treatment.[2] In August 2008, an Avahan-funded project released a book *Aids-Sutra* that chronicled AIDS in the lives of many of the worst affected populations – prostitutes, devdasis, hijras, and gays. The launch of this book, with chapters written by literary and cultural stars such as the author Salman Rushdie, received great publicity in the national and international media and extended the conversation about AIDS in India in new and thoughtful ways. A project that showcases short films about those living and dying with AIDS by different directors spearheaded by acclaimed director Mira Nair has also garnered publicity. India, hence, appears to be poised at the brink of looking at the disease with the compassion and understanding that arrived in the West almost two decades ago rather than the revulsion and rejection that has been its hallmark since the beginning.

India's gay community has also come into its own in the last decade, emboldened by this socio-economic liberalization. In 2008, the largest gay rights parade in India's history was held in New Delhi. Community activists are becoming more outspoken about their rights and in the latter half of 2008, a debate has raged about article 377 of the Indian Penal Code, a hold-over from British days that identifies homosexual acts as crimes punishable by up to 10 years in prison. Manvendra Singh Gohil, a scion of a princely family from Rajpipla, Gujarat, made national and international headlines when he came out to the world, especially on the Oprah Winfrey Show in October 2007 as India's "gay prince." Since that time, he has established a foundation, Lakshya Trust, that is devoted to HIV-AIDS-related issues. In many ways, these high-profile actors have engaged in tearing down the taboos related to discussions of HIV-AIDS.

As television audiences swell and the channels available to Indians have risen to over a hundred, commercials highlighting the help available for HIV-positive individuals have become increasingly visible. For instance, these commercials target HIV-positive mothers and educate about the availability of nephrapine, a drug that could reduce the possibility of mother–infant HIV transmission. Other commercials target treatment for those with HIV who are suffering from tuberculosis. Government agencies such as the National Rural Health Mission or NGOs sponsor these commercials (as seen on NDTV, 2008).

Finally, on the political level, the Congress government of Manmohan Singh (in office since 2004, re-elected in 2009) has been a responsible voice in addressing the pandemic. For the first time, an Indian Prime Minister has appeared to take a personal interest in spreading the word about the disease and its prevention to the people. He has engaged in many public events over his years in office, including meetings with non-profits

(Manmohan Singh ..., 2008), youth, and media (Singh, 2006), lending his voice and considerable stature as a politician most Indians respect highly, to the AIDS message. Congress party president Sonia Gandhi has also been an advocate for prevention programs, often representing India at international conferences with world leaders like Bill Clinton and Nelson Mandela (Sonia Gandhi ..., 2006) and speaking urgently about the crisis at home. Gandhi, the widow of the former Prime Minister Rajiv Gandhi and bearer of the Gandhi dynasty, is a national figure of great heft and her involvement certainly enhances the AIDS movement. As opposition leader during prior to 2004, she urged the government to pay special attention to those areas still not on the AIDS radar (Pasricha, 2003).

RUSSIA

The first official case of HIV infection in the USSR was acknowledged by the Soviet government in early March 1987. Allegedly, the infection was the result of bisexual practices on the part of a military translator working in Africa; after returning to the USSR, the translator's continued sexual relations resulted in another dozen men, women, and children being infected with the virus (Feshbach, 2005).[3] Reports of AIDS diagnoses sporadically appeared in Soviet newspapers, journals, and broadcast media throughout the late 1980s. Invariably, such reports highlighted that these infections were either the result of contact with Westerners or the "depraved" practices of prostitutes and IDUs, the official acknowledgement of whom had only recently come to light under Gorbachev's policies of *glasnost* and *perestroika*.

As with India, the government's reluctance to inform and educate the citizenry about the growing HIV/AIDS problem – the domestic scale of the problem and specific avenues of virus transmission – made the situation worse. This official non-response lulled Soviets who did not have contact with foreigners, homosexuals, or prostitutes into a false sense of security. But, in fact, according to a government bulletin released in 1997, the primary means of HIV transmission between 1987 and 1990 was not through contact with Westerners, prostitutes, or IDUs, but through medical errors that took place during hospital stays.

Also as in the Indian case, the Soviet government's reluctance to address the topic and traditionalist elements in Russian society contributed to extreme social stigmatization of those increasing numbers falling victim to the virus. As the Soviet system collapsed in December 1991, a number of factors converged to bring about a sharp increase in new infections.

The implosion of the Soviet health care system, particularly its formerly highly touted preventive care and epidemiological branches, contributed to this upsurge. In addition, relaxed restrictions on citizens traveling abroad also abetted the spread of HIV infection. Added to this mix was the failure of the now post-communist government of Boris Yeltsin to inform the populace of the growing dangers or develop measures to combat the spread of HIV. Mirroring the Indian case, difficulties in training adequate numbers of nurses, doctors, and other medical professionals in HIV/AIDS care and ensuring ample supplies of disposable syringes, testing kits, and sterilization equipment continued to afflict the country throughout the post-communist period (Santibanez et al., 2005).[4]

Until very recently, official government statistics revealed that since 1987, approximately 5,000 persons had died from AIDS. However, we now know that the late Soviet and post-communist death toll from HIV and AIDS was considerably higher; indeed, in August 2006, the Federal Service for Supervision of Consumer Rights and Human Welfare (Rospotrebnadzor) posted on its website a figure 140% higher than previously recognized, that is, approximately 12,000 AIDS deaths since 1987 (Health Agency, 2006).

Approximately 362,000 Russians were registered with authorities as HIV-positive in 2006; reportedly, about 60% of these cases were located in just 13 of Russia's 89 regions (On AIDS Day ..., 2006).[5] However, experts contend that the real number of HIV carriers in Russia *may* have been significantly higher due to under-reporting. Evidence given by a senior member of Russia's Federation Council, Valentina Peterenko, and under-lined by the Central Research Institute of Pandemics concurred that Russia had between 800,000 and 1,100,000 HIV carriers in 2006, with 100 new infections on average being reported daily (One Hundred New HIV ..., 2006). Others argued that the real figure may be closer to 1.5 million HIV carriers (Russia Finds Money Alone ..., 2006).

In the new millennium, despite a continued and increasing rate of HIV prevalence among IDUs[6] and prostitutes, heterosexual contact is becoming a significant new route of human immunodeficiency virus infection in Russia today, a development that is mirrored in India. The percentage of all Russians receiving transmission of the virus through unprotected sexual contact has increased from 6% to 45% since 2001 (*Canadian Medical Association Journal*, 2005; Health Agency, 2006).

Another disturbing recent trend noticed by Russian and foreign epidemiologists is the increasingly youthful visage of persons living with HIV/AIDS (PLWHA) in Russia; indeed, the overwhelming majority (80%)

of those infected with HIV or AIDS are youths between the ages of 15 and 30 years. Since 2001, more than 80% of new Russian HIV cases were found in those in the 15–29-year age group (*Canadian Medical Association Journal,* 2005; Twigg, 2007).

As well, in yet another portentous warning, women are beginning to comprise a larger percentage of those persons newly infected with HIV. Indeed, in 2000 women accounted for just 20% of new infections; however, within five years, women accounted for 40% of all new HIV infections in the Russian Federation. And, in Moscow, more than one-half of the 28,000 registered HIV cases today are women (*Canadian Medical Association Journal,* 2005; Gorst, 2006; Osadchuk, 2008). These data mirror UNAIDS data that suggest 38% of AIDS cases in India in 2007 were women.

Projections of the growth of HIV/AIDS in Russia vary widely according to which source is consulted. However, experts all concur that the future scourge in Russia will be quite severe. According to the National Intelligence Council's (2002) report on "The Next Wave of HIV/AIDS," intelligence analysts believe Russia's HIV/AIDS adult prevalence rate could soar from approximately 1.30–2.50% to between 6% and 11%; this estimate would place the number of Russian infected at between 5 and 8 million by 2010 (National Intelligence Council, 2002).[7] As well, recently released official data are equally discouraging, as Russian government sources indicated a "five percent surge" in new HIV infections in the January–September 2006 period over the same nine-month period in 2005.

Given these disturbing trends and projections and the potential disastrous consequences that may ensue, one might think that the Russian people would consider the present HIV/AIDS situation as an urgent issue. However, public opinion polls prove this is not the case.

According to a survey conducted by Theodore P. Gerber and Sarah E. Mendelson, Russian society ranked the burgeoning problem of HIV/AIDS as a much less important issue than a number of other societal ills. Overall, the "spread of HIV/AIDS" ranked 13th on a list of 24 items, with poverty, price increases, unemployment, corruption and bribery, the growing cost of higher education, the lack of prospects among the young, and others ranking before it. And, according to the authors, successive surveys demonstrate that concern with HIV/AIDS in Russia is not increasing, but *decreasing* among the population. Additional surveys indicate that even medical professionals in the field and government officials in health ministries discount the significant risk of HIV/AIDS in Russia today (Gerber & Mendelson, 2005). Although such surveys are not available in the

Indian case, one wonders whether the results would be substantially different given its place in the recent social limelight.

What has the Russian government been doing to stem the looming problem? According to many analysts, the HIV/AIDS crisis did not even appear on the Kremlin's agenda until 2003, when President Putin referred to the disease – in connection with Russia's demographic decline – in his "State of the Union" address (Gorst, 2006). Until late 2005 the Putin administration had been doing little to evaluate the limitations of previous government measures in this area.

Since mid-2006, though, considerable government attention and, more importantly, government resources have been committed to fighting the spread of HIV/AIDS. The Director of the Open House Institute, Elena Zaitseva, a non-governmental organization active in fighting HIV/AIDS, commented that finally, "we are seeing a breakthrough in the government's understanding of what is required to fight AIDS." Speaking before a group of government officials in April 2006, President Putin himself told the audience that the struggle against AIDS could only succeed if federal agencies and government ministries work together to fight the disease and increase public awareness. Stating that "So far, there is no general strategy for such work," Putin concluded by asking for assistance from non-governmental organizations,[8] political parties, and private businesses to help authorities with raising funds and organizing a nationwide HIV/AIDS program; to that end, the Russian government appointed a commission to develop a national anti-AIDS strategy (Gorst, 2006).

To address the issue of treatment of those infected with HIV/AIDS, the government in 2006 began to sequester funds in order to quintuple the number of Russians who in 2005 (4,000 persons) received anti-retroviral therapies from public health agencies. However, this increase resulted in only 20,000 Russians receiving these life-saving therapies, or a mere 6% of those *officially* registered as HIV-positive in that year (*The Economist*, September 2006; On AIDS Day..., 2006).

In a significant change in policy, the government declared in late 2005 that it would spend a part of the oil stabilization fund for overall HIV/AIDS treatment and prevention programs, totaling approximately 3.3 billion rubles (or $124 million) through the first three quarters of 2006 (*The Economist*, 2006). In November 2006, the Russian government announced a doubling of the allotment in 2007, or $289 million (7.7 billion rubles) to be spent on fighting HIV and AIDS; portions of this were to be spent on building new AIDS clinics in under-served areas of the country,[9] upgrading existing ones, and informing young people about the dangers of

HIV/AIDS (Nowak, 2006). Weeks prior to the announcement, Dmitry Medvedev, then the Deputy Prime Minister of the Russian government, confessed that government authorities had minimized the risks of an AIDS outbreak and stated that total government spending on all health care needs in 2007 would again increase, this time to 130 billion rubles or approximately $5 billion for the year (Russian Government to Allocate ..., 2006). However, of the total monies spent in 2007 on HIV/AIDS, only 3.6% (400 million rubles or $15.4 million) was spent on prevention (Russia's Chief Medical Officer ..., 2008). Reasons for this include a late start in developing a comprehensive national AIDS policy and the necessity to create the critical infrastructure needed for its implementation from scratch.

CONCLUSION – THE TWO GOING FORWARD

It appears that while both countries have recently woken up to the realities of a potentially devastating AIDS crisis, the response has been more heartfelt particularly on the societal level in the Indian case, whereas in Russia the response is still primarily bureaucratic and governmental. While it is too early to evaluate Medvedev, Putin did not become a crusader for AIDS awareness in the same way as Manmohan Singh or Sonia Gandhi, and Russian society does not appear to have mobilized around its celebrities and well-known personalities to personify the crisis and give workers in the field the support they need to infiltrate traditionally unresponsive conservative cultures. Indeed, its government needs to marshal its forces to mount a comprehensive public awareness campaign making substantial use of its considerable influence over mass media organs in the country.[10] On the other hand, it appears to have spent more money on the crisis in recent years.

In Russia, besides restructuring the health care sector and ramping up production of anti-retroviral therapies for all those already infected with HIV,[11] the government needs to spend significantly more on prevention, as still a minority of governmental funds is currently spent on such efforts with "no large-scale HIV-prevention programs in existence" at the regional or federal levels of government (Twigg, 2007). Additionally, the Russian government could begin to reconsider effective policies in harm prevention that it has previously found objectionable; such programs, for example, needle exchange plans and methadone program treatments, have been found to be exceedingly effective in reducing HIV rates in IDUs elsewhere in the world (Schwirtz, 2008).

In the area of infrastructure, India seems to be ahead of Russia and much of this difference might lie in the enormous role that the Gates Foundation has played, which in turn has spawned many dedicated NGOs. Russian authorities need to dramatically expand their outreach capabilities for those at risk through creating more regional and local government AIDS centers. As well, Russia today does not have a satisfactory surveillance program that can monitor the progress of the HIV/AIDS epidemic (Burns, 2007).

In both countries, the governments need to do a better job to reduce the severe discrimination felt by PLWHA. In Russia, there should be measures to end the forced segregation of PLWHA when seeking medical attention by merging regional AIDS centers with ordinary polyclinics, allowing both the patients to feel less stigmatized and non-specialist doctors and nurses the opportunity to increase their awareness and knowledge of HIV/AIDS (Burns, 2007). In India, many misconceptions about the disease still abound and some doctors even today refuse to treat AIDS patients. There are many stories that highlight the tragic plight of AIDS patients shunned by society and children shunned by their schools and playmates. No national laws currently exist to protect positive children and the government is being lobbied for the enactment of such laws (India's AIDS Children Shunned, 2004).

Both governments must work to engage state-owned and private businesses in their anti-AIDS efforts. Where they already exist, health education schemes in the Russian workplace tend to focus on the dangers of smoking and alcohol dependency, rather than HIV/AIDS (Gorst, 2006). Now the government should encourage hitherto uninterested business to introduce specific anti-AIDS-discrimination and confidentiality policies (Twigg, 2007). The same is largely true in India, where to date only a few businesses have signed a voluntary non-discrimination code against its HIV-positive workers that is being promoted by an industry NGO.

Both countries do not make it easy for international NGOs or experts to lend their expertise in alleviating the crisis. The Medvedev administration needs to take another look at amending a 2005 law on foreign NGO operations in Russia. This law may put severe barriers in the path of well-intentioned Western non-governmental organizations and anti-AIDS advocacy and assistance groups, as all foreign NGOs have to re-register as Russian entities. In India's case, it has never been easy to navigate the infamous bureaucratic tangles in order to get the requisite permits and licenses to set up organizations.

It is seen, hence, that both countries face considerable challenges as they move forward. While both governments have come some ways in their recognition of greater resources due to the crisis, the Indian Prime Minister's personal role has not been echoed in Russia. The growing positive involvement of Indian society's most visible players – Bollywood actors and actresses, and other celebrities – promises to play a substantial role in the future fight and could be a model that Russia could seek to replicate.

NOTES

1. See, for instance, Mira Kamdar's *Planet India* and Edward Luce's *In Spite of the Gods: The Strange Rise of Modern India.*
2. Indeed, while the Indian government's health budget is about $160 million annually, the Gates foundation has provided more than $200 million and continues to fund AIDS programs.
3. In actuality, however, according to Feshbach earlier infections had occurred in the USSR at least two to three years prior to 1987. For example, Russian scientists have reportedly acknowledged that a teenage girl was diagnosed with AIDS as early as 1984, one year before Gorbachev's rise to power; the teenager allegedly obtained HIV through a blood transfusion nine years earlier.
4. One of the most important reasons for the shortage in medical professionals in the Russian Federation is the extremely low salaries that they typically earn.
5. According to the Russian government, the cities of Moscow and St. Petersburg and the regions of Sverdlovsk, Moscow, Samara, and Irkutsk lead the country in the percentage of persons infected with the virus (On AIDS Day..., 2006).
6. In some cities, for example, Moscow and St. Petersburg, the level of HIV prevalence among IDUs has reportedly reached 30%, placing these cities among the worst urban areas in the world on this indicator.
7. In comparison, between 1.039 and 1.185 million persons in the United States were living with HIV/AIDS in 2003 (Protocol: Surveillance of HIV-Related Events ..., 2006).
8. At the same time, the government's attempt to more directly control the activities of foreign NGOs by passing a 2006 law on NGO re-registration is certainly not timed well to assist the state struggle with growing health crises.
9. In 2006 it was estimated that barely 100 AIDS clinics existed throughout all of the Russian Federation, excluding Moscow (Nowak, 2006).
10. According to Russia's chief public health official, government and the media are both culpable in the failure to prevent widescale infections, saying "We are reaping the fruit of naïve approaches to prevention, when the media has formed a negative image of an HIV-positive person, or has frightened the population with the threat of being infected with AIDS" ("Russia's Chief Medical Officer ..., 2008).
11. Although Russia has quite recently devoted significant new funds to provide anti-retroviral drugs to those infected with the disease, the 2008 UNAIDS report on the global AIDS epidemic argues that the country is still among the 55 countries in the world in which less than 25% of adults and children with advanced HIV are receiving these therapies (Report on the Global AIDS Epidemic, 2008).

REFERENCES

Bollywood. (2006). TV stars to spread awareness as AIDS cases mount. *The Body*, June 5, viewed December 4, 2008. Available at http://www.thebody.com/context/art23567.html

Burns, K. (2007). Russia's HIV/AIDS epidemic. *Problems of Post-Communism, 54*(1), 28–36.

Canadian Medical Association Journal, April 12, 2005.

Feshbach, M. (2005). Potential social disarray in Russia due to health factors. *Problems of Post-Communism, 52*(4), 22–27.

Gerber, T., & Mendelson, S. (2005). Crises among crises among crises: Public and professional views of the HIV/AIDS epidemic in Russia. *Problems of Post-Communism, 52*(4), 28–41.

Goodspeed, P. (2006). Epidemic reveals north–south divide. *National Post*, August 8.

Gorst, I. (2006). A problem with patriarchal society. *The Financial Times*, December 1, p. 10 (Special Report).

Gunther, M. (2004). A crisis business can't ignore. *Fortune, 150*(5). Available at: http://money.cnn.com/magazines/fortunes/fortune_archive/2004/09/06/380315/index.htm. Accessed on 1 Decemcer 2009.

Health Agency. (2006). Nearly 12,000 people died of AIDS in Russia since 1987. *Johnson's Russia List*, August 9, #180.

India's AIDS Children Shunned. (2004, July 28). Viewed October 15, 2008. Available at http://www.cbsnews.com/stories/2004/07/28/world/main632654.shtml

Manmohan Singh meets with Coalition for AIDS Treatment. (2008, February 23). Viewed on May 30, 2009. Available at http://www.thaindian.com/newsportal/india-news/manmohan-singh-meets-with-coalition.html

Misra, N. (2005). *HIV cases show huge drop in India but it's a glitch*, May 30, Associated Press Worldstream. Available at: http://www.aegis.org/news/ads/2005/AD051053.html. Accessed on 1 April 2009.

National Intelligence Council (2002). The next wave of HIV/AIDS: Nigeria, Ethiopia, Russia, India, and China. ICA 2002-04D, National Intelligence Council, Washington, DC, September 2002. Available at: www.cia.gov/nic/PDF_GIF_otherprod/HIVAIDS/ICA_HIVAIDS20092302.pdf. Accessed on 15 October 2006.

NDTV AIDS-Prevention Commercial, National Rural Health Mission. (2008). Viewed November 30.

Nowak, D. (2006). *Moscow Times*, November 15.

On AIDS Day Russia Admits Problem Cannot Be Resolved Shortly. (2006). *Johnson's Russia List*, December 1, #271.

One Hundred New HIV Cases Reported in Russia Every Day. (2006). Johnson's Russia List, October 17, #233.

Osadchuk, S. (2008). The new face of an epidemic. *The Moscow Times,* May 21.

Pasricha, A. (2003). Indian politicians urge greater action on AIDS. Available at http://www.voanews.com/english/archive/2003-07/a-2003-07-27-india.htm

Pembry, G. (2005). *Overview of HIV and AIDS in India*. Viewed November 6, 2006. Available at http://avert.org/aidindia.htm

Report on the Global AIDS Epidemic. (2008). UNAIDS, Geneva, July.

Ruehl, C., Pokorovsky, V., & Vinogradov, V. (2002). *The economic consequences of HIV/AIDS in the Russian Federation*. Report 192. The World Bank.

Russia Finds Money Alone Will Not Stem HIV. (2006). *Johnson's Russia list*, August 7, #178.

Russia's Chief Medical Officer Calls for More AIDS Funding at Moscow Forum. (2008). *BBC Worldwide Monitoring*, May 3.

Russian Government to Allocate 250 Billion Rubles. (2006). *Russia business list*, October 26, #2064.

Santibanez, S., Abdul-Qader, S., Broyles, A. S., Gusseynova, L. N., Sofronova, N., Molotilov, R., et al. (2005). Expansion of outreach through government AIDS centers. *Drugs: Education, Prevention and Policy, 12*(1), 71–74.

Schwirtz, M. (2008). Russia scorns methadone for heroin addiction. *New York Times*, July 22, p. F5.

Singh, J. (2006). HIV/AIDS prevention and creating awareness: Role of media. Available at http://www.boloji.com/society/086.htm

Sonia Gandhi and Bill Clinton launch AIDS Programme for Children. (2006). Available at http://www.unicef.org/infobycountry/india-37179.html

Surveillance of HIV-Related Events Among Persons Not Receiving HIV Care (2006). Never in care (NIC) project. Atlanta, GA: Centers for Disease Control and Prevention publication (Unpublished paper).

The Economist. (2006). September 9–15.

Twigg, J. (2007). *HIV/AIDS in Russia: Commitment, resources, momentum, challenges.* Washington, DC: Center for Strategic and International Studies.

Zaheer, K. (2006). HIV/AIDS epidemic to dent India's progress. July 20. Available at: www.globalhealth.org/news/article/7682. Accessed on 9 September 2008.

PART II
THE SIGNIFICANCE AND PROCESS
OF EMERGENCE

THE CONCEPT OF EMERGING INFECTIOUS DISEASE REVISITED

Márcia Grisotti and Fernando Dias de Avila-Pires

ABSTRACT

Purpose – *To analyze the concept of emerging infectious diseases, departing from the accepted definitions adopted by the Centers for Disease Control and Prevention (CDC, USA) and the now classical definition suggested by Grmek (1993, 1995). The emphasis of this chapter is on the roles that socio-economic and cultural changes play on the emergence of diseases.*

Methodology – *Bibliographical research.*

Findings – *Current definitions fail to address all instances of the emergence of disease. In order to illustrate the concept of emergence, we discuss two case studies. The first describes the constitution of abdominal angiostrongyliasis in Costa Rica. The second concerns an outbreak of Chagas disease that took place in 2005 in the state of Santa Catarina, Brazil.*

Contribution – *As a result of our analyses we propose a new classification of instances of emergence and emphasize the importance of an inter-disciplinary approach for the understanding of diseases.*

Understanding Emerging Epidemics: Social and Political Approaches
Advances in Medical Sociology, Volume 11, 61–75
Copyright © 2010 by Emerald Group Publishing Limited
All rights of reproduction in any form reserved
ISSN: 1057-6290/doi:10.1108/S1057-6290(2010)0000011008

INTRODUCTION

The decline in the incidence of certain diseases such as tuberculosis preceded the findings of Pasteur's microbiology, and was ascribed by historians of medicine to the improvement in the general conditions of housing, sanitation, and hygiene. The post-war belief that exogenous infections were on the wane proved to be premature. The expectations surrounding the conquest of infectious and parasitic diseases, with the advent of the theory of the microbial origin of infectious diseases followed by the production of serums and vaccines at the end of the 19th century and by the discovery of sulfa-based and other antibiotics in the 20th century, did not fulfill our optimistic expectations. The emergence of HIV/AIDS and of a number of zoonotic diseases at the end of the 20th century disproved the concept of an epidemiological transition where infectious and parasitic diseases would give way to endogenous, chronic, and degenerative conditions as the main causes of human morbidity and mortality.

Microorganisms are versatile, and display a wide array of adaptations to adverse environmental conditions both in the external world and in the internal milieu of their hosts. Advances in our understanding of their biological processes, in the production of new generations of antimicrobial drugs and vaccines, and in the improvement of effective barriers to their dispersal are actually slower than the possibilities of mutation, recombination, and dispersal shown by microorganisms (Ochman, Lawrence, & Groisman, 2000).

Furthermore, the supposedly chronic nature of several diseases is currently being questioned, since the description, in 1979, of *Helicobacterium pylori*, a bacterium that proved to be associated with gastric ulcers. Peptic ulcers, formerly thought to originate mainly from stress, may result from the colonization of the stomach and duodenum by *H. pylori*, which survives the extremely acidic environment of the stomach, being the only organism capable of doing so. Antibiotics are now used to treat ulcers (Relman, 1998; Ewald, 2002; O'Connor, Taylor, & Hughes, 2006).

This is the context in which the concept of emerging infectious disease arose. However, an analysis of the literature points to existing ambiguities in this concept, especially when viewed from a historical perspective. Different points of view lead to distinct meanings of this expression, resulting in confusion. What does a new disease mean? When can we recognize it as an emergent one? Is a given disease the same in distinct hosts, human and non-human, or even in different individuals (Sournia, 1984; Delaporte, 1998)?

Emerging diseases include both infectious and chronic/degenerative conditions. Our objective is to analyze the concept of emerging infectious diseases, departing from the accepted definitions adopted by the Centers for Disease Control and Prevention (CDC, USA) and the now classical definition suggested by Grmek (1993, 1995). The emphasis of this chapter is on the roles that socio-economic and cultural changes play on the emergence of diseases, with respect to changes in the factors that determine the natural history of disease.

In order to illustrate the concept of *emergence*, we present two case studies. The first describes the constitution of abdominal angiostrongyliasis in Costa Rica, where it is considered an *endemic disease* diagnosed as part of routine tests performed on patients with tumors and negative appendectomies. In Brazil, however, it is considered an emerging infectious disease, unknown to both medical doctors and the general public, and controversial as to its diagnosis and incidence. The second concerns an outbreak of Chagas disease that took place in 2005 in the state of Santa Catarina, Brazil, a disease that is endemic in most areas of Brazil and other countries in the American continent but ignored in this state.

HOW HUMAN INFECTIOUS DISEASES EMERGE AND SPREAD

In order to understand the emergence of diseases we must learn something about the nature of diseases, the role of biological and sociocultural interventions and predisposing factors regarding incidence, the nature of parasitism, and the importance of the geographical distribution and dispersal of pathogenic organisms across the globe. To this end, we borrow some concepts from biogeography. A combination of biological and sociocultural factors is found at the root of all human infectious and parasitic diseases. As to their evolutionary origins, the great majority of such conditions were acquired from non-human reservoirs along our evolutionary history. Some became so well adapted to humans as to lose the ability to infect their former hosts (Sournia, 1984; Karlen, 2001). Among these we find measles, rubella, and falciparum malaria. A few others originated from a normal endogenous microbe, as *Escherichia coli* strayed from its normal microhabitat in the colon.

From a scientific evolutionary point of view, we may be interested in the investigation of a novel association between a pathogen and a host.

Along the history of *Homo sapiens* and its ancestors, there were many occasions for the acquisition of new parasites, following with the changes in diet, level of activity, domestication of plants and animals, farming, and urbanization (Karlen, 2001); paleopathologists, paleoarcheologists, and paleoparasitologists are involved in this type of investigation. Besides, historians of medicine search for the routes of dispersal of diseases across the globe. The American continent, Australia, and the oceanic islands offer a good field for this type of investigation (Crosby, 1994) because many diseases emerged in these places that did not exist there prior to the arrival of European colonizers.

Regarding geographical origin, for instance, bubonic plague originated in Mongolia, with steppe marmot hunters, and followed the dispersion of the black rat, *Rattus rattus*, across Asia, Europe, Africa, and the Americas. Syphilis originated in Europe and not in Central America as was previously believed. The search for the geographical origin or source of the influenza pandemics that periodically occur points to southern China, where an ingenious system of rice cultivation leads to an epidemiological chain involving ducks and pigs, enabling non-human influenza strains to infect humans.

Before the advent of paleoparasitology, we were restricted to the often inaccurate or mythic description of symptoms by traveling medical doctors and naturalists. Recently, the search for parasites in coprolites became an important tool to pinpoint the advent of a given parasite to a given region as well as the parasite's provenance. In the case of old European colonies, paleoparasitology indicates if a parasite existed before the arrival of the colonizers.

Where emergence is concerned, it may be helpful to adopt the definitions used in the field of biogeography. Simpson (1953) defines an *autochthonous* organism as one that has evolved in the same place where it now exists. A *native* organism is one that exists naturally in a region, not having been introduced there by accident or purpose. Dubos, Shaedler, Costello, and Holt (1955) and Dubos (1965) adopted Simpson's definitions, and Hershkovitz (1958) equated *native, autochthonous,* and *indigenous* to be equivalent to Simpson's *autochthonous.* Simpson's, Dubos', and Hershkovitz' suggestions as applied to animal evolution and geographical distribution are useful in our present context of emerging diseases.

Schistosomiasis mansoni (also known as bilharzia or snail fever), for instance, is autochthonous in Africa and is now native in Brazil, where it was first introduced with the slave traffic and found local viable intermediate snail hosts (*Biomphalaria* spp.) as well as alternative mammal reservoirs.

Changes in the physical environment or changes in social mores can also facilitate the emergence of infectious diseases. The expansion of schistosomiasis that resulted from the building of the Aswan reservoir has been widely reported. Scientists had predicted and expected an increase in the incidence of schistosome infection (snail fever) in consequence of the damming of the Nile River. Predictions were proved true when the annual floods became perennial. The Aswan High Dam and the Nile itself became a suitable habitat for year-round undisturbed populations of the snails that transmit the parasite to humans. Before the construction of the dam, irrigation canals dried up as there was an enforced period of 40 days of closure. During the ensuing flood of the river Nile, the silt with the snails and the weeds deposited on the dry beds were washed away. Population displacements and social disorganization resulting from revolutions or wars have given rise to well-publicized epidemics. Floods, earthquakes, and natural disasters always are followed by a rise in morbidity and mortality rates, and trade, travel, and deliberate or unexpected transportation and introduction of plants, animals, and microorganisms aid the worldwide dissemination of diseases.

CURRENT DEFINITIONS

Emerging infectious diseases, according to the CDC definition, are those infections that appeared recently in a population, or those that already existed but are spreading rapidly, in terms of both incidence and geographical distribution (Lederberg, Shope, & Oaks, 1992). Such spread may be due to the recent introduction of a new etiological agent or to a mutation arising in an existing agent, followed by its rapid dissemination in the population (Morse, 1995).

Throughout human history, many diseases have appeared and vanished, but it has not always been possible to ascertain if they were actually new or if they had been present but undetected. For this raison, Grmek (1993) substituted the idea of *emergence* for that of *novelty* and proposed five distinct historical instances for the recognition of emergence and novelty. In the first four, diseases may be considered emergent, and in the last one, as new.

1. It existed before being recognized, but escaped medical attention because it went unrecognized as a nosological entity of its own.

A seemingly new disease may have been confused with another disease for a long time or may simply not have been diagnosed and recognized by medical science. In this sense we agree with Latour and Woolgar (1979), accepting that social facts are socially constructed and, therefore, a disease is a social construct. We disagree with those authors in recognizing the objective reality of *lesions, vectors, and parasites.* They exist and have existed long before the appearance of humans, independent of the observer and of their official taxonomic, scientific, or popular recognition. *Diseases,* on the contrary, are collective descriptions of signals and symptoms as they affect different individuals mediated by culture (Avila-Pires, 2008). The highly subjective expressions "fever is high in most cases" and "many patients develop a rash, which may be absent in others" are clear evidence of the constructed character of diseases.

The case of Chagas disease is seminal. This disease actually emerged twice. The first time in 1909 when Carlos Chagas, a Brazilian medical researcher, described what he considered a new disease. Unfortunately, he gave a composite description of its symptoms and called it a "parasitic thyroiditis." The second emergence occurred after bitter arguments among researchers and was due to the Argentinean researcher Romaña who showed that Chagas had combined the real American trypanosomiasis and goiter in a nosological chimera (Delaporte, 1999).

Ensuing epidemiological investigations revealed that Chagas disease was widespread on the American continent, affecting millions of people before it was recognized by scientists.

2. It existed, but was only detected after a qualitative and quantitative alteration of its characteristics made it noticeable.

Biological evolution is a law of life. Pathogens evolve as do their vectors, hosts, and reservoirs. Changes in microorganisms may be rapid, enabling the invasion and colonization of new hosts, or leading to an increase or reduction of virulence. Hosts and reservoirs of pathogens act as biological filters, selecting genomic lineages among the vast array of natural polymorphic variants, which are capable of surviving the host's body defenses. Avian influenza viruses, for instance, do not infect humans, but if they are passed on to pigs, they may acquire that ability. Before this can happen, pigs and birds must coexist, allowing viruses to adapt to mammalian hosts before they can mutate and pass on to humans. In this category, life style and social behavior and the organization of public health services are fundamental to the emergence of infectious diseases.

A good example is the widespread use of air conditioning in houses, hotels, and hospitals with poor maintenance, providing the necessary conditions for legionellosis (Legionnaire's disease) outbreaks to emerge. Another example, presented by Grmek (1993), is toxic shock syndrome. Although described in 1978 as a new disease, it is actually a particular expression of the pathogenic action of the old staphylococcus, which results from the increased use of high-capacity tampons by women, which allow for an increase in the bacteria's virulence.

Our present concern also lies with the forecasts based on the possible consequences of global warming. The rise in global average temperatures may affect the geographical distribution of existing vectors and reservoirs of infectious diseases, thus widening the prevalence of zoonotic diseases in humans.

3. It was introduced in a region where it did not occur previously.

Migrations, wars, and the movement of people are chief factors in the spread and emergence of diseases (Thomas, 1956), as Crosby (1986) illustrated with respect to the role of colonialism. European expansionism was responsible for the introduction of several infectious and parasitic diseases across the world. Migratory waves from Europe, and the introduction of slaves from the African continent into the Americas, accounted for the eruption of epidemics and for the subsequent endemization of Old World diseases in the New World. However, length of travel and distance prevented many diseases from spreading far. Either the sick or the non-human hosts, vectors, or microorganisms would die in route. Today, the speed of travel, tourism, and international trade contributes to the globalization of many infectious diseases.

4. The emergence of a disease acquired from a non-human reservoir.

The term *zoonosis* was incorrectly credited to the German pathologist Virchow. In 1951, a Joint Committee of Experts from the World Health Organization (WHO) and the Food and Agriculture Organization (FAO) of the United Nations adopted the current official definition: it applies to the transmissible diseases that naturally affect humans and other vertebrate animals.

Hemorrhagic fevers such as Ebola, Hanta, Nipah, Lassa, and Marburg, as well as severe acute respiratory syndrome (SARS) and bird flu, are good examples of viruses that caused epidemics in recent times. Not all epidemiological chains have so far been elucidated and, for some diseases, the original sources are not known. Outbreaks due to the importation of animals for laboratory research, surgical transplants or organs, and for the production of drugs occurred. Nipah virus passed from flying fox bats to pigs and to humans, in a chain of events propitiated by the special conditions where pigsties were located. Lassa and Hanta are passed from rodents to humans, and Ebola was transmitted from apes to humans.

5. A new disease, when the causal agent or the necessary environmental conditions for its occurrence did not exist before the first clinical observations identified its presence.

There is also the possibility that as the result of laboratory manipulation of pathogenic organisms intended for research, biological warfare, or genetic engineering of agricultural products, a new disease emerges and spreads. In this fifth instance, Grmek recognizes the existence of a certain continuity with the past, as no organism may originate from spontaneous generation.

6. In addition to the categories proposed by the CDC and by Grmek we add the role of under-notification of those conditions presented by official lists of diseases subjected to compulsory notification, and also the failure to recognize and notify uncommon diseases.

Our knowledge about the incidence and prevalence of diseases depends on a reliable system of notification. There are lists of notifiable diseases at different levels of health administration and control: international, national, and regional (state, province, county, and municipality). International health regulations adopted by the WHO established smallpox, poliomyelitis due to wild-type poliovirus, human influenza caused by a new subtype, and SARS as notifiable diseases. They also include the following diseases because they have demonstrated the ability to cause serious public health impact and to spread rapidly and internationally: cholera, pneumonic plague, yellow fever, viral hemorrhagic fevers (Ebola, Lassa, and Marburg), and West Nile fever.

However, under-notification is at the basis of many emergent diseases. These cases occur and are diagnosed, but doctors and health authorities ignore or fail to report them. To justify this category we present two case studies illustrating the role under-notification plays in the characterization of emerging infectious diseases.

THE CASE OF ANGIOSTRONGYLIASIS

From a medical point of view abdominal angiostrongyliasis is a disease in which the symptoms are vague, for which there is no cure, and which can usually only be diagnosed by viewing and isolating the parasite through biopsies or detecting it through serological tests, when the result indicates an infection. There may be crossed reactions with other simultaneous or past parasitic infections and the treatment with anti-helminthics; drugs that kill pathogenic worms may result in the parasite migrating to other organs. The clinical manifestations occur in sites where such symptoms as severe abdominal pain, vomiting, and general weakness progressing to fever may be erroneously diagnosed as those of other diseases such as appendicitis or abdominal tumors.

In 1967, in Costa Rica, Céspedes et al. described a clinical case of a new disease for the medical science. In the same year Morera (1967) recognized its parasitic nature. In 1970 the intermediate (slugs) and definitive hosts (rodents) of the parasite were identified, and in 1971 Morera and Céspedes (1971), Morera (1971), and Morera and Ash (1971) described in greater detail the etiology, biological cycle, pathology, and the clinical characteristics of the disease.

In Brazil, a medical pathologist (Agostini, Marcolan, Lisot, & Lisot, 1984) described the first findings of the parasite and identified the characteristic intestinal lesions and was instrumental in expanding the study of this disease in the country. His former student and collaborator, Graeff-Teixeira became one of the foremost experts of angiostrongyliasis. In his doctoral thesis Graeff-Teixeira (1991) considered whether it was a new human parasitic disease or one that had been under-diagnosed, deciding in favor of the latter alternative. His own field research showed that the disease is commonly asymptomatic. His findings differ from those published in Costa Rica, where the disease seemed to be endemic. For Morera, the lack of medical knowledge was the main obstacle to showing the high prevalence of the disease, but for Graeff-Teixeira, the apparent rarity of this parasitosis in Brazil was due to the fact that, despite impressions that the disease occurs frequently, it is actually rare and, in most cases, asymptomatic. These differing conclusions derived from the different approaches taken by the researchers. Morera concentrated on individual case studies and anatomopathological (physically evident morbidity) results of tests, while Graeff-Teixeira (1991) relied on seroepidemiological (population-level clinical study) investigations in populations exposed to contamination, in areas where intermediate hosts were present using a test he developed.

Several articles reported the occurrence and distribution of cases in Brazil, although the disease went unreported in many states. In spite of the Graeff-Teixeira's conclusions regarding the possibility of under-diagnosis, we can neither rely on the prevalence of angiostrongyliasis nor dismiss the possibility of its wide presence, undetected, because of the lack of investigation.

Graeff-Teixeira's research indicated the need to revise the accepted diagnosis of the disease as described by Morera and the accompanying prophylactic procedures. Despite their differing conclusions, both Graeff-Teixeira and Morera agree that angiostrogyliasis is not a new disease but is under-diagnosed. From these facts, we conclude that this disease is endemic in Costa Rica and emergent in Brazil.

To be able to characterize a disease as emergent in a certain place and time, we depend on the following criteria: the ability to diagnose, and the medical outlook in a given place, at a given time; the state of the art concerning research in the relevant field and the available techniques at the disposal of medical doctors and scientists; and the priorities established by health authorities.

A LOCALIZED OUTBREAK OF POSSIBLY EMERGING CHAGAS DISEASE

In 2005 an unknown disease struck the members of a family from the municipality of Penha, northern Santa Catarina state, Brazil. It was eventually identified as Chagas disease. Early symptoms may not be easily recognized and include fever, anemia, swelling of lymphatic glands, and headaches, evolving to a pathological enlargement of certain organs as the esophagus, colon, and heart. A characteristic swelling of the site of the insect-vector bite is present. This disease has been considered, at different times, to be emergent, endemic, and under-notified, in view of the absence of official records of previous such cases in Santa Catarina.

A literature search showed that, since 1959, reports of the presence of the insect vectors of the disease have been on file in the official state health institute. In 1961, a scientific paper divulged the results of field investigations showing that in the state capital, Florianópolis, 40% of the insect vector *Panstrongylus megistus* and 70% of *Rhodnius domesticus* from natural environments, including nests of rodents and marsupials, were infected with a *Trypanosoma cruzi*-like protozoan. *P. megistus* is the most common species of the Chagas bug in Santa Catarina and is found living around houses and in chicken pens and other outbuildings in urban areas (Galvão, Mello, Ferreira Neto, & Leal, 1961).

By 1971, experts recognized that the situation of autochthonous Chagas disease was little known in Florianopolis and in the state of Santa Catarina. In 1985, a new study showed that 23.5% of all captured opossums and 5.2% of rodents found near human habitations were infected and reported two new cases of Chagas disease from Santa Catarina, one probably from Florianopolis. Although several papers reported new findings, no action was taken in order to investigate the occurrence of the disease in humans in the state (Schlemper et al., 1985).

In 2002, a doctoral dissertation (Silva, 2002) used the records at the Blood Bank (HEMOSC) of Florianopolis to show that there were prospective blood donors in the state of Santa Catarina, who were – or had been – infected with *T. cruzi*.

Current maps of the occurrence and geographical distribution of Chagas disease in Brazil show the state of Santa Catarina as free of this disease, in spite of the confirmed presence of infected animal reservoirs and vectors within its political borders. In consequence, there is no system of health surveillance for Chagas disease. The distribution of a disease can only be understood in terms of the ecology and environmental requirements of animal reservoirs, vectors, and parasites, which seldom coincides with political borders, as national, state, or municipal limits.

Chagas disease may also be present in large numbers of individual carriers that show no symptom of the infection. They are *infected* but not *sick*, or *clinically ill*. That was the situation in March 2005, when three deaths in the same family were officially recorded, soon to be followed by further cases in the area. At that time, a meeting on tropical medicine was taking place at Florianopolis, in which a paper on the possibility of oral transmission of Chagas disease in northeastern Brazil was read (Shikanai-Yasuda et al., 1991). The members of the affected family blamed sugar cane juice they had consumed at a roadside establishment. As the first tentative diagnosis of that unknown condition had been of leptospirosis, a water-borne infection, discarded when no contaminated source was found and laboratory tests showed presence of the parasite of Chagas disease in the blood of patients, the investigators assumed that the origin of the epidemic was the sugar cane juice.

Anyway, if the patients were contaminated orally or through the conventional pathway (an insect vector), the disease would be classified as emergent in Santa Catarina on the account of under-notification of this disease in this state.

CONCLUSION

It is time for us to reconsider the possibility of adopting a single, all-embracing definition of emergent diseases for the following reasons.

From a philosophical point of view, the alternative conceptions of infectious diseases as independent entities or as physiological alterations of subjects are of fundamental importance. Also of significance is the argument raised by Delaporte concerning the identity of diseases as they affect human or non-human hosts: what passes from a non-human host to the human species is a pathogen or parasite, not a disease. For that reason, Delaporte (1998) discounts Grmek's fourth category, the passage of a pathogen from a non-human reservoir to a human one as an emergent disease. Can we say, for example, that Chagas disease in an armadillo is the same as in humans? For that matter, what about different persons with the same disease but showing different symptoms? We are aware that the movement of a pathogen along a biological/epidemiological chain produces organic modifications. The introduction of organisms into a new environment may change the genetic composition of its populations. Dobzhansky (1941) described this phenomenon as a *balanced polymorphism*, as he observed the variation in the genetic composition of a population of *Drosophila* flies in the Amazons, and verified that certain genes were dominant at certain times of the year, according to changes in microclimatic conditions.

This issue involves the definition of disease and the conception of diseases as constructs, which also depends on the sociocultural context in which the researcher works (Avila-Pires, 2008). If we follow the CDC definition of emerging infectious diseases as infections that appeared recently in a population, or those that already existed but are spreading rapidly, we adopt a pragmatic point of view. It may be useful in the realm of public health administration, where actions do not always depend on the investigation of the origins and evolution of diseases. Controlling measures are often a generic nature, regardless of the specific identity of the pathogen, and are directed toward the manipulation of environmental factors and conditions, and to the adoption of sanitary measures concerning the quality of air, soil, water, wastes, vectors, and reservoirs. Those measures are intended to block the roads of disease transmission. Manson (1900) showed that it was possible to control a disease – malaria – without attacking the disease directly, or treating patients, but by using a model to estimate risk, and controlling the populations of mosquito vectors. Strategies are the same for groups of diseases, according to their ecology and means of dissemination, and are seldom – if ever – specific.

For a practicing physician who is required to arrive at a precise diagnosis and prescribe a proper treatment, these philosophical issues are both academic and immaterial. For historians and epidemiologists, however, the search for the index case in an epidemic is a valid endeavor, as it is also the search for the original non-human reservoirs and vectors of new human pathogens. For recent examples, see the searches for the non-human sources of hemorrhagic fevers and HIV.

On the other hand, if we adopt Grmek's proposal, we end by considering almost every infectious disease to be emergent. For instance, seasonal common influenza *emerges* every year. Diseases that are endemic within the confines of a given geographical region would be considered emergent when introduced elsewhere, which happens all the time. Children's diseases, such as measles and mumps, reemerge every seven or eight years in places where vaccination is not the rule, as a new generation reaches school age.

Another source of confusion when we try to adopt a single definition arises from the fact that different researchers may define and classify diseases in different ways or even use the term "disease" ambiguously. For example, the history of medicine records three major pandemics of plague: the first began during the 14th century, the second in the 17th century, and the third in the 19th century. The pathogen was *Yersinia pestis* in all cases, but, with respect to clinical symptoms, they were distinct diseases. The first epidemic was bubonic plague, which is not airborne and requires a flea vector to be transmitted from one human to another. The 17th-century epidemic, which became known as the Black Death, was pneumonic plague, which is one of the most contagious airborne diseases known and necessitates the isolation of patients and the institution of quarantine. For a bacteriologist they are the same disease, but for the practicing medical doctor they require different approaches and treatments, while for the public health official they demand different responses and controlling measures. Another disease that provokes distinct symptoms in its hosts is rabies. Rabies is a *viral zoonotic neuroinvasive* disease that causes acute *encephalitis* and has a lethality of 100% in humans. It affects several species of mammals and the infected saliva of a diseased animal transmits it through a deep bite. In carnivores and in humans, an incontrollable excitation is characteristic, while in ruminants it causes paralysis. Bats may become infected without any apparent symptoms or they may suffer an acute infection, followed by unusual behavior when insectivorous and herbivorous species attack mammals.

Such considerations demonstrate the conflation of situations which are clearly distinct under a single definition without making a distinction between diseases and their pathogens. We may continue to do so, for logistical reasons, but it is crucial that we consider, as social scientists, policy makers, and medical practitioners, what the political and practical implications of such conflation might be.

REFERENCES

Agostini, A. A., Marcolan, A. M., Lisot, J. M. C., & Lisot, J. U. F. (1984). Angiostrongilíase abdominal. Estudo anátomo-patológico de quatro casos observados no Rio Grande do Sul, Brasil. *Memórias do Instituto Oswaldo Cruz, 79*(4), 443–445.

Avila-Pires, F. D. (2008). On the concept of disease. *Revista de Historia & Humanidades Medicas, 4*(1). Available at: http://www.fmv-uba.org.ar/histomedicina/index1024x768.htm (accessed 12 October 2008).

Céspedes, R., Salas, J., Mekbel, S., Troper, L., Mullner, F., & Morera, P. (1967). Granulomas entéricos y linfáticos con intense eosinofilia tisular producidos por un estrongilídeo. I Patologia. *Acta Médica Costarricense, 10*(3), 235–255.

Crosby, A. W. (1986). *Ecological imperialism.* Cambridge: Cambridge University Press.

Crosby, A. W. (1994). *Germs, seeds & animals. Studies in ecological history.* Armonk: Sharpe.

Delaporte, F. (1998). La nouveauté en pathologie. In: D. Lecourt (Ed.), *Vers des nouvelles maladies* (pp. 9–37). Paris: Puf.

Delaporte, F. (1999). *La maladie de Chagas.* Paris: Payot.

Dobzhansky, T. (1941). *Genetics and the origin of species.* New York: Columbia University Press.

Dubos, R. (1965). *Man adapting.* New Haven: Yale University Press.

Dubos, R., Shaedler, R. W., Costello, R., & Holt, D. (1955). Indigenous, normal, and autochthonous flora of the gastro-intestinal tract. *Journal of Experimental Medicine, 192,* 67–76.

Ewald, P. (2002). *Plague time. The new germ theory of disease.* New York: Anchor.

Galvão, A., Mello, L., Ferreira Neto, J., & Leal, H. (1961). Sôbre a distribuição geográfica e infecção natural do *Rhodnius domesticus* Neiva e Pinto, 1923. *Revista Brasileira de Malariologia e doenças tropicais, 13*(1–2), 57–60.

Graeff-Teixeira, C. (1991). Contribuição ao conhecimento da epidemiologia da angiostrongilíase abdominal no sul do Brasil. *Tese de Doutorado* em Medicina Tropical, Instituto Oswaldo Cruz, Rio de Janeiro.

Grmek, M. D. (1993). Le concept de maladie émergente. *History and Philosophy of the Life Sciences, 15,* 282–296.

Grmek, M. D. (1995). Declin et émergence des maladies. *História, Ciências, Saúde-Manguinhos, II*(2), 9–32.

Hershkovitz, P. A. (1958). Geographic classification of neotropical mammals. *Fieldiana Zoology, 36*(6), 583–620.

Karlen, A. (2001). *Plague's progress. A social history of man and disease.* London: Phoenix.

Latour, B., & Woolgar, S. (1979). *Laboratory life: The social construction of scientific facts.* Los Angeles: Sage.

Lederberg, J., Shope, R. E., & Oaks, S. C., Jr. (1992). *Emerging infectious: Microbial threats to health in the United States.* Washington: National Academy Press.

Manson, P. (1900). Experimental proof of the mosquito-malaria theory. *British Medical Journal, 2,* 949–951.

Morera, P. (1967). Granulomas enteericos y linfáticos con intensa eosinofilia tisular producidos por un estrongilideo. II aspecto parasitologico. *Acta Médica Costarricense, 10*(3), 257–265.

Morera, P. (1971). Investigación del huésped definitivo de Angiostrongylus costaricensis. *Boletin Chileno de Parasitologia, 15,* 133–134.

Morera, P., & Ash, L. R. (1971). Investigación del huésped intermediario de *Angiostrongylus costaricensis. Boletin Chileno de parasitologia, 25,* 135.

Morera, P., & Céspedes, R. (1971). *Angiostrongylus costaricensis* n, sp. (Nematoda: Metastrongyloidea), a new lungworm occurring in man in Costa Rica. *Revista de Biologia Tropical, 18*(1), 173–185.

Morse, S. S. (1995). Factors in the emergence of infectious diseases. *Emerging Infectious Diseases, 1*(1), 7–15.

Ochman, H., Lawrence, J. G., & Groisman, E. A. (2000). Lateral gene transfer and the nature of bacterial innovation. *Nature, 405,* 299–304.

O'Connor, S. M., Taylor, C. E., & Hughes, J. M. (2006). Emerging infectious determinants of chronic diseases. *Emerging Infectious Diseases, 12*(7), 1051–1056.

Relman, D. A. (1998). Detection and identification of previously unrecognized microbial pathogens. *Emerging Infectious Diseases, 4*(3), 1–10.

Schlemper, B. R., Jr., Steindel, M., Gargioni, R., Farias, C., Oliveira, R., & Trianon, J. (1985). Reservatórios e vetores silvestres de *Trypanosoma cruzi* e suas relações com o domicilio humano na Ilha de Santa Catarina. *Arquivos Catarinenses de Medicina, 2*(14), 91–95.

Shikanai-Yasuda, M., Brisola, M. C., Guedes, L. A., Siqueira, G. S., Barone, A. A., Dias, J. C. P., et al. (1991). Possible oral transmission of acute Chagas disease in Brazil. *Revista do Instituto de Medicina Tropical de Sao Paulo, 33*(5), 351–357.

Silva, A. M. (2002). *Sobre a transmissão da doença de Chagas por transfusão sanguínea no Estado de Santa Catarina, Brasil.* Tese de Doutorado (Departamento de Epidemiologia da Faculdade de Saúde Pública da Universidade de São Paulo), São Paulo.

Simpson, G. G. (1953). *Evolution and geography.* Eugene: Condon Lectures Publications.

Sournia, R. (1984). *Les épidémies dans l'histoire de l'homme.* Paris: Flammarion.

Thomas, W. L., Jr. (1956). *Man's role in changing the face of the earth.* Chicago: The University of Chicago Press.

SOUNDING A PUBLIC HEALTH ALARM: PRODUCING WEST NILE VIRUS AS A NEWLY EMERGING INFECTIOUS DISEASE EPIDEMIC

Maya K. Gislason

ABSTRACT

Purpose – *The purpose of this chapter is to illustrate that when produced through relations of power, West Nile virus (WNV), as it exists on the Public Health Agency of Canada's (PHAC) website, is an effect of the kinds of knowledge, techniques of power, and disciplinary apparatuses that operate on the website and in society.*

Methodology/approach – *The approach used in the in-depth research project which informs this chapter is an elaboration of Michel Foucault's work on relations of power which offers an effective way of studying the PHAC's website as a collection of authoritative knowledges and as a product of a set of systems, structures, and processes which have helped to assemble and distribute knowledge about WNV.*

Findings – *The findings discussed in this chapter offer a critical reading of the PHAC's overall production of WNV, focusing particularly on its initial emergence starting in 2001. Cumulatively, this chapter*

Understanding Emerging Epidemics: Social and Political Approaches
Advances in Medical Sociology, Volume 11, 77–99
Copyright © 2010 by Emerald Group Publishing Limited
All rights of reproduction in any form reserved
ISSN: 1057-6290/doi:10.1108/S1057-6290(2010)0000011009

argues that myriad relations of power have produced WNV as a bio-socio-administrative construct.

Contribution to the field – *This research illustrates one way that Foucault's theories of power can be used to conduct a critical analysis of both the discursive and material dimensions of the production of contemporary public health issues. Such an approach is useful to scholars who wish to place the emergence of a disease phenomenon within political, institutional, economic, cultural, and social relations of power; thereby drawing attention to how specific spaces, places, individuals, and institutions contribute to the production of contemporary health alarms.*

INTRODUCTION

In this chapter a study of how the Public Health Agency of Canada (PHAC) has used its website to develop and distribute a very specific set of messages about West Nile virus (WNV) is presented. Official public health websites are ideal data sources for the study of how authoritative knowledge about newly emerging, re-emerging, and surging diseases is being produced by scientific, medical, and public health practitioners within the public sphere. Analytically, the value of the these official websites is that each text posted contains discursive information about the kinds of ideas that inform the organization's responses to new disease phenomena as well as offer insight into how disease emergences are produced as public health alarms within the public health context. The theoretical work of Michel Foucault is used to frame this social construction analysis and does so through an analysis of how power is enacted in particular relations of power in order to "produce" specific effects. The methodological use of power allows for an analysis of the "production" of WNV by paying attention to three key activities: first, locating the production of WNV within political, institutional, economic, cultural, and social relations of power is made possible. Second, highlighting the fact that techniques of power have both discursive and material dimensions – an observation which draws attention to the discursive and material aspects of the PHAC's production of WNV – is enabled. Third, emphasizing the importance of power relations within the production of WNV draws attention to the generativity of power/knowledge relations and to how specific spaces, places, individuals, and institutions have contributed to the production of WNV.

In the first section of this chapter I discuss the phenomenon of disease emergences and how emergence is interlinked with the organizations and structures which respond to these novel events. I then introduce features of Foucault's theories of power, placing the focus on discipline, discourse, and power/knowledge, and describe how I place these concepts at the center of my study. A brief introduction of Foucault's theoretical understanding of techniques of power is also offered as is an explanation of how and why I employ these conceptual mechanisms, identified as surveillance, individualization, totalization, classification, normalization, exclusion, regulation, and distribution, to analyze the PHAC's website. Key findings of this study are discussed in the following section. Insight one describes how WNV is a bio-social–administrative phenomenon while the second one makes the observation that WNV is a product of the PHAC as it was in the current historical moment. The third insight suggests that WNV is a justification for the PHAC's new pro-active public health care delivery system. The chapter concludes with comments on how this study of WNV draws attention to specific ways in which institutional responses to biological entities are inextricably linked to relations of power and to the value of studying the production of diseases in an age where health risks are proliferating both inside and outside of Canada.

THE EMERGENCE OF DISEASES AND STRUCTURES OF RESPONSE

In February 2000, two years before the first WNV infections in humans were detected in Canada, Health Canada – the *department* of the government of *Canada* responsible for national *health* – established a West Nile Virus Steering Committee (PHAC, 2005a). Since 2000, although the remit of public health has been shifted out of Health Canada and been placed under the auspices of a newly formed public health agency, the WNV committee continues to stand today and is comprised of representatives from organizations such as Health Canada, various Provincial Ministries of Health, Conservation, Environment, and Natural Resources, the Department of National Defence, Environment Canada, the Canadian Food Inspection Agency, and the Canadian Cooperative Wildlife Health Centre (PHAC, 2008). In 2000 the federal government instructed this steering committee to develop a pan-Canadian strategy for controlling the spread of WNV in Canada and to ameliorate its impacts once it arrived (Health Canada, 2003a, 2003b, 2003c). On September 24, 2004, amid growing concern about infectious disease epidemics in Canada, and a lack of confidence in the government's ability to respond to them through Health

Canada,[1] the federal Liberal government announced the creation of the PHAC (PHAC, 2004a). The government presented the PHAC as a pro-active pan-Canadian public health agency that would address WNV as one of the many newly emergent infectious diseases placed under this new agency's jurisdiction (Privy Council Office, Canada, 2004; Treasury Board of Canada Secretariat, 2005). This announcement marked not only a new era of newly emerging infectious disease challenges to public health both nationally and internationally, but also a new era of public health governance in Canada.

Although citizen and media activity (Morshed, 2002; Hawaleshka, 2003; CBC, 2006) helped to maintain the PHAC's awareness on WNV, it is ultimately through the PHAC organizational mandate that a systematized, authoritative health promotion response to WNV has been administered. As such, the PHAC has played a central role in constructing what kind of a health threat WNV is perceived to be as well as in articulating its relevance to Canadians. One place of significant interface between the PHAC and the Canadian public is its website which is the most comprehensive information resource about WNV in Canada. The texts compiled on this site define WNV (PHAC, 2003, 2004b), explain how it arrived in Canada (PHAC, 2005a), describe the ways in which WNV is a health threat (PHAC, 2004c), convey statistics on who is more likely to fall seriously ill from WNV (PHAC, 2004d, 2004e), and instruct people in how to protect themselves against infection (PHAC, 2004f). The website also contains health advisories for public servants (PHAC, 2004g), diagnostic protocols for laboratory technicians and medical practitioners (Office of Laboratory Security, PHAC, 2003; PHAC, 2004g), information for people who work with animals or have pets (PHAC, 2004h), and an epidemiological database titled *The MONITOR*, which provides up-to-date reports, statistics, and satellite images of WNV infection in birds, mosquitoes, and humans across Canada (PHAC, 2005b).

FOUCAULDIAN PERSPECTIVES IN POWER

As an empirical site, WNV can be studied using an array of theoretical approaches; however, I have identified Michel Foucault as a theorist who offers an effective way of studying the PHAC's website as a collection of authoritative knowledges about WNV and as a product of a set of systems, structures, and processes which have helped to assemble and distribute this knowledge. In particular, it is Foucault's theories of power that are useful as he sees power as an overarching physics or technology, enacted in the empirical world (see 1980b, p. 140) through specific techniques. Examples of

Foucault's techniques at work in the PHAC's texts are evident across the website. In some texts the health promotion messages seem like they are not only intended to educate the reader, but also designed to change the reader's behaviors vis-à-vis WNV. In other passages the techniques are less visible, as is the case with the website's exclusion of "inferior" preventative strategies. Specifically, on the WNV website specific forms of knowledge are the entities that are most often excluded. The PHAC does not tend to actively exclude ideas by discussing the concepts that are being rebuffed, or by offering a rationalization for the rejections; instead, more covert means are used, such as not mentioning the existence of alternatives. Therefore, although competing scientific and popular perspectives exist as to what WNV is, only one perspective – that of the PHAC – is promoted. In order to accomplish such a task, the PHAC has even excluded information produced by organizations that agree with the PHAC's basic conception of the virus yet have been opposed to aspects of the PHAC's proposed method of remediation, for example, the use of specific chemicals in WNV treatment programs. This is the case with literature produced by medical and scientific organizations which expresses concerns about the health impacts of larvicides and pesticides, such as a report by Toxics Action Centre and the Maine Environmental Policy Institute (Sugg & Wilson, 2001) and the World Research Institute (see Repetto & Baliga, 1996). As a result, one of the uncontested and central messages promoted on the website is that using chemicals is an effective preventative strategy even though this is a highly contested issue and a subject that in recent years the PHAC has also started to reconsider (see CBC, 2008). Still other times, there is a noteworthy overlap between the vocabulary Foucault uses to describe techniques of power and the terminology the PHAC uses to describe its own activities. For example, the terms surveillance, regulation, and classification often appear on the website.

In this study I place WNV at the center of the grid of relationships, structures, and effects by using the concepts of: (1) discourse, (2) power/knowledge, (3) discipline, and (4) techniques of power to investigate how relations of power shape what is known about WNV as a viral public health alarm.

DISCOURSE

On the PHAC website discourses are at once a medium through which the PHAC produces ideas about WNV and simultaneously a mechanism that reveals the construction process (Foucault, 1980b, p. 101). This is possible because discourses materialize through "social practices and specific activities that sustain and reproduce [their] discursive formations"

(Moss & Dyck, 2002, p. 15). Since discourses are loosely structured combinations of concerns, themes, and types of assertions, they can be thought of as reflecting the epoch within which they emerge (Marshall, 1998, p. 163). In a sense not only do discourses reformulate a body of heterogeneous ideas from diverse disciplines into a single collection of texts, but they are also embodied in "technical processes, in institutions, in patterns for general behavior, in forms for transmission and diffusion, and in pedagogical forms which, at once, impose and maintain them" (Foucault, 1995, p. 2000). Examples of this weaving together of heterogeneous ideas, disciplinary orientations, and political processes abound on the website. The discourses about WNV presented on the website are produced through a bringing together of a variety of organizations each concerned with their own jurisdiction including the *Centre for Food-borne, Environmental and Zoonotic Infectious Disease, the PHAC*, provincial and territorial Ministries of Health, the Canadian Cooperative Wildlife Health Centre, Health Canada's First Nations and Inuit Health Branch (FNIHB), the Canadian Blood Services, and Héma-Québec (PHAC, 2010a). There is also a notable continuity between the key organizations involved in monitoring WNV in Canada and the themes presented as relevant to the general public by way of the main menu on the WNV website which directs visitors to information under the headings: symptoms, protect yourself and your family, First Nations, animals, surveillance, maps & stats, and public education resources (PHAC, 2010b). The discourses produced on the PHAC website are distributed widely across Canada via provincial public health organizations and through public health promotion literature and through this process become the authoritative knowledge on WNV. What is more, in order to assemble specific aspects of its WNV construction, texts on the PHAC website repeatedly rely on a variety of external discourses pertaining to disease, risk, fear, and discipline. For example, the PHAC uses discourses to define WNV as a virus-causing illness and to strategically produce responsible individuals who are expected to enact the PHAC's prevention plans. The discourses the PHAC draws upon to produce "good, healthy citizens" include medical, governmental, and scientific discourses about health, risk, and prevention, which the PHAC links to discourses of responsibility and self-discipline.

POWER/KNOWLEDGE

On the PHAC website, official knowledge is both drawn upon and produced within discourses relating to WNV. Foucault suggests that it is "in discourse that power and knowledge are joined together"(1980b, p. 100). In addition, through its construction of WNV, the PHAC also participates in the delineation of some forms of knowledge as "popular" and therefore dismissible. For example, information relating to insect repellents that do not contain DEET as well as a variety of "alternate" forms of natural insect repellents (such as citronella) suffers from such a dismissal. In place of identifying specific kinds of knowledge as an alternative to the website's official discourse the PHAC actually subjugates many forms of knowledge it has labeled as "popular." The PHAC justifies the subjugation of ways of knowing and sets of knowledge not developed within mainstream scientific contexts on the basis that they are "located low down on the hierarchy, beneath the required level of cognition or scientificity" (Foucault, 1980a, p. 81). The PHAC sends the message to the Canadian public that it would be irresponsible for a governmental agency to distribute or endorse such knowledge.

The concept of power/knowledge and the identification of official and subjugated knowledges enable me to think about the production of WNV as a disciplinary practice (discussed in more detail in the next section). Together the PHAC's texts (the discourses) and the techniques of power found within them produce WNV as a social construct that is more than a biological entity and more than an educational or public health entity as well. I can see power/knowledge most clearly within texts on the PHAC website where the production of WNV is linked to efforts to generate specific outcomes, especially the production of healthy citizens who know enough to voluntarily adhere to the PHAC's public health prevention strategies. When power/knowledge sets the parameters of possibility for the construction of WNV in this particular historical moment, it is then possible to see the various milieus within which knowledge about WNV is produced. This holds true not only for the material, but also for the conceptual milieus, which in the case of the PHAC's production of WNV is a context contoured by the principles of governmentality, the view that knowledge produced through scientific positivism is authoritative, the neo-liberal political context of an era characterized as a risk culture where notions of fear, threat, and disharmony circulate widely, and a worldview that links pandemics to global health insecurity.

POWER AND DISCIPLINE

Foucault characterizes modern societies as disciplinary societies because they achieve social regulation and control through the production and discipline of individuals. The power/knowledge nexus governs disciplinary societies, and the enactment of force often occurs simply through shaping people's thoughts, concerns, interests, and motivations. These dynamics are played out in informal settings between people who know each other well and in formal settings such as institutional relationships. Once people understand this, the disciplinary practices at work within the relations of power in which they are enmeshed begin to become visible.

Relations of power are inextricably linked to the discipline of populations because relations of power form the mediums through which discipline is imagined, its technologies developed, and its practices enacted. This linkage also exists because relations of power form the institutions, procedures, analyses, reflections, calculations, and tactics through which discipline is exercised (Foucault, 1991, p. 102). Foucault observed that governmental activities often justify disciplinary practices by invoking the notion of the welfare of the population (1991, p. 100). In accordance, organizations such as the PHAC employ disciplinary practices to manage populations both on the larger scale of the "the people" as an undifferentiated population and on the smaller scale of groups and individuals. The more discrete the grouping, the more intensive and detailed the PHAC's disciplinary strategies for managing the population can be (see Foucault, 1991, p. 102; Petersen & Lupton, 1997).

In order to see the management of populations at work at the scale of both individuals and groups one must look for moments when the techniques of "individualization" and "totalization" are being employed. By the technique of individualization, Foucault is referring to the role individuals play in the circulation of power. Individualization refers to the process where physical form is characterized, made visible, and set up as a conduit of power. For example, individualization is a mechanism that enables the PHAC to test the efficacy of its WNV prevention program. In this case, individuals are produced as discrete units of measurement. In 2004 a Canadian Communicable Disease Report on WNV published data from a statistical survey of individual's impressions about the efficacy of the PHAC's response to WNV and the degree to which the response had shifted people's thoughts about and behaviors toward WNV. In producing the individual, the PHAC had created another method for reproducing and refining its own practices. Totalization on the other hand is a specification of collectivities (Gore, 1995, pp. 179–180). A collectivity is totalized when it is made tangible, recognizable, and solid enough to be interacted with. An effect of totalization is that collectivities are made readily recognizable and can then be taken up within other techniques of power. Predominantly, totalization is a technique of power used for governing and regulating groups as well as for producing knowledge. A very clear technique of totalization is the PHAC's grouping of "First Nations and Inuit peoples" as distinct (and separate) from the "general population" in order to systematize its distribution of information to a wide range of community groups.[2] Most generally it is a grouping expressed by placing WNV information for the two groups on separate websites and by customizing the prevention message to each group. Comparing the material produced for the two groups demonstrates that totalization is a technique that not only produces groupings and characterizes them, but also serves an instrumental purpose within the distribution of the WNV campaign material. Once totalized and characterized, groupings can be submitted to other techniques of power such as regulation, classification, and exclusion.

The concept of discipline sensitizes me to three ideas in particular. First, because the PHAC is the administrator of the WNV response, the agency's production of WNV is linked to governmental approaches to promoting the welfare of the population. Second, given this governmental affiliation, the subtle disciplining of the individual must be at work in the production of WNV. I am suggesting here that relations of power not only depend on disciplinary tactics to keep people safe, but also use discourses surrounding WNV as a tool within their disciplinary practices designed to protect people and the nation-state. Finally, given the variety of individuals, institutions, practices, and agendas involved in the production of WNV, WNV's meaning must be permutated by each relationship of power involved in its production. In this case, WNV is an instrument of, but also instrumental to, both the practice of discipline within relations of power and their roles within the PHAC's production of healthy Canadians.

TECHNOLOGIES OF POWER AND TECHNIQUES OF POWER

In the *History of Sexuality, Vol. 1*, Foucault suggests that the exercise of power is a technology that assembles various techniques into a single machinery (technology) (1980b, p. 140). Technologies operate on the scale of institutions and governments by combining various elements of social and economic reality, according to specific sets of rules, and in order to control populations (Ewald, 1991, p. 197). Techniques, on the other hand, are mechanisms, procedures, tools, and skills that turn discipline into the art of delicate and detailed transformations. Though there are multiple techniques through which power as a technology is enacted, Foucault's work draws particular attention to the techniques of surveillance, individualization, totalization, classification, normalization, exclusion, distribution, and regulation (see Gore, 1995). Although each technique of power functions in a unique way, when they work together these mechanisms form "a closely linked grid of disciplinary coercions whose purpose is in fact to assure the cohesion of the social body" (Foucault, 1980a, p. 106). As I read the techniques of power as producing WNV, it was possible to see how specific disciplinary coercions are central to the PHAC's institutional responses to infectious diseases and how these responses are dependent on a cohesive representation of WNV as a public health threat. The central tenet of this chapter – that it is possible to study mechanisms of power through noting how they function within relations of power (see Foucault, 1980a, p. 39) – is also substantiated by Foucault's observation that techniques of power are at work throughout (disciplinary) society because they operate across scales that range from the macro- or structural scale to the micro- or individual scale (see Rouse, 1994, p. 95). Perhaps for this reason, Foucault describes a swarming effect that transforms "local exercise[s] of force within the confines of a particular institution into far-reaching relationships of power" (Rouse, 1994, p. 106). Therefore, whether by way of his notions of discourse, power/knowledge, or discipline, Foucault emphasizes that the social world both shapes and is shaped by specific activities that can be observed (Turner, 1997, pp. ix–xxi).

METHODOLOGY

In order to conduct a Foucauldian analysis of the role of power relations in the production of WNV it was essential to stop thinking about WNV as a biological viral entity and to engage the idea that, on the PHAC website, WNV is something other than a biological entity; it is a product of social relations. Foucault's theories of power draw attention to the mechanisms that produce social phenomena. Congruently, on the PHAC website, techniques of power empirically reveal how WNV has been produced because techniques of power are both conceptual abstractions and concretely enacted within the social world. As such, the texts on the PHAC website must be viewed as the products of specific activities by PHAC personnel as well as by scientists, medical practitioners, public health officials, and governmental administrators. The mixed elements that have been used by the PHAC to assemble its WNV response include institutional mandates, technological innovations, social response patterns to fear, cultural expectations about health, architectural expressions of governmental administration, regulatory decisions, public health administrative practices, and scientific research into WNV. A result of thinking about WNV as the product of a mélange of concrete acts and specific forms of knowledge is that WNV becomes not only an effect of power, but also the entire process of constructing WNV.

The methodological use of power in this research occurs in three ways. First, placing power at the center of the study locates the production of WNV within political, institutional, economic, cultural, and social relations of power. Second, highlighting the fact that techniques of power have both discursive and material dimensions draws attention to the discursive and material aspects of the PHAC's production of WNV. Third, emphasizing the importance of power relations within the production of WNV draws attention to the generativity of power/knowledge relations and to how specific spaces, places, individuals, and institutions have contributed to the production of WNV.

The analytical strategy I use for thinking about power as a conceptual tool is based on the work of Jennifer Gore (1995; Gore & Gitlin, 2003) who identifies, categorizes, and operationalizes power in terms of the eight techniques of power that she sees as central to Foucault's work: surveillance, individualization, totalization, classification, normalization, exclusion, regulation, and distribution. Her definitions, and examples of how she uses the techniques, offer an analytical strategy for working with data that is responsive to the various contexts, participants, and disciplinary agendas being studied because it constantly draws the attention back to an analysis of the techniques and not the actors or the mediums of exchange.

FINDINGS

Three key insights emerge from this study about how Foucault's eight techniques of power work together on the PHAC's website to produce WNV: (1) WNV is more than simply a viral entity, it is a biological, social, and administrative construct; (2) WNV is a product of the PHAC as it exists in our current historical moment; and (3) WNV is a justification for the PHAC's new type of pro-active public health care delivery system.

Insight One: WNV as a Bio-social–administrative Phenomenon

On the PHAC website, the production of WNV is premised on the idea that WNV is a biological phenomenon. However, on the website, it is not the biological dimensions of WNV but rather their social significance that is the focus of most of the texts assembled. By weaving discourses about the biology of WNV and WNV infection into its public health response, the PHAC produces texts that highlight the social implications of WNV infection. In that the construction of WNV also occurs within the context of the PHAC as a public health agency, WNV is conceptualized as an administrative event. Therefore, on the PHAC website, WNV is produced as a biological, social, and administrative phenomenon. At times, these three conceptualizations of WNV are kept separate, as is the case when various individuals and branches of the PHAC work separately, but simultaneously, to define WNV as a discrete biological, social, and administrative event. In these moments, individuals and branches endeavor to keep their own discourses, and the relations of power that produced them, separate. For example, many scientists exclusively define WNV as a virus and draw on concepts such as epidemic, outbreak, prevalence, cure, vaccine, and transmission to describe the relevance of WNV to science. These framings are found in the diagnostic literature for doctors and the laboratory protocols for diagnosis. In contrast, PHAC personnel developing "Fight the Bite!" campaign material define WNV in terms of its social relevance. Finally, governmental administrators produce WNV as a policy, fiscal, human resources, national security, research, public health programming, or election campaign issue.

At other times, the biological, social, and administrative discourses are folded into one representation referred to as WNV. The technique of folding disparate discourses into one form is most obvious within the PHAC's administrative response to WNV. WNV becomes an administrative construct when the PHAC considers how the virus infects people, how it is transmitted, evaluates the kinds of illness it produces in people, and estimates, according to region, the number of severe cases of WNV infection that will emerge. Once WNV takes on the form of an entity to be administered, the PHAC can then respond by assessing its responsibilities and resources vis-à-vis particular populations and regions. Clearly, the PHAC's organizational apparatus requires that WNV become something other than simply a viral entity because it is an agency designed to react politically, socially, and economically to "newly emergent infectious diseases." For example, within branches of the PHAC that deal with national health security issues, WNV is produced both as a virus and as a viral threat to national security and over time comes to be referred to using the short-hand "a viral threat" or "a viral invader." WNV as the "viral invader" is then linked to various administrative infectious disease response protocols. Another way of stating this is to say that administratively, WNV is a product of power/knowledge relations that are at work within the PHAC's public health infrastructure.

The practice of defining WNV simultaneously as a bio-social–administrative entity is evidenced in other responses, such as within the production of material for the "Fight the Bite" campaign where WNV is presented as a virus transmissible by mothers to their fetuses and breastfeeding infants or as a virus that preys on families more generally. Within these framings, WNV forms an indiscriminate biological risk to the Canadian public writ large and poses, therefore, a significant challenge to the public health infrastructure. As this example shows, the assembly of WNV as a bio-social–administrative construct reveals the mutuality between relations of power within the PHAC and the circulation of discourses about WNV through these relations of power.

Insight Two: WNV as a Product of the PHAC in this Current Historical Moment

The heterogeneity of WNV and the variety of arenas within which it has currency make it difficult to pull together a comprehensive definition of WNV. This is because the PHAC website gives significance variously to WNV as an administrative, a biological, and a social phenomenon. In short, the PHAC has produced a multitude of WNV constructs – a heterogeneous entity – and each assemblage has its own discursive composition, relevance to society, definition of risk, and ties to specific disciplinary apparatuses involved in its production. Each apparatus, in turn, is embedded within particular relations of power. One meaningful way to read WNV, therefore, is as a product of its historical, political, and social context. To illustrate, the information presented on the PHAC's website is constructed from knowledge produced through negotiations between governmental employees, public health administrators, and scientists and medical practitioners. The content of the negotiations, the contexts within which these various groups respond to WNV, and the conditions surrounding these collaborations all shape the production of WNV and, hence, the information about this new disease that is presented on the PHAC's website. Stated differently, within collaborations between experts, the contingencies that all parties can respond to limit the scope and definition of what WNV "is" and thus contour the PHAC's WNV responses.

WNV, in the forms that it eventually takes, obviously did not exist before the production of the PHAC's website. I am not suggesting, however, that the PHAC's response is not connected to, or even reflective of, the biological realities of the disease nor am I dismissing all warnings about WNV posted on the website. Rather, I am suggesting that the PHAC website says more about the organizations, disciplines, mandates, timeframes, legal expectations, power struggles, role of positivist science, kinds of surveillance technologies, budgets, the governmental organization of ministries, conceptualizations of health and illness, governmental and social responses to the unknown, the role of notions of risk, and practices of prevention in public health structures than it does about the RNA virus called West Nile. I am also offering the insight that WNV is an effect of power/knowledge relations and can serve, therefore, as a conceptual tool for the reader of other PHAC websites who wants to place the role of PHAC, and the information presented on its website, within a larger social and administrative context. Through the act of critical contextualization, the production of WNV can be explored in relation to the socio-administrative milieus within which the disease has been constructed. As Foucault observes, the social world is discursively constructed through power/knowledge relations and, through these associations, power and the effects of power are distributed throughout society (1995, p. 215).

Insight Three: WNV as a Justification for the PHAC's New Pro-active Public Health Care Delivery System

The WNV that the PHAC produces has little to do with its biological composition or actual pathogenesis (WNV as entity) and a lot to do with the images and responses to WNV that are produced by governmental, social, public, scientific, medical, and media relations. To this end, the PHAC brings into relationship various institutions and people and sets them the task of producing various aspects of the WNV response. Once set in motion, these "working groups" produce relations of power, and it is through these relations that WNV is produced. By questioning how these groups do their work, I have been able to focus on the role techniques of power play in the production of WNV. What I have found is that techniques of power can assemble myriad WNV constructions, some of which are used for educational purposes. However, there are other constructed ideas about WNV that are useful when trying to influence people's behaviors vis-à-vis WNV.

The most evident form of WNV as a valuable disciplinary tool for the PHAC appears in instances where the PHAC defines WNV as a threat that the agency must respond to, regardless of the measures it must take, on account of the agency's mandate to protect the health of Canadians. In the name of "control" and "prevention," therefore, the PHAC has enacted various interventions which have not necessarily been approved unanimously by science nor by the public such as the use of adulticides and other pesticides in marshes and in residential areas, even in the face of widespread community protest. What is more, on the website the PHAC does not present WNV as posing a clear and imminent danger to large numbers of people. Rather, the website's authors represent WNV as a virus that introduces the possibility that some people will become seriously ill. In this sense, the PHAC website presents WNV as a risk. Within the nefariousness of WNV risks, there is room to propagate disciplinary activities.

The PHAC's administrative mandate is to respond pro-actively to infectious diseases risks such as WNV. On the website the development of a pro-active public health response is presented as an enhancement of the Canadian public health system. Following on from this, the construction of WNV plays a role in the production of the new PHAC organizational framework by defining WNV as risk and developing a complementary framing of the PHAC as the agency that has the mandate, expertise, and infrastructure to pre-empt infectious disease risks. Given the frequency of the conceptual linkage made between risks and strategies of prevention, throughout this analysis I have referenced the "risk/prevention scheme" to describe this public health strategy. The risk/prevention scheme is used strategically by the PHAC in its WNV campaign because pro-active responses work by imagining, anticipating, hypothesizing, and speculating about health risks as possible dangers. Techniques of power are mechanisms that produce knowledge, practices, and effects. Therefore, depending on the tasks to which the techniques are applied and material supplied, techniques of power produce both hypothetical and empirically tangible outcomes. In this case techniques of power produce theoretical ideas about risk and, hence, are not always used to produce or respond to pre-existing social facts. In this sense, through techniques of power the PHAC not only constructs what WNV appears to be in the present moment, but also anticipates what WNV will do in the future. One effect of this production is that the PHAC is beginning now to build the mechanisms and infrastructures of its future responses both to WNV and to other newly emerging infectious diseases.

An example of the PHAC's response to a hypothetical WNV future is the production of pro-active surveillance technologies which not only place under observation areas where WNV has already been detected, but also use data, predictive models, and virtual images to develop a spatial image of the "possible factors" that are "liable" to produce a risk of WNV infection (see Castel, 1991, p. 288). Horizon scanning, for example, investigates disease activities and emergence patterns in areas that already have WNV in order to make suggestions about where WNV may next emerge are activities that are conducted in the name of prevention. These activities (based on a *scientific* hypothesis and virtual modeling) construct a theoretical image of WNV that can become more real than the real outbreak and for that reason make it difficult to ascertain the actual levels of danger WNV poses to the Canadian public in the present. In this sense, the PHAC is engaged in producing knowledge that may be articulated with disciplinary techniques. An effect of the production of these new techniques and (disciplinary) practices is that through them, the PHAC introduces an arbitrary element to the processes and protocols used to determine when something is an empirical danger and when it is a statistically sound, yet hypothetical, risk. This strategy also leaves fewer avenues of recourse, or even inquiry, to those people, for example, citizens or non-experts, who question public health responses to WNV and the actual threats posed by other newly emerging, re-emerging, and surging infectious diseases.

CONCLUSION

In June 2006 personnel at PHAC altered the visual presentation of the WNV website by condensing the formerly extensive WNV website menu into a small menu box with small print and placing it on the right-hand side of the screen alongside the other top reportable communicable diseases in Canada. The changes to the website impacted the PHAC's overall message about WNV because today this disease appears to be just one of the many infectious diseases that falls under the PHAC's jurisdiction. Aside from shifts in the visual presentation of the WNV website, however, the texts themselves have been only lightly edited since 2006, although some claims about the dangers of WNV have been lessened while others remain the same. New scientific information appears in some documents while a few of the more speculative and sensationalized statements about the WNV risk have been removed. The edits to the website in the summer of 2006 mean that this is a study of the production of a new infectious disease emergence and an example of the fact that governmental and public perception of infectious disease outbreaks shift over time.

Diminishing the importance of one health threat while concurrently beginning to address another also draws attention to the speeds at which an infectious disease transitions from being new and emergent to endemic and naturalized. The speeds of transition point not only to the capabilities and characters of many of the newly emerging diseases, but also to the discontinuity within the public health system between high-intensity, resource-rich responses conjured during times of crises and the challenges of gathering resources post-crisis to carry on research and development that is dedicated to long-term planning. In addition to WNV, since 2000, Canadians have experienced a quick succession of new disease emergences cast as public health threats such as variant Creutzfeldt–Jakob disease (variant CJD), found for the first time in a Canadian in April 2002 (see PHAC, 2006a); severe acute respiratory syndrome (SARS), first detected in a person in Canada on February 23, 2003 (PHAC, 2006b); avian influenza, still anticipated by Canadian health officials to be a possible cause of a global pandemic (PHAC, 2006c, 2009a); and H1N1 (swine flu) which as of the end of August 2009 had been detected in 71 humans and led to 4 deaths (PHAC, 2009b). In the social sphere this has resulted in an interplay between real threats to human well-being and perceived dangers which are not ameliorated by public health claims of having developed increased control and prevention competencies. Rather, there is a growing awareness that along with rapid disease emergences come transformations in the biological, social, social, cultural, and institutional aspects of the interrelationship between humans, vectors, diseases, and environments. New questions are arising, therefore, about the roles and responsibilities of agencies such as the PHAC in responding to disease phenomenon whose behaviors illustrate that they are in fact not easily organized, categorized, and disciplined. However, rather than tackling these emerging issues, the speed of change allows for a quick refocusing away from disease such as WNV and toward the last health alarm.

Beginning in 2006, the simultaneity of the PHAC's decision to highlight the importance of avian influenza (H5N1) to human health while at the same time shifting its attention away from WNV and in 2009 making another shift away from H5N1 in favor of attending to the fervor surrounding H1N1 (swine flu) suggests that governmental activity plays a role in the production and management of the "emergence" of infectious diseases. Paying attention to the shift in status of WNV on the PHAC website raises questions about the relationship between the novelty of a health risk, the rapidity of its emergence, and the correlative intensity of governmental and citizen responses to the disease. The shifts within the PHAC's response to WNV over time reinforce my observation that WNV is an effect of the institutional infrastructure of the PHAC and that it has variously and simultaneously been produced as a bio-socio-administrative construct. I have come to understand that the emergence of WNV is linked to the development and promotion of Canada's new public health infrastructures as well as to the practice of linking disease outbreaks to national security responses (Privy Council Office, Canada, 2004).

Throughout this study, I have seen that power comes into play when various knowledge producers, administrators, and social subjects work together to produce the PHAC's WNV response. The role of the PHAC as administrator of Canada's WNV response and as the creator of the WNV website is substantiated within Canada due to the PHAC's authority as the governmental agency responsible for WNV and its affiliation with scientific research on the subject. As a result, the links between government and science form the basic power/knowledge nexus through which the WNV response has been produced in Canada. The PHAC has relied heavily on scientific knowledge about WNV and the authority it gives the PHAC as an administrator of an infectious disease epidemic to determine the parameters of the kinds of knowledge used within the PHAC's response and distributed to Canadians via its website.

Through its response the PHAC has not only determined what is visible and sayable, but also decided what WNV is on the website. Most obvious is the PHAC's production of WNV as a bio-social–administrative construct. Consequently, to the PHAC, WNV is not simply a biological entity or an entity around which to educate people about an illness, but is a social construct that rationalizes, justifies, and perpetuates certain relations of power and forms of knowledge both within the public health system and more broadly within systems of which the public health agency is but one constituent part. Among the uses to which the PHAC has put the WNV construct are the PHAC's legitimization of the authority of positivist scientific ways of knowing and forms of knowledge, the expansion of the breadth of technological determinism within public health programming in Canada, the promotion and proliferation of the surveillance, regulation, and administration of people and places in the name of health and safety, as well as the production of new kinds of risks and the propagation of fears about them within Canadian society.

To shift current ideas about WNV would require a shift in the composition of the administrative structures, resources, and mandates of the PHAC and the fields of knowledge harnessed within the PHAC's working groups. In other words, a critique of the PHAC's production of WNV is an assessment of the PHAC's physical, operational, administrative, and philosophical infrastructures. In order to change how the PHAC, and as a result how the Canadian public, respond to WNV it is important that Canadians, both on the scale of the institution and on the scale of the individual, reflect on how they relate to and with one another across a broad spectrum of relations of power – including the contexts within, and mechanisms through which lay people and experts collaborate.

While the scope of this chapter is limited to an investigation of the PHAC's production of WNV on its public information website, the findings in this chapter may be relevant to the analysis of other public health public information portals as these virtual spaces now play a central role in producing public health issues, distributing authoritative sets of information about diseases, informing citizens about how they can best protect themselves against serious health threats, and, perhaps ironically, raising anxiety about the proliferation of new health risks. In short, studying public health websites, such as the PHAC's, is valuable because of the role virtually accessed information plays in producing not only authoritative knowledge, but also concerned citizens with a vested interest in specific public health campaigns. Clearly more work is needed. First, in the arena of theory, using relations of power as a method for studying the production of social phenomena can be extended through linking this approach with theories of fear, risk, health, disease, and lived experience (embodiment) as well as through theories on practices of governmental regulation and control. The analytical techniques could be further refined and adapted to other empirical settings. It would also be valuable to see if the PHAC's production of WNV is reflective of its production of other disease epidemics and if it is reflective of the approach used by public health agencies in different countries. Most importantly, however, this research should raise questions about how health promotion strategies can work through the traditional risk/prevention schemas while also venturing into new, more ethically driven public health arenas, where novel disease emergences are approached as opportunities to build a public health system where the conditions of emergence are addressed long before there is a breakdown in or a catastrophic event that radically alters the stability and resilience of the natural, social, and cultural systems that directly and indirectly determine human health and well-being.

NOTES

1. For example, in 2002, a civil action lawsuit was filed by a group of 49 Ontario residents against the Ontario provincial government. The case was built around the allegation that the government had neglected to inform people of the seriousness of the new WNV threat, a failure that the group claimed led to the death of 17 Canadians in 2002 alone (O'Connor, 2002). This was a precedent setting court action that opened up the ability of citizens to hold the provincial and federal governments legally responsible, "within reason," for the public health of Canadians (CTV, 2004).

2. The categorization of First Nations, Inuit and Aboriginal peoples as distinct from the general Canadian public reflects most immediately the organizational structure of the Federal Government's Public Health Ministry which maintains a separate FNIHB. The precedent for this was set in 1945 when Indian Affairs transferred the First Nations health portfolio to Health Canada (it was not until 1962 that Health Canada provided direct health services to First Nations peoples on reserves and Inuit in the North) (Health Canada, 2010).

ACKNOWLEDGMENTS

I would like to thank Professors Pamela Moss, Martha McMahon and Bill Carroll of the University of Victoria for their counsel on the larger study upon which this chapter is based.

REFERENCES

Canadian Broadcasting Corporation. (2006, October 10). *Indepth West Nile virus facts.* Retrieved October 20, 2006, from http://www.cbc.ca/news/background/westnile/
Canadian Broadcasting Corporation. (2008, September 23). *Indepth. West Nile virus facts.* Retrieved August 20, 2009, from http://www.cbc.ca/news/background/westnile/
Castel, R. (1991). From dangerousness to risk. In: G. Burchell, C. Gordon & P. Miller (Eds), *The Foucault effect: Studies in governmentality* (pp. 281–298). Chicago: University of Chicago Press.
CTV. (2004, July 19). *West Nile lawsuits can proceed against Ontario.* Retrieved May 28, 2006, from http://www.ctv.ca/servlet/ArticleNews/story/CTVNews/1090253318946_85662518.
Ewald, F. (1991). Insurance and risk. In: G. Burchell, C. Gordon & P. Miller (Eds), *The Foucault effect: Studies in governmentality* (pp. 197–210). Chicago: University of Chicago Press.
Foucault, M. (1980a). *Power and knowledge: Selected interviews and other writings, 1972–1977* (C. Gordon, L. Marshall, J. Mephar, & K. Sopher, Trans.). New York: Pantheon.
Foucault, M. (1980b). *The history of sexuality, volume 1: An introduction.* New York: Vintage Books.

Foucault, M. (1991). Governmentality. In: G. Burchell, C. Gordon & P. Miller (Eds), *The Foucault effect: Studies in governmentality* (pp. 87–104). Chicago: The University of Chicago Press.

Foucault, M. (1995). *Discipline and punish: The birth of the prison* (2nd ed., A. Sheridan, Trans.). New York: Vintage Books.

Gore, J. M. (1995). On the continuity of power relations in pedagogy. International Studies in Sociology of Education, 5(2), 165–188.

Gore, J. M., & Gitlin, A. D. (2003). [Re]Visioning the academic–teacher divide: Power and knowledge in the educational community. *Teachers and Teaching: Theory and Practice, 10*(1), 35–58.

Hawaleshka, D. (2003). Waiting for West Nile. *Maclean's, 116*, 16–23.

Health Canada. (2003a). *Health Canada is coordinating a national approach to West Nile virus.* Retrieved July 8, 2005, from http://www.hc-sc.gc.ca/english/media/releases/2003/2003_22.htm

Health Canada. (2003b). *Health Canada launches national West Nile virus public education campaign.* Retrieved July 8, 2005, from http://www.hc-sc.gc.ca/english/media/releases/2003/2003_57.htm

Health Canada. (2003c). *News release: Health Canada launches national West Nile virus public education campaign.* Retrieved July 31, 2003, from www.hc-sc.gc.ca/english/media/releases/2003/2003_57.html

Health Canada. (2010). West Nile virus and first nations. Retrieved on 10 January 2010, from http://www.hc-sc.gc.ca/fniah-spnia/diseases-maladies/wnv-vno/index-eng.php

Marshall, G. (1998). *Oxford dictionary of sociology.* Oxford: Oxford University Press.

Morshed, M. G. (2002, Winter). The West Nile virus in North America: Coast-to-coast? *CMPT Connections, 6*(4). Retrieved July 20, 2005, from http://www.hc-sc.gc.ca/pphb-dgspsp/wnv-vwn/

Moss, P., & Dyck, I. (2002). *Women, body, illness: Space and identity in the everyday lives of women with chronic illness.* Lanham, MD: Rowman and Littlefield Publishers.

O'Connor, R. E. K. (2002). *Roy Elliott Kim O'Connor West Nile virus group action.* Retrieved May 28, 2006, from http://www.reko.ca/westnile.html

Office of Laboratory Security, Public Health Agency of Canada. (2003). *Material safety data sheet – Infectious substances.* Retrieved July 7, 2005, from http://www.phac-aspc.gc.ca/msds-ftss/msds175e.html

Petersen, A., & Lupton, D. (1997). *The new public health: Health and self in the age of risk.* London: Sage.

Privy Council Office, Canada. (2004). *Securing an open society: Canada's national security policy.* Ottawa, Canada: National Library of Canada.

Public Health Agency of Canada. (2003). *Brochure for the general population.* Retrieved July 7, 2005, from http://www.phac-aspc.gc.ca/wn-no/materials/general-grandpublic_e.html

Public Health Agency of Canada. (2004a). *News release: Government of Canada appoints first chief public health officer to head public health agency of Canada.* Retrieved May 19, 2006, from http://www.phac-aspc.gc.ca/media/nr-rp/2004/phac_nr_e.html

Public Health Agency of Canada. (2004b). *General overview.* Retrieved July 7, 2005, from http://www.phac-aspc.gc.ca/wn-no/gen_e.html

Public Health Agency of Canada. (2004c). *Symptoms, diagnosis and treatment.* Retrieved July 7, 2005, from http://www.phac-aspc.gc.ca/wn-no/symptom_e.html

98   MAYA K. GISLASON

Public Health Agency of Canada. (2004d). *Surveillance, education, prevention and response.* Retrieved July, 7, 2005, from http://www.phac-aspc.gc.ca/wn-no/surveillance_e.html#5

Public Health Agency of Canada. (2004e). *Pregnancy and breastfeeding.* Retrieved July 7, 2005, from http://www.phac-aspc.gc.ca/wn-no/preg-gros_e.html

Public Health Agency of Canada. (2004f). *Protect yourself from West Nile virus – Transcript.* Retrieved July 7, 2005 from http://www.phac-aspc.gc.ca/wn-no/materials/video1_transcript_e.html

Public Health Agency of Canada. (2004g). *Workplace health and public safety programme.* Retrieved July 7, 2005, from http://www.phac-aspc.gc.ca/wnv-vwn/work_wnv_e.html

Public Health Agency of Canada. (2004h). *Frequently asked questions.* Retrieved May 18, 2006, from http://www.phac-aspc.gc.ca/media/nr-rp/2004/faq_e.html

Public Health Agency of Canada. (2005a). *History.* Retrieved July 7, 2005, from http://www.phac-aspc.gc.ca/wn-no/hist_e.html

Public Health Agency of Canada. (2005b). *West Nile virus monitor.* Retrieved July 7, 2005, from http://www.phac-aspc.gc.ca/wnv-vwn/mon_e.html#nsr

Public Health Agency of Canada. (2006a). *First Canadian case of variant Creutzfeldt–Jakob disease (variant CJD).* Retrieved on May 19, 2006, from http://www.phac-aspc.gc.ca/cjd-mcj/vcjd-ca_e.html

Public Health Agency of Canada. (2006b). *SARS (severe acute respiratory syndrome) outbreak period.* Retrieved on May 19, 2006, from http://www.phac-aspc.gc.ca/sars-sras/sars.html#numbers

Public Health Agency of Canada. (2006c). *Avian influenza.* Retrieved on May 19, 2006, from http://www.phac-aspc.gc.ca/influenza/avian_e.html

Public Health Agency of Canada. (2008). *The monitor.* Retrieved October 20, 2008 from http://www.phac-aspc.gc.ca/wnv-vwn/index-eng.php

Public Health Agency of Canada. (2009a). *Current avian influenza (H5N1) affected areas.* Retrieved 21 August, 2009 from http://www.phac-aspc.gc.ca/h5n1/

Public Health Agency of Canada. (2009b). *Surveillance: Deaths associated with H1N1 flu virus in Canada.* Retrieved 21 August, 2009 from http://www.phac-aspc.gc.ca/alert-alerte/h1n1/surveillance-eng.php

Public Health Agency of Canada. (2010a). *What organizations are involved in planning Canada's response to the threat of West Nile virus?* Retrieved on January 10, 2010, from http://www.phac-aspc.gc.ca/wn-no/role-eng.php#1

Public Health Agency of Canada. (2010b). *West Nile virus – Protect yourself!* Retrieved on January 10, 2010, from http://www.phac-aspc.gc.ca/wn-no/index-eng.php

Repetto, R., & Baliga, S. S. (1996). *Research report: Pesticides and the immune system: The public health risks.* Washington, DC: World Resources Institute.

Rouse, J. (1994). Power/knowledge. In: G. Gutting (Ed.), *The Cambridge companion to Foucault* (pp. 95–122). Cambridge: Cambridge University Press.

Sugg, W. C., & Wilson, M. L. (2001). *Overkill: Why pesticide spraying for West Nile virus may cause more harm than good.* Retrieved on July 12, 2006, from http://www.toxicsaction.org.

Treasury Board of Canada Secretariat. (2005). *RPP 2005–2006 Public Health Agency of Canada – Infectious disease prevention and control.* Retrieved May 20, 2006, from http://www.tbs-sct.gc.ca/est-pre/20052006/PHAC-ASPC/PHAC-ASPCr5602_e.asp

Turner, B. S. (1997). Forward: From governmentality to risk, some reflections on Foucault's contribution to medical sociology. In: A. Petersenm & R. Bunton (Eds), *Foucault, health and medicine* (pp. vii–xix). London: Routledge.

EMERGING AND CONCENTRATED HIV/AIDS EPIDEMICS AND WINDOWS OF OPPORTUNITY: PREVENTION AND POLICY PITFALLS

Shari L. Dworkin

ABSTRACT

Purpose – *The purpose of this chapter is to use the particulars of a single case study (Vietnam) to underscore common pitfalls that several governments have made during the emerging and concentrated stages in their policy responses to the HIV/AIDS epidemic and to underscore much needed actions in the HIV/AIDS prevention realm.*

Methods – *Literature syntheses, policy reports, interviews with in-country stakeholders, and a case study approach are used to explore key issues regarding common government missteps at the concentrated epidemic phase.*

Findings – *These include coverage of the history of social ills in the country and how these intersect with – first, myths about the spread of HIV within a given region; second, inadequate intervention with high-risk groups and lack of consideration of the ways in which high-risk groups*

Understanding Emerging Epidemics: Social and Political Approaches
Advances in Medical Sociology, Volume 11, 101–124
ISSN: 1057-6290/doi:10.1108/S1057-6290(2010)0000011010

interact with the general population (neglect of bridge populations); and third, poor emphasis on women and young women, who are disproportionately affected by key epidemic transitions, particularly the transition from emerging to the concentrated epidemic phase.

Contribution to the field – *Documenting policy lessons in emerging and concentrated epidemics is urgent and can assist within and across nations to help control the spread of HIV/AIDS.*

INTRODUCTION

Current estimates suggest that there are 33 million people in the world living with HIV/AIDS (UNAIDS, 2008). Approximately one-half of these are women. At present, there is a partially effective vaccine, female-initiated methods such as microbiocides and diaphragms have not shown successful trial results as had been hoped for (Global Campaign for Microbiocides, 2008), and there are myriad challenges associated with male circumcision trial results and scale-up (Dowsett & Couch, 2007; Sawires et al., 2007), including recent results that there is an increase in HIV risk among female partners whose male partners have been circumcised (Gray et al., 2009). Therefore, behavioral prevention and government and political leadership around HIV policies are central to slowing the epidemic. Fatalla and Rashad adeptly underscored the need for such leadership particularly during emerging and concentrated HIV epidemics in the Middle East and North Africa region. Their comments about the urgency of leadership applies to numerous other regions and governments around the world that are also facing emerging and concentrated HIV/AIDS epidemics: "we have a window of opportunity to prevent what will otherwise be an epidemic, when the disease spreads beyond high risk groups. The costs of ignoring this window of opportunity will be high" (2008, p. 817).

The purpose of this chapter is to use the particulars of a single case study (Vietnam) to underscore common pitfalls that several governments have made during the emerging and concentrated stages in their policy responses to the HIV/AIDS epidemic and to underscore much needed actions in the prevention realm. Special attention is paid in this work to common government missteps including (1) myths about the spread of HIV within a given region; (2) inadequate intervention with high-risk groups and lack of consideration of the ways in which high-risk groups interact with the general population (neglect of bridge populations); (3) poor emphasis on women and young women, who are disproportionately affected by key epidemic transitions, particularly the transition from emerging to the concentrated epidemic phase. Literature syntheses, policy reports, experiences from the author's participation in think tanks and policy working groups, and a case study approach are used to explore these key issues.[1]

Policy analysis is particularly important for regions and countries that are in a concentrated epidemic phase, where less than 1% of the general population but more than 5% of any "high-risk" group is HIV-positive. Within a concentrated epidemic, there is the risk that the epidemic becomes exacerbated and shifts increasingly in scope and size to impact the general population. To be clear on terms, "general population" refers to members of the population that are not located in high-risk groups (such as MSM, intraveneous drug users, and sex workers). However, some have problematized these distinctions in terms of both the categories themselves and the lack of attention to interactions between "high-risk" groups and "the general population," for example, see Treichler (1988, 1999). Additionally, for critical analysis on the ways that epidemiological and biomedical classifications of "risk groups" can produce erroneous conceptions of who is surveilled and/or at risk in the epidemic, see Dworkin (2005), Patton (2002), and Treichler (1988, 1999). Simultaneously, research recognizes that shifts from emerging to concentrated HIV/AIDS epidemics are complex and are generally due to numerous contextual risks (e.g., social inequalities, norms of early marriage, gender relations, violence, migration movements, economic contexts, and consistency between "rights" on paper and in practice), the degree to which government commitment to fighting HIV/AIDS is expressed and carried out, the strength of health care systems, and the degree of disjuncture between national plans and their implementation (World Bank, 2006).

What Fatalla and Rashad are referring to is that it is necessary to ensure that low and concentrated epidemics receive intensive policy and programmatic attention so that these epidemics do not progress to the next stage. To be clear on terms, when a country is said be in a "low" or "emerging" stage of the epidemic, this means that the country is in a stage where the virus has never spread to a significant level to any sub-population and is largely confined to "high-risk" individuals such as injection drug users, men who have sex with men, and sex workers. Concentrated epidemics are those where less than 1% of the general population but more than 5% of any "high-risk" group is HIV-positive (Lyerla, Gouws, Garcia-Calleja, & Zaniewski, 2006). Finally, "mature" or "generalized" epidemics are those where more than 1% of the population is HIV-positive – in this stage, HIV is referred to as having transferred well into the "general population" (or beyond the "high-risk groups" to include married couples and partners who do not engage in classic high-risk behaviors). Given that concentrated epidemics involve a relatively high seroprevalence rate among high-risk groups, and high-risk groups have sexual partners, it is likely that there has already been some or even substantial transference to the general population in this phase. Hence, simply because it is named a "concentrated" epidemic does not mean that HIV has not already transferred to the general population.

Concentrated epidemics are especially important to focus on from a policy perspective to ensure that critical windows of opportunity in which to act are not missed. Regions of the world in which there are countries experiencing concentrated epidemics include: Asia, parts of Eastern Europe and Central Asia, parts of the Caribbean, Latin America, and some segments of the Middle East and North Africa region. Other parts of the world have transitioned from a concentrated epidemic to a more generalized one (e.g., many countries in sub-Saharan Africa, especially the southern portion, parts of Asia, parts of Eastern Europe, Central America, and the Caribbean). Through government commitments, policies, and implementation efforts, some countries have been able to put the brakes on a concentrated epidemic such that it does not progress. What is vital is that there are ample lessons learned across several countries and regions to draw upon that would help governments who are at emerging and concentrated stages to work toward halting the epidemic.

There are many factors that contribute to an exacerbation (or slowing) of epidemics in various regions of the world – and the complexity of these factors and space requirements here do not allow for in-depth coverage of these. The main goal of this chapter is to examine some common government policy missteps in the early and concentrated state of epidemics. Before delving into this, it is undoubtedly worth first asking why some countries are successful at halting/slowing HIV epidemics while others are not. It is, for example, worth asking why Uganda was able to share "success stories" of reduced seroprevalence rates through government leadership, frequent, open national discussions about HIV, *and* intensified prevention efforts and national-level ABC prevention strategies (abstinence, be faithful, and condom use), while the neighboring countries of Zambia and Malawi were not. Similar questions have been asked about different countries on the African continent and elsewhere; these types of questions have already been the subject of much research and debate (a few of these include Boerma, Gregson, Nyamukapa, & Urassa, 2003; Ntozi & Ahimbisibwe, 1999; Stoneburner & Carballo, 1997; Stoneburner & Low-Beer, 2004).

Many scholars and students alike might argue that it is poverty and resources which shape the response to an HIV/AIDS epidemic or its progression, but this would be simplistic. For example, Uganda showed substantial reductions in seroprevalence rates while South Africa, which had HIV/AIDS soaring in the same time period, did not. South Africa is the richer country and is even considered the richest country in sub-Saharan Africa while Uganda is among one of the world's poorest countries. While South Africa's health care system is enormously overburdened and there are large inequities in health care in the country, the change of government in South Africa in 1994 inherited a much better established and functional health care system than did Uganda (Parkhurst & Lush, 2004). Still, it was the South African government, and not Uganda, which had many troubles implementing its national-level HIV/AIDS programs, including its reliance on AIDS denialism and former President Mbeki's role in the nation's slow response (Kalichman, 2009; Schneider, 2002).

President Museveni of Uganda is credited with speaking openly about HIV/AIDS in his country, rallying Ugandans to work together, successfully enlisting massive international donors, rallying non-governmental organizations (NGOs) and other institutions to work across sectoral lines, reaching out to churches and women's groups, and more to make up for initial deficits in the health care system response (Ehrhardt, Dworkin, & White-Gomez, 2004; Parkhurst & Lush, 2004). Thus, in any region, it is important to remember that a nation's response to the epidemic is not simply shaped by government commitment or political leadership alone, although this is important – but is also shaped by the unique historical, governmental, social, and contextual features of that nation, as well as its economic resources, health care systems, institutional capacities, political commitments, attention to human rights, civil society organizations, and mobilization (Berkman, Garcia, Munoz-Laboy, Paiva, & Parker, 2005; Schneider & Stein, 2001; Robins, 2008).

While research has already emphasized numerous success stories such as those in Thailand, Senegal, and Uganda (Celentano et al., 1998; Konde-Lule, 1995; Stoneburner & Low-Beer, 2004), there are some important comparisons to make concerning what worsens epidemics in some areas while others are eased. Many published policy analyses on HIV/AIDS are carried out in regions of the world which are already at a *mature* epidemic phase where a substantial proportion of the adult population is HIV/AIDS infected and it is much more difficult to change course. It is much less common for countries that are in the concentrated epidemic phase to receive policy analysis in the published literature. This is unfortunate, and this policy report/case study approach is viewed as a step to fill that gap to think further about government actions in the critical window of opportunity.

Indeed, in order to succeed at preventing the spread of HIV/AIDS, while it is important to understand success stories and "what works," it is just as important to underscore and understand what does not work. As has been noted by Ehrhardt et al. (2004) in their policy analysis of HIV/AIDS in various countries, there has been:

> a horrible repetition where we have observed different governments – large and small – making the same mistakes and therefore being unable to control the HIV/AIDS epidemic in their societies and communities. The national responses have proven to be usually unsuccessful because they are based on *myths* rather than *facts* about HIV/ AIDS, they are too slow and are typically reactive rather than proactive, without a comprehensive strategic plan, and HIV/AIDS is usually not sufficiently prioritized over other public health issues. Most frustrating and deeply troubling is the fact that the success stories that *do exist* do not become integrated into strategic plans for countries with new or emerging epidemics. Instead, the same ineffective measures get repeated over and over again as if countries and governments have to reinvent the same mistakes and follow the same ineffective script.

But what are these ineffective measures? What are some of these missteps? Understanding what not to do is just as important as determining the key elements of what to do.

Providing an in-depth case study of Vietnam, which is now in a concentrated epidemic in Southeast Asia, is instructive in fleshing out and contextualizing some of these common missteps. Southeast Asia is a very important context in which to examine this question because very tiny increases in prevalence rates can means millions of people given the very large population sizes in countries in this region. Southeast Asia has the second highest burden of HIV on the globe, after sub-Saharan Africa (UNSW & HMU, 2009). Additionally, as the background information on Vietnam below will show, Vietnam has experienced enormous change and progress both socially and economically, and hence the context in which HIV/AIDS emerged was one that appeared to have all of the signs of producing a very successful response to the HIV/AIDS epidemic. And indeed, Vietnam has been hailed by many as having the most impressive response to the epidemic in the (Southeast Asia) region. However, as is the case within many countries, government contributions to myths about HIV/AIDS and the attendant actions that surrounded these myths need to also be carefully analyzed in order to fully understand a nation's response to this epidemic.

In particular, I will focus on a relatively unexamined set of subjects such as the Vietnamese government's emphasis on drug use, sex work, and HIV/AIDS as "social ills/vices/evils" (which will be explained in-depth), the creation of "05" and "06" "rehabilitation centers" for sex workers and drug users in the country, and the lack of prevention, care, and treatment activities in the centers (and reintegration activities following release from the centers). "Social ills/vices/evils" as an ideology and set of social practices have a long history in Vietnam (for a nuanced history, see Robert, under review) and were embraced by the government to "contain" perceived moral and cultural threats to the nation at large. HIV/AIDS was not the first to be added to the list of social ills/vices that were identified in the country (prostitution, drug use, and gambling were identified first).

Coverage of "social vices" or "ills" is commonly referred to within most of the Western literature as a campaign against "social evils" – however, within Vietnam, some argue that this is in fact a radical mistranslation, and that "social vices" or "social ills" are the correct terms – hence, I will use the term social vices/ills throughout. Campaigns to crack down on social vices led to local laws which called for roundups by the police (street sweeps and sex work establishments) that were coupled with mandatory time for sex workers and drug users in 05–06 rehabilitation centers. These state-run centers, and the way that HIV/AIDS prevention, treatment, and care – and health care more generally – was/is lacking there, help to exacerbate the epidemic among high-risk groups who then finish their terms (sometimes also called sentences) and are "released" into their communities and the general population. The assumptions that undergird "social ills" and the attendant range of responses to these by the Vietnamese government will be critically examined, particularly for how these contribute to myths about HIV, drug use, and sex work. Before delving into these specific responses to the HIV/AIDS epidemic, it is important to become more clear on numerous contextual details within the country.

THE VIETNAMESE CONTEXT

Vietnam is a socialist country in Southeast Asia, located on the east coast of the Indochine Peninsula, with a population of 85 million. It is the 2nd largest country in Southeast Asia and the 13th most populous nation in the world. Currently, three-quarters of the Vietnamese population lives in rural areas and one-quarter lives in urban areas. More than half of the country is under 25 years old. Vietnam is undergoing rapid urbanization. Nearly half of the Vietnamese population is expected to live in urban areas by 2020, which represents a doubling of the urban population.

Vietnam has undergone dramatic social and economic transformation, particularly since *Doi Moi* (renovation), a policy package passed by the Vietnamese government in the mid-1980s to transform prospects for economic growth, and to open up markets and participation in trade. The United States is now in the number one place, in dollar amounts, to which exports are sent from Vietnam (albeit this may have changed recently given the recession that the United States is now facing). This is a fairly remarkable transformation given that the United States did not lift its economic embargo against Vietnam until 1994 and did not normalize diplomatic relations or open the doors of trade until Bill Clinton signed the 2000 U.S.–Vietnam trade agreement. In a rather short period of time, then, the country has changed from a centrally planned and directed economy to a market economy with a major role for state-owned enterprises. There has been a fundamental shift in foreign policy from relations primarily with other socialist countries to dramatic integration into the international community and a substantial bolstering of relationships around the world. Finally, in 2006, Vietnam was accepted into the WTO.

Vietnam scores quite well in human development indicators despite the fact that it is not a rich country. It has one of the highest female literacy rates in the world (92%) and the child mortality rate is very low – less than many middle-income countries (UNICEF, 2007). Almost all children are enrolled in primary school, and girls are only a fraction behind boys, although there are larger secondary school and urban–rural gaps that remain (Khuat, 2003). Similar to countries that are considered much wealthier, life expectancy is high and remains among the highest in the world. Additionally, there are very high labor force participation rates (at around 85%, with women constituting half of that) (UNDP, 2000) and economic growth has been steady, with GDP growing at a healthy clip of 8% a year for several years in a row (Open Society Institute, 2007).

Gender and sexuality norms in the country have changed rapidly in the past several decades. While formal documents emphasize women's equality, the government does consider that women's roles as wife and mother are central to the stability of the nation, and mass organizations place much responsibility on women to maintain it (Gammeltoft, 2002; Schuler et al., 2006). The Vietnamese Women's Union, an important mass organization in the country concerning women's issues, makes it clear that women should contribute to the ideals of a "happy and harmonious family," a formal ideology they help to put forward at the national, provincial, and local commune levels. The burden of holding the family together and tolerating its lack of harmony (many women are said to tolerate men's infidelity and domestic violence out of economic need) is coupled with women's high percentage of participation in the labor force, which means that women's spare time is largely spent taking care of household and family needs (Go et al., 2002; Phinney, 2008; Rydstrom, 2006; Schuler et al., 2006).

Gender and sexuality relations have changed before and after Doi Moi. Prior to Doi Moi, premarital sex was considered highly punishable and lacking in morality (Rydstrom, 2006; Population Council, 2007). Premarital sex is still not condoned, but the age at sexual debut has dropped over the past several years and HIV/AIDS rates among the young are on the rise (Mensch, Clark, & Anh, 2002). Age gaps between partners, early marriage, and contraceptive availability play important roles in shaping premarital sex trends (Cu Le, Magnani, Rice, Speizer, & Bertrand, 2004). The abortion rate in Vietnam is the highest in the world, and has more than doubled in the last decade among young women, indicating that discussions of sexuality are still off limits and that there is a lack of access to health care and reproductive health information and low levels of sexual and reproductive health knowledge (Khuat, 2003). Rural–urban gaps only exacerbate this, with studies showing that less than half of females adolescents in rural areas have ever heard the term "family planning" (Rydstrom, 2009; Le, 2000). Finally, some women do not use contraceptives and stress their own sexual inexperience to male partners, in part to adhere to feminine constraints of sexual innocence (Khuat, 2003).

Additionally, sexual norms are that men are the knowers and doers in sex while women are oriented to meet their partner's needs – this means that negotiating safe sex can be difficult for women, and economic disenfranchisement and/or dependencies can dramatically complicate this (UNAIDS, 2004, 2008). Major shifts in gender and sexuality relations are in part due to the opportunities and vulnerabilities presented by economic and social changes under Doi Moi (Phinney, 2008). Along with these changes, there have also been increasing levels of drug use, prostitution, and a large and growing urban–rural poverty gap that has stimulated massive internal mobility of young people to cities looking for work (Hien, Long, & Huan, 2004).

Vietnam has acted to make several improvements in development terms, including closing gender inequality gaps and improving well-being, making improvements in poverty rates overall (while in the 1980s, two-thirds of the population was under the poverty line, currently less than one-third is), maintaining high labor force participation rates, and having the highest percentage of women in the National Parliament in the region (World Bank,

2006). At the same time, women constitute only 5–7% of the executive decision making in bodies such as the People's Committee, constitute an increasing proportion of those who are HIV-positive, and constitute the majority of those who are trafficked people or who are landless. The country is also experiencing increased economic inequality – a large and growing gap between urban and rural incomes, health care, and well-being (and growing gaps on the same variables between the rich and the poor – and minority and ethnic majorities), negative impacts of Doi Moi on women's land ownership, high rates of violence against women (OMCT, 2005; Rydstrom, 2003), and a very high burden of family care on women (Go et al., 2002; Rydstrom, 2006), and still ranks 80th out of 136 countries on its gender development index (World Bank, 2006). Some argue that gender inequality has worsened post-Doi Moi, including an exacerbation of the feminization of poverty (Goodkind, 1995).

The above details underscore how Vietnam has experienced enormous change and progress both socially and economically, and hence many would assume that the nation was especially well poised to offer a successful response to an emerging HIV/AIDS epidemic. Indeed, on several fronts, Vietnam as a nation has had a successful response and is in the process of continuing to make intensive progress. Next, this chapter will emphasize how, within an emerging HIV/AIDS epidemic, government missteps can contribute to myths about HIV that lead to specific actions that require nuanced analysis.

The first case of HIV was reported in 1990, in Ho Chi Minh City, and HIV has since spread to all 64 provinces of the country. Currently, it is estimated that there are 293,000 people living with HIV (UNAIDS, 2008) and the epidemic has doubled in the last six years. The largest proportion of HIV-positive people are under age 30, 85% of cases are among men, and 62% of HIV-positive people are intravenous drug users (IDU), a group with very high infection rates among IDU (a large range is presented in research reports, up to 65%, with an average across studies of nearly 30%) (Ghys et al., 2003; Hammett et al., 2005; Hien et al., 2004; UNSW & HMU, 2009).

Seroprevalence rates among commercial sex workers (CSW) are also high. Research shows a range of rates here as well, ranging from 4 to 33% among sex workers but can be quite variable depending on the area (Ghys et al., 2003; Hien et al., 2004; Nemoto et al., 2008; UNAIDS, 2008; UNSW & HMU, 2009). There is also a high proportion of sex workers who are also IDU, and the rates of HIV in those who are both CSW and IDU are very high – approximately 50% (Tran, Detels, Hien, Long, & Nga, 2004; UNAIDS, 2008). Sex worker visits are common among married men in the general population, and the combination of CSW–IDU interactions and this fact are thought to be two major factors that can contribute to the future spread of HIV within the general population. Sex worker visits may not pose challenges to the stability of marriage, which is often based largely on economic providership for men and family care for women (Hirsch, Higgins, Bentley, & Nathanson, 2002; Hirsch et al., 2007; Phinney, 2008).

There is increasing recognition that MSM exist in Vietnam (as they do in all countries) – some are associated with minority sexuality communities that are in formation, some are drug users and/or sex workers themselves, and some are married men – all of whom are at risk of HIV/AIDS as are their partners (AMFAR, 2006; Vu, Girault, Do, Colby, & Tran, 2008; Clatts, Giang, Goldsant, & Yi, 2007; Colby, Cao, & Doussantousse, 2004). In sum, rates of HIV/AIDS are high among high-risk groups in Vietnam and are spreading to the general population. Recent work reveals that nearly one-half of new cases are outside of the classic high-risk categories, and 70% of new infections are sexually transmitted (Open Society Institute, 2007).

The epidemic is referred to as concentrated and has shown signs of transferring to the general population for some time. Over the past several years, there have been rapid increases in the general male population, military recruits, pregnant women, partners of IDU, and partners of sex workers (UNAIDS, 2008). There has been significant heterosexual spread and the prevalence of HIV among women is rising (Open Society Institute, 2007; Khuat, 2003; UNSW & HMU, 2009).

It is true that the Vietnamese government has made good progress in responding to the HIV/AIDS epidemic. The government first responded to the epidemic in 1993, surveillance data were collected on most groups since 1994 (although MSM surveillance was left out and MSM were not formally acknowledged until more recently), and the latest version of the national plan is known as the National Strategy on HIV/AIDS Prevention and Control until 2010 with a Vision to 2020 and was approved in 2004. Some of the early political barriers to responding adequately to the epidemic were overcome with the recent National Strategy on HIV/AIDS (Socialist Republic of Vietnam, 2004). Most recently, Vietnam has been commended for implementing a national month of action on HIV/AIDS, where the Deputy Prime Minister Truong Vinh Trong (who is also Chairman of the National Committee on AIDS, Drugs and Prostitution Prevention and Control) "called upon the Vietnamese people to launch a grassroots, community-based response to the challenge of HIV" (UNAIDS, 2008).

Much international funding has been offered to Vietnam in order to respond to the epidemic. In June 2004, Vietnam was named as the 15th country to receive PEPFAR funds approved into existence by President Bush (President's Emergency Plan for AIDS Relief) (PEPFAR, 2008). In 2005, PEPFAR funds provided $27.6 million to fight HIV/AIDS in Vietnam; in 2006 this rose to $34.1 million, and in 2007 this support rose to $65.8 million. In the year 2009, $88.9 was expected from PEPFAR to support these efforts (PEPFAR, 2008), although a large proportion of the money was spent on treatment and not on prevention. As has been noted, the response to the epidemic has been highlighted as one of the finest in the Southeast Asia region, and the National Plan identifies nine priority areas for action: information, education, and communication (IEC), harm reduction; care and support; treatment; prevention of mother to child transmission, management of sexually transmitted infections (STIs); blood safety; capacity-building; and monitoring and evaluation (M&E).

MORALITY, POLITICS, AND SOCIETY

Despite all of the positive momentum, there are numerous difficulties with implementing the national plan as there are in many nations, and some of these include resource constraints and a dispersed, localized response that is not centralized, wide reaching, or intensive enough (UNAIDS, 2008). Far less has been written about government stances on social vices/ills, 05–06 rehabilitation centers, and the prevention, treatment, and care opportunities and reintegration activities that are available to individuals who (are in and) leave the centers and return to their communities. In fact, there is very little published information on the rehabilitation centers and there has been even less work that has been peer reviewed in journals on this topic (UNSW & HMU, 2009).

The government first responded to the epidemic in 1993 and launched a series of intensified activities in 1995 to fight "social ills," or those actions/ people that were thought to harm the morality of society. Literally translated, social "vices" or "ills" (*ten an xa hoi*) did not have to do with individual social problems, individual moralities, or individual actions or behaviors. Rather, social vices carried a responsibility to society and indicated failure toward one's family and the nation as a whole (Robert, under review). This point is made more clear by examining a 1999 version of a Vietnamese government handbook which stated that "social evils are social phenomenon comprising behaviors which deviate from common social standards, and which have serious negative consequences on morality, and on economic, cultural, and social life" (as cited in Robert, under review, p. 16). These are defined as "violations of the principles of [Vietnamese ways] of life, cultural traditions, social morality," and "against customs, and established fine social values" (as cited in Robert, under review, p. 16). In summary, the characterization of social vices/ills is not one that necessarily refers to individual behaviors, but rather, the impact that these ills have on collective values, collective norms, and collective well-being.

Some find that the campaign against social vices in the Vietnamese government was a response to the perception that Vietnamese society at large was experiencing increases in crime, violence, and the consumption of porn, increases in homosexuality (or its visibility), drug addiction, and the harassment of young women (Rydstrom, 2006). Other scholars find that the "fight" against "social vices" coincided directly with Doi Moi and the cultural and economic changes that took place as Vietnam increasingly integrated with the world community. Specifically, some scholars suggest that such campaigns may be a reaction against Vietnam's fear that integration into the global community involved "foreign influences" and a weakening of traditional values, hence putting forward a resurgence of Vietnamese culture (Robert, under review). Whatever the case may be, the government intensified its surveillance of social vices on a widespread basis by cracking down on prostitution, gambling, and drug use through arrests using "Local Law 87," in addition to taking pornographic items out of view in stores, and more (Rydstrom, 2006).

The fight against HIV/AIDS became integrated into the campaign against social ills, as was particularly evident in 2000 when it was formally structured into the national organizing body that was assembled to respond specifically to social vices and HIV. This organizing body was formally named the National Committee for AIDS, Drugs, and Prostitution. Thus, strategies to fight HIV/AIDS became intimately linked to the emphasis on "social evils" within the country. This emphasis in fact prevented many good programs from being implemented early in the response to the epidemic because these were viewed as conflicting with the aim of "social evils" programming (Ngyuen, Giang, Binh, & Wolffers, 2000). The emphasis has also resoundingly exacerbated HIV/AIDS-related stigma and discrimination (Busza, 2001; Khoat, Hong, An, Ngu, & Reidpath, 2005).

One can tell by its name that HIV/AIDS was placed into the tripartite of "vices" which designated members of these groups as contributing to a lack of collective good and were viewed as contributing to a sense of collective moral degeneracy (Robert, under review). While deeply rooted in moral ideals in the country and not intending to harm the population in ways that Westerners might easily assume (and the term should not take attention away from moralizing or denial of rights in the West concerning its own populations), this stance meant that very complex social problems were simultaneously collectivized and individualized in powerful ways, with riveting effects. That is, if the collective is harmed by the moral degeneracy of social ills, and such vices are carried out as behaviors that are not simply from the West but are also found within Vietnam, then the nation can rally around rehabilitating society through a recommitment to traditional Vietnamese values. This meant that drug use and sex work were not necessarily seen solely as crimes but resulted in the need for "rehabilitation" in 05–06 centers which required labor, halting sex work and drug use, and re-engaging with what it means to abide by Vietnamese values (e.g., termed "re-education").

The government-run centers where sex workers and drug users were/are brought are known as 05–06 rehabilitation centers – with 05 referring to (largely female) sex workers (many of whom are also drug users) and 06 referring to (largely male) drug users. The 06 center translates to "labor and social education" center, and the central means of rehabilitation measures here are education on the dangers of drug use and HIV transmission, mandatory detoxification, and labor. Those caught selling sex are sent to re-education centers known as 05 centers, state-run centers that are administered at the provincial level. While precise numbers are not available on how many sex workers have been in the centers, policy reports internal to the country state that approximately 235,000 drug users went through the 83 state-run centers from 2001 to 2006 (MCNV & DOLISA, 2007). Despite the facts that these centers are not supposed to be analogous to prison or prison terms and that the Vietnam's Ministry of Health is supposed to be providing guidance on health-related issues within the centers, the health-related services within the 05 and 06 centers are provided by MOLISA – the Ministry of Labour, War Invalids and Social Affairs, and the Ministry of Public Security (MOPS) – which oversees drug control measures in the country (Open Society Institute, 2007). Additionally, the centers are said to be a mix of "voluntary" and "involuntary" residents, but some argue that even "voluntary" entry into rehabilitation centers can mean that the family has "volunteered" members of their family against their wishes and pays for them to spend time there (Oosterhoff & Nguyen, 2006).

Needless to say, despite the positive intentions that a desire to adhere to a collective good can have, and despite the solid intentions that undergird attempts to reintegrate those on the margins of society at large, the emphasis on social vices and the creation of 05–06 centers has produced a vast degree of stigmatization of high-risk groups. Previous societal stigmas about sex workers and drug users were linked/combined in new ways toward people living with HIV/AIDS (ICRW, 2003; Ogden & Nyblade, 2005). Unfortunately, the state has neglected the prevention, treatment, and care needs of high-risk groups in rehabilitation centers (and them and their partners on release). The centers also serve to partition off "bad" members of society and stimulate the perception among those in the general population that certain groups within society are putting Vietnamese values at risk (and are the only ones at risk of HIV/AIDS). It also overlooks that high-risk groups regularly interact with each other sexually (in the rehabilitation centers, with low condom availability – among men and between women and men) – and with the general population upon release. While the precise contribution of these factors to the epidemic is impossible to ascertain and data are truly not available from inside of state-run rehabilitation centers, my own informal interviews with at least 40 HIV/AIDS workers, policy makers, researchers, and members of NGOs, community-based organizations (CBOs), and international NGOs (INGOs) within Vietnam point to how these factors can contribute substantially to an exacerbation of the epidemic for several reasons:

1. Many HIV-positive people who are released from 05–06 centers choose not to disclose their status due to high levels of stigma and discrimination and high degrees of shame and guilt that result from being socially marginalized and placed in a rehabilitation center. Many HIV-positive individuals may not engage in a reduction of high-risk sexual practices as a result. Additionally, only 7% of HIV-positive people from rehabilitation centers were even informed of their status, making risk reduction for them and their partners next to impossible (UNSW & HMU, 2009).

2. Prevention, treatment, and care activities were/are very limited in the settings, and even UNAIDS (2008) has identified that "providing prevention, treatment, and care in closed settings [in Vietnam] remains a challenge." HIV prevalence ranges between 40 and 50% in the centers and people living with HIV in the centers account for nearly 20% of the reported HIV cases in Vietnam. While research already shows that there are very high rates of HIV among drug users and sex workers, if there is little to no prevention, treatment, or care in the centers, this increases the possibility that an exacerbation of the epidemic is occurring within relatively high seroprevalence populations, only to be reintegrated on release into a lower seroprevalence setting. That is, similar to migratory flows that move from higher to lower seroprevalence areas – and back again – this is a surefire epidemiological recipe for increased rates of HIV/AIDS in the general population.

3. As has been explained, drug use was not seen as a medical condition that required treatment – it was seen as a social vice/ill that required rehabilitation. The steps in drug rehabilitation that were offered were: behavior education, detoxification, relapse counseling, and vocational training. However, the lack of perception that drug use is an addiction has meant that no methadone was provided in the centers. There was a recent pilot project approving the testing of methadone for drug users in Vietnam, and this started in 2007. This means that drug users who did not receive treatment were forced to stop taking drugs during rehabilitation, and went without real drug rehabilitation. Hence, most drug users went back to taking drugs once they left the center – some report that the relapse rate among drug users will be about 90% (see Martin et al., 2009). This fact also helps to guarantee a migratory loop in and out of rehabilitation centers (where HIV rates are very high) – and back into the general population (where HIV rates are lower) – which could further exacerbate the epidemic. Furthermore, as the large majority of drug users are young men who, according to the published research, do not often use condoms (and drug use decreases the probability that they will) and who have multiple sexual partners, this will increase infections among their partners (Ngyuen et al., 2000).

4. Policing drug use means that injectors are carrying out new, rushed injection practices (often in the streets, where many inject) which put them at increased risk of HIV, including paying less attention to cleaning or preparing needles, and increasing the probability of sharing needles for fear of being stopped by the police (Clatts et al., 2007; Hien et al., 2004). Additionally, drug users are very slow to access voluntary counseling and testing for HIV given fears that they will be identified as a drug user, and arrested, or sent (or re-sent) to rehabilitation centers (Murphy, 2007).

5. For both sex workers and drug users, an emphasis on social vices denies sufficient attention to the root causes of increased drug use among young men and women and sex work among young women. Poverty helps to produce these behaviors, and worsening income inequalities between the rich and the poor may exacerbate these behaviors. Some sex workers and drug users who have time in rehabilitation centers have been offered income generation programs to assist with reintegration into their communities. However, these programs are not wide reaching, and it is difficult to know if the income generation programs being deployed can be successful in a country where the microfinance industry varies widely in its quality and is being newly regulated. Finally, the impact of income

generation programs is unclear in Vietnam, and these programs may offer only minor increases in income as alternatives to sex work or the sale of drugs.

6. The government recently acknowledged that the use of social vices/ills as a strategy to fight HIV was not productive and changed their position on this. However, drug use and sex work currently remain in the campaigns against social vices/ills, which means that levels of stigma against sex workers and drug users in (and outside of) the HIV/AIDS epidemic is very high (ICRW, 2003) (and since homosexuality was also viewed as a social vice, it is also highly stigmatized). Sex workers and drug users who attempt to access ARV treatment and care have also been met with much stigma and high degrees of stigma are also found in the health care system (ICRW, 2003; Khuat, Nguyen, & Ogden, 2004). NGOs and CBOs are increasingly trying to reach these populations, as treatment, prevention, and care are desperately needed, as are reintegration activities within families and communities. Aside from the clear urgency of community-level anti-stigma programs, improved efforts to carry out prevention with positives and negatives is also urgently needed not just among high-risk groups, but with their partners.

7. The strong emphasis on social vices/ills leads to the perception in broader Vietnamese society that HIV/AIDS is a cause for concern only within high-risk groups due to their (marginalized status and) perceived to be immoral behavior. This leads numerous people in the "general population" in a position of underestimating their own risks and an avoidance of HIV risk reduction behaviors, and testing (UNSW & HMU, 2009).

CONCLUSION

At this time, the Vietnamese government is making intensive progress with its response to the epidemic. Of importance, there is increasing emphasis on taking HIV/AIDS out of the moral realm and placing it into the public health realm. Furthermore, there is increasing emphasis on ensuring that HIV/AIDS is not only viewed in the health realm but, rather, is viewed as a more cross-cutting issue that will require a multi-sectoral response. There are some new programs being designed to fill the gaps that are mentioned in this chapter, such as pilot reintegration programs that emphasize support groups among those who have ended their terms at rehabilitation centers.

There are also collaborations, such as those between FHI and Health Systems 2020 that are focused on evaluating pilot transitional programs with case management/drug counseling pre- and post-release focused on individuals returning from drug rehabilitation facilities in several target districts. This program is also focused on services offered in communities post-release, and selected clients will also receive methadone. Should these programs be successful, it is hoped that these are rapidly taken to scale.

Additionally, the country has begun to move to implement "the three ones" principles which will hopefully allow for better coordination of national responses to HIV/AIDS through: (1) one agreed-upon HIV/AIDS Action Framework that provides the basis for coordinating the work of all partners; (2) one National AIDS Coordinating Authority with a broad-based multi-sectoral mandate; and (3) one agreed country-level Monitoring and Evaluation System. These "pillars" of the response are said to help to make the most efficient and effective response possible (UNAIDS, 2005). Each time the Vietnamese government is faced with a challenge, it has embraced change, taken action to improve, and sought advice. These efforts and programs have been impressive.

However, the early and sustained historical and cultural history/emphasis on social vices and ills, and the prevention, treatment, and care activities inside and outside of 05–06 centers for high-risk groups, has meant that the structural drivers of the epidemic – such as gender inequality, economic contexts, and migration movements – do not get enough attention. Unfortunately, a stance on vices/ills also drives underground the very behaviors it is trying to "protect" society against (Hien et al., 2004). Furthermore, prevention activities tend to focus on sex worker and drug user interventions as separate populations when in fact the two frequently merge in the region. And, despite strong legislation on rights, researchers have found that the rights of people living with HIV are often violated through stigma and discrimination, and Vietnam has a long way to go before rights are fully realized (UNSW & HMU, 2009). The same can be said for the sexual and reproductive health needs of residents in rehabilitation centers (UNSW & HMU, 2009). Current projections of HIV in Vietnam indicate that much more intensive prevention efforts are needed – present estimates are that the number of people living with HIV in Vietnam by 2010 will represent a doubling in the number of cases since 2001 (Ministry of Health, 2005). UNAIDS is now reporting the risk that the epidemic can move to a generalized stage if prevention efforts are not pursued more aggressively.

This particular case study analysis underscores several common myths that numerous countries embrace and that existed in Vietnam concerning the spread of HIV/AIDS. First is the belief that HIV/AIDS is caused by individual or collective vices that can be morally and educationally resolved. Second, given an emphasis on vice and "rehabilitation," adequate intervention has not been scaled up with high-risk groups and there has been a lack of consideration of how high-risk groups interact with the general population (neglect of bridge populations such as IDUs and CSWs). This is particularly the case given the high regularity with which married men and IDU have CSW engagements here and elsewhere in the region. Third, given assumptions about "high-risk" groups and the lack of attention to interaction between high-risk groups and the general population, there is also a resoundingly poor emphasis on women, who are disproportionately affected by key epidemic transitions, particularly at the concentrated epidemic phase. Some scholars argue that women are increasingly at risk and that the prevalence of HIV infection among women is strongly underestimated given gender-biased data collection and a lack of prevention programs that target women (Nguyen et al., 2008). Additionally, several scholars report that HIV-positive women are more stigmatized than men since men have their HIV care generally provided by wives, girlfriends, or mothers, while women are often neglected or abandoned by families (Khuat et al., 2004; UNSW & HMU, 2009).

Numerous countries in Southeast Asia and elsewhere focus primarily on high-risk groups, without much consideration for bridge populations, and this typically means that women become invisibly and increasingly infected with HIV/AIDS. Recent policy analysis of Vietnam recognizes that the current National Plan "fails to address the prevention of sexual transmission of HIV and the vulnerability of women and girls," an alarming omission given the recent increases in the number of female infections. In addition, although fighting stigma and discrimination against people living with HIV/AIDS prominently features in the policy framework, there is little mention of efforts to address stigma and discrimination against marginalized groups, such as drug users and sex workers (Open Society Institute, 2007, p. 12). While this chapter has outlined some interaction between ideologies and actions that the government has taken that have both helped and exacerbated the epidemic, only time will tell us whether the "window of opportunity" to prevent a more explosive HIV/AIDS epidemic will be closed. Documenting policy lessons such as these in emerging and concentrated epidemics can assist within and across nations to help control the spread of HIV/AIDS.

NOTES

1. Lessons are drawn from synthesis of the current literature and policy reports that I have authored and coauthored, including Dworkin, S. L., Gambou, S., Sutherland, C., Moalla, K., & Kapoor, A. (2009). Gendered empowerment and HIV/ AIDS prevention: Policy and programmatic pathways to success the MENA region. *JAIDS*, *51*, S111–S118. Policy presentation prepared as a policy report for a think tank on gendered empowerment and HIV/AIDS titled "Gender and HIV/AIDS" think tank "Policy Lessons for Low Seroprevalence Scenarios"; Sawires, S., Dworkin, S. L., & Coates, T. (2007). *Report on male circumcision and HIV/AIDS prevention: Social, medical, and ethical debates.* Report prepared for the Ford Foundation from the UCLA Program for Global Health with Columbia University, HIV Center; Coates, T., Fiamma, A., Dworkin, S. L., et al. (2007). *Reflections on the XVI international AIDS conference, Toronto, Canada, with emphasis on themes of leadership, accountability, and equity.* Report prepared for the Ford Foundation from the UCLA Program for Global Health and with Columbia University, HIV Center; Ehrhardt, A. A., Dworkin, S. L., & White-Gomez, M. (2004). *A blueprint for action: Global progress in the fight against HIV/AIDS.* Prepared for the Ford Foundation, Hanoi, Vietnam. Some case study themes are also drawn from travels carried out to lay the groundwork for future research in Vietnam, South Africa, and the Middle East. In Vietnam, in 2005, thanks to the HIV Center for Clinical and Behavioral Studies at the New York State Psychiatric Institute and Columbia University, I carried out 40 informal interviews with policy makers, heads of NGOs, researchers at think tanks, foundation program officers, university professors, INGOs, and CBOs. I kept in touch with several of these key informants since then to keep abreast of the latest developments, policy reports, and publications internal to the country.

ACKNOWLEDGMENTS

This work was supported by the HIV Center for Clinical and Behavioral Studies, New York State Psychiatric Institute, and Columbia University. Support was from Center grant P30-MH43520 and P50-MH43520 from the National Institute of Mental Health to the HIV Center for Clinical and Behavioral Studies (Anke A. Ehrhardt, Ph.D., Principal Investigator).

REFERENCES

AMFAR. (2006). *MSM and HIV/AIDS risk in Asia: What is fueling the epidemic among MSM and how can it be stopped?* Available at http://www.amfar.org/binary-data/AMFAR_PUBLICATION/download_file/47.pdf (accessed November 2, 2008).

Berkman, A., Garcia, J., Munoz-Laboy, M., Paiva, V., & Parker, R. (2005). A critical analysis of the Brazilian response to HIV/AID: Lessons learned for controlling and mitigating the epidemic in developing countries. *American Journal of Public Health, 95*, 1162–1172.

Boerma, J. T., Gregson, S., Nyamukapa, C., & Urassa, M. (2003). Understanding the uneven spread of HIV within Africa: Comparative study of biologic, behavioral, and contextual factors in rural populations in Tanzania and Zimbabwe. *Sexually Transmitted Diseases, 30*, 779–787.

Busza, J. R. (2001). Promoting the positive: Responses to stigma and discrimination in Southeast Asia. *Aids Care, 13*, 441–456.

Celentano, D. D., Nelson, K. E., Lyles, C. M., Beyrer, C., Eiumtrakul, S., Go, V. F., et al. (1998). Decreasing incidence of HIV and sexually transmitted diseases in young Thai men: Evidence for success of the HIV/AIDS control and prevention program. *AIDS, 12*, F29–F36.

Clatts, M., Giang, L. M., Goldsant, LA., & Yi, H. (2007). Male sex work and HIV risk among young heroine users in Hanoi, Vietnam. *Sexual Health, 4*, 261–267.

Colby, C., Cao, N. H., & Doussantousse, S. (2004). Men who have sex with men and HIV in Vietnam: A review. *AIDS Education & Prevention, 16*, 45–54.

Cu Le, L., Magnani, R., Rice, J., Speizer, I., & Bertrand, W. (2004). Reassessing the level of unintended pregnancy and its correlates in Vietnam. *Studies in Family Planning, 35*, 15–26.

Dowsett, G., & Couch, M. (2007). Male circumcision and HIV prevention: Is there really enough of the right kind of evidence? *Reproductive Health Matters, 15*, 33–44.

Dworkin, S. L. (2005). Who is epidemiologically fathomable in the HIV/AIDS epidemic? Gender, sexuality, and intersectionality in public health. *Culture, Health, and Sexuality, 7*, 16–23.

Ehrhardt, A. A., Dworkin, S. L., & White-Gomez, M. (2004). *Blueprint for action: Global progress in the fight against HIV/AIDS.* Hanoi, Vietnam: Institute of Journalism and Communication and Ford Foundation.

Fathalla, M., & Rashad, H. (2008). Sexual and reproductive health of women. *BMJ, 333*, 816–817.

Gammeltoft, T. (2002). Seeking trust and transcendence: Sexual risk taking among Vietnamese youth. *Social Science & Medicine, 55*, 483–496.

Ghys, P. D., Saidel, T., Vu, H. T., Savtchenko, I., Erasilova, I., Mashologu, Y. S., et al. (2003). Growing in silence: Selected regions and countries with expanding HIV/AIDS epidemics. *AIDS* (Suppl. 4), S45–S50.

Global Campaign for Microbiocides. (2008). *Trial results and updates.* Available at http://www.global-campaign.org/trial-updates.htm (accessed November 4).

Go, V., Vu Minh, Q., Chung, A., Zenilman, J., Vu Thi Minh, H., & Celentano, D. (2002). Gender gaps, gender traps: Sexual identity and vulnerability to sexually transmitted diseases among women in Vietnam. *Social Science & Medicine, 55*, 467–481.

Goodkind, D. (1995). Rising gender inequality in Vietnam since reunification. *Pacific Affairs, 68*, 342–359.

Gray, R., Kigozi, G., Serwadda, D., Makumbi, F., Nalugoda, F., Watya, S., et al. (2009). The effects of male circumcision on female partners genital tract systems and vaginal infections in a randomized trial in Rakai, Uganda. *American Journal of Obstetrics and Gynecology, 200*, E1–E7.

Hammett, T. M., Johnston, P., Kling, R., Doan, N., Tung, N. D., Binh, K. T., et al. (2005). Correlates of HIV status among injection drug users in a border region of southern China and Northern Vietnam. *Journal of Acquired Immune Deficiency Syndromes, 38*, 228–235.

Hien, N. T., Long, N. T., & Huan, T. Q. (2004). HIV/AIDS epidemics in Vietnam: Evolution and responses. *AIDS Education & Prevention*, *16*(Suppl. A), 137–154.

Hirsch, J. S., Higgins, J., Bentley, M. E., & Nathanson, C. A. (2002). The social constructions of sexuality: Marital infidelity and sexually transmitted disease – HIV risk in a Mexican community. *American Journal of Public Health*, *92*, 1227–1237.

Hirsch, J. S., Meneses, S., Thompson, B., Negroni, M., Pelcastre, B., & del Rio, C. (2007). The inevitability of infidelity: Sexual representation, social geographies, and marital HIV risk in rural Mexico. *American Journal of Public Health*, *97*, 987–996.

International Center for Research on Women. (ICRW) (2003). *Understanding HIV-related stigma in two Vietnamese cities. Preliminary insights.* Available at http://www.icrw.org/docs/stigma_vietnam_researchupdate_1003.pdf (accessed November 10, 2008).

Kalichman, S. (2009). *Denying AIDS: Conspiracy theories, pseudoscience, and human tragedy.* New York: Springer.

Khoat, D. V., Hong, D., An, C. Q., Ngu, D., & Reidpath, D. D. (2005). A situational analysis of HIV/AIDS related discrimination in Hanoi, Vietnam. *AIDS Care*, *17*(S2), S181–S193.

Khuat, H. T. (2003). *Study on sexuality in Vietnam: The known and unknown issues.* South and East Asia regional working paper series. Population Council, Hanoi.

Khuat, H. T., Nguyen, A. T. V., & Ogden, J. (2004). *Understanding HIV and AIDS related stigma in Vietnam.* International Center for Research on Women. Available at www.icrw.org/ppt/hong-stigma-vietnam.ppt

Konde-Lule, J. K. (1995). The declining HIV seroprevalence on Uganda: What evidence? *Health Transition Review*, *S5*, 27–33.

Le, Q. N. (2000). *Case study, Vietnam: Communication and advocacy strategies adolescent reproductive and sexual health.* Hanoi: UNFPA.

Lyerla, R., Gouws, E., Garcia-Calleja, M., & Zaniewski, E. (2006). The 2005 workbook: An improved tool for estimating HIV prevalence in countries with low level and concentrated epidemics. *Sexually Transmitted Infections*, *82*, iii41–iii44.

Martin, G., Stephens, D., Burrows, D., Vu, U. N., Nguyen, L. T., Tran, S. X., et al. (2009). *Does drug rehabilitation in closed settings work in Vietnam?* Available at http://www.unodc.org/documents/eastasiaandpacific//presentation/2009/hiv-aids/ihra-conference/Does_drug_rehabilitation_in_closed_settings_work_in_Viet_nam_Duc.pdf

Medical Committee Netherlands–Vietnam (MCNV) & DOLISA (Department of Labor, Invalids, and Social Affairs). (2007). *Hanoi B93 clubs evaluation.*

Mensch, B. S., Clark, W. H., & Anh, D. N. (2002). *Premarital sex in Vietnam: Is the current concern with adolescent reproductive health warranted?* Population Council. Available at http://www.popcouncil.org/pdfs/wp/163.pdf

Ministry of Health. (2005). *HIV/AIDS estimates and projections 2005–2010.* Available at http://www.inthealth.ku.dk/reach/resources/hivestimatesvn2005-10.pdf/

Murphy, E. (2007). *Evidence to action: The new era of implementation.* Available at http://www.unaids.org.vn/othersupport/cmhcm/docs/071107/Speech_11_Oct_EMurphy_%2019 Oct.pdf

Nemoto, T., Iwamoto, M., Colby, D., Witt, S., Pishori, A., Le, M. N., et al. (2008). HIV-related risk behaviors among female sex workers in Ho Chi Minh City, Vietnam. *AIDS & Behavior*, *20*, 435–453.

Ngyuen, T. A., Giang, L. T., Binh, P. N., & Wolffers, I. (2000). The social context of HIV risk behavior by drug injectors in Ho Chi Minh City, Vietnam. *Aids Care*, *12*, 483–495.

Nguyen, T. A., Oosterhoff, P., Hardon, A., Tran, H. N., Coutinho, R. A., & Wright, P. (2008). A hidden HIV epidemic among women in Vietnam. *BMC Public Health, 8,* 1303–1305.

Ntozi, J. M., & Ahimbisibwe, F. E. (1999). Some factors in the decline of HIV/AIDS in Uganda. In: I. O. Orubuloye, J. C. Caldwell & J. P. M. Ntozi (Eds), *The continuing African HIV/AIDS epidemic* (pp. 93–107). Canberra: Australian National University, National Centre for Epidemiology and Population Health, Health Transition Center.

Ogden, J., & Nyblade, L. (2005). *Common at its core: HIV-related stigma across contexts.* Available at http://www.icrw.org/docs/2005_report_stigma_synthesis.pdf (accessed November 3, 2008).

OMCT. World Organization against Torture. (2005). *Violence against women in Vietnam.* Report prepared for the Committee on the Elimination of Discrimination against Women. Available at http://www.unhcr.org/refworld/publisher,OMCT,,VNM,46c19 1170,0.html (accessed October 30, 2008).

Oosterhoff, P., & Nguyen, N. T. (2006). *Reintegrating residents of rehabilitation camps in Northern Vietnam.* Available at http://www.kit.nl/net/KIT_Publicaties_output/ showfile.aspx?e = 1057

Open Society Institute. (2007). *HIV/AIDS policy in Vietnam: A civil society perspective.* Available at http://www.soros.org/initiatives/health/focus/phw/articles_publications/ publications/vietnam_20071129/vietnam_20071129.pdf (accessed November 14, 2008).

Parkhurst, J. O., & Lush, L. (2004). The political environment of HIV: Lessons from a comparison of Uganda and South Africa. *Social Science & Medicine, 59,* 1913–1924.

Patton, C. (2002). *Globalizing AIDS.* Minneapolis: University of Minnesota Press.

PEPFAR (President's Emergency Plan for AIDS Relief). (2008). *Country profile: Vietnam.* Available at http://www.pepfar.gov/documents/organization/81672.pdf (accessed November 14, 2008).

Phinney, H. (2008). Rice is essential but tiresome; you should get some noodles: Doi Moi and the political economy of men's extramarital sexual relations and marital HIV risk in Hanoi, Vietnam. *American Journal of Public Health, 98,* 650–660.

Population Council. (2007). *A study of Vietnamese youth's decision-making for health and HIV/ AIDS prevention in Kien Gang and Quang Ninh provinces.*

Robert, C. (under review). 'Social evils' and the threats of the market economy in contemporary Ho Chi Minh City. November 2008.

Robins, S. (2008). *From revolution to rights in South Africa: Social movements, NGOs and popular politics after apartheid.* Durban: UKZN Press.

Rydstrom, H. (2003). Encountering "hot" anger: Domestic violence in contemporary Vietnam. *Violence against Women, 9,* 676–697.

Rydstrom, H. (2006). Sexual desires and 'social evils': Young women in rural Vietnam. *Gender, Place, and Culture, 13,* 283–301.

Rydstrom, H. (2009). Moralising female sexuality: The intersections between morality and sexuality in rural Vietnam. In: M. Heintz (Ed.), *The anthropology of moralities* (pp. 118–135). New York: Berghahn Press.

Sawires, S., Dworkin, S. L., Peacock, D., Fiamma, A., Szekeres, G., & Coates, T. (2007). Male circumcision and HIV/AIDS: Challenges and opportunities. *Lancet, 369,* 708–713.

Schneider, H. (2002). On the fault line: The politics of AIDS policy in contemporary South Africa. *African Studies, 61,* 146–167.

Schneider, H., & Stein, J. (2001). Implementing AIDS policy in post-apartheid South Africa. *Social Science & Medicine, 52,* 723–731.

Schuler, S. R., Tu Anh, H., Song Ha, V., Minh, T. H., Thanh Mai, B. T., & Thien, P. V. (2006). Constructions of gender in Vietnam: In pursuit of 'three criteria'. *Culture, Health, and Sexuality, 8,* 383–394.

Socialist Republic of Vietnam. (2004). *National strategy on HIV/AIDS prevention and control in Vietnam till 2010 with a vision to 2020.* Available at http://www.unaids.org.vn/sitee/index.php?option = com_content&task = view&id = 26&Iteid = 72

Stoneburner, R. L., & Carballo, M. (1997). *An assessment of emerging patterns of HIV incidence in Uganda and other East African countries.* International Center for Migration and Health. Available at http://nzdl.sadl.uleth.ca/cgi-bin/library?e = d-00000-00—off-0mhl–00-0–0-10-0—0—0prompt-10—4————0-1l–11-en-50—20-about—00-0-1-00-0-0-11-1-0utfZz-8-00&cl = CL2.5&d = HASH01ff4994f4498075f63cdcc4.2&x = 1

Stoneburner, R. L., & Low-Beer, D. (2004). Population-level HIV declines and behavioral risk avoidance in Uganda. *Science, 304,* 714–718.

Tran, T., Detels, R., Hien, N., Long, H., & Nga, P. (2004). Drug use, sexual behaviors and practices among female sex workers in Hanoi, Vietnam – A qualitative study. *International Journal on Drug Policy, 15,* 189–195.

Treichler, P. (1999). AIDS, homophobia, and biomedical discourse: An epidemic of signification. In: R. Parker & P. Aggleton (Eds), *Culture, society, and sexuality: A reader* (pp. 190–266). London: Taylor & Francis.

Treichler, P. A. (1988). AIDS, gender, and biomedical discourse: Current contests for meaning. In: E. Fee & D. M. Hox (Eds), *AIDS: The burdens of history* (pp. 190–266). Berkeley: University of California Press.

UNAIDS. (2004). *Women in Mekong region face higher rates of HIV infection than men.* Available at http://data.unaids.org/media/press-releases02/PR_UNIFEM-UNAIDS_08Mar04_en.pdf (accessed October 17, 2008).

UNAIDS. (2005). *The "three ones" in action: Where we are and where we go from here.* Available at http://www.unfpa.org/upload/lib_pub_file/506_filename_jc935-3onesinaction_en_pdf.pdf

UNAIDS. (2008). *Report on the global AIDS epidemic.* Available at http://www.unaids.org/en/KnowledgeCentre/HIVData/GlobalReport/2008/

UNDP. (2000). *Human development report.* Available at http://hdr.undp.org/en/media/HDR_2000_EN.pdf

UNICEF. (2007). *State of the world's children.* Available at http://www.unicef.org/sowc07/ (accessed November 10, 2008).

University of New South Wales. (UNSW) and Hanoi Medical University (HMU). (2009) *HIV/AIDS and rehabilitation centers in Vietnam: Sexual and reproductive health needs, care, and choices of current and former detainees and their sexual partners.* Available at http://www.ihhr.unsw.edu.au/images/Publications/Tech%20Review%20Eng.pdf

Vu, B. N., Girault, P., Do, B. V., Colby, D., & Tran, L. T. (2008). Male sexuality in Vietnam: The case of male-to-male sex. *Sex Health, 5,* 83–88.

World Bank. (2006). *Vietnam: Country gender assessment.* Available at http://www-wds.worldbank.org/external/default/WDSContentServer/WDSP/IB/2007/01/24/000310607_20070124141846/Rendered/PDF/384450ENGLISH0VN0Gender01PUBLIC1.pdf (accessed November 13, 2008).

THE SOCIAL POLITICS OF PANDEMIC INFLUENZAS: THE QUESTION OF (PERMEABLE) INTERNATIONAL, INTER-SPECIES, AND INTERPERSONAL BOUNDARIES

Ananya Mukherjea

ABSTRACT

Purpose – *This chapter considers the social politics of H5N1 ("avian influenza"), the 2009 H1N1 pandemic, and the response to it within the context of the history of pandemic influenzas and the continuing need for robust preventative public health systems more generally. In particular, the author considers how the borders between nations, species, and individuals are thrown into relief and called into question by influenza outbreaks and their management.*

Methodology/approach – *This work relies on literature review, media research, and critical and interpretative sociological methods.*

Findings – *While panic surrounding new and potentially highly virulent influenza strains is reasonable, such panic is not sustainable and belies the*

Understanding Emerging Epidemics: Social and Political Approaches
Advances in Medical Sociology, Volume 11, 125–141
Copyright © 2010 by Emerald Group Publishing Limited
ISSN: 1057-6290/doi:10.1108/S1057-6290(2010)0000011011

fact that every year presents the danger of a pandemic. This chapter argues that, if public health systems only respond to immediate panic and fail to consider how quickly airborne diseases can cross all sorts of borders, they do not attend to the real need for far-seeing, long-term, internationally collaborative disease prevention and disaster preparedness.

Contribution to the field – *The author offers a critical and wellness- and prevention-oriented perspective on what priorities should be emphasized in the rapidly growing fields of disaster studies and disaster preparedness, which, by their nature, tend to be crisis oriented and focused on the micro-term, with planning done on a case-by-case basis. Such a narrow focus can render preventative health systems inflexible and unable to rise to the challenge of a disease that can spread easily through casual contact.*

INTRODUCTION

This chapter is a consideration of the politics and public health implications of responding to and preparing for a potentially deadly global influenza, in light of the devastating 1918–1919 influenza pandemic, the threat of avian influenza since the first recorded H5N1 outbreak in humans in 1997, and the 2009 H1N1 pandemic. Many critics (Garrett, 2000; Rhodes, 1998, e.g.) have argued that we put ourselves at great risk – in the United States and internationally – by continuously deprioritizing what is already an insufficient public health infrastructure. The rush to provide sufficient vaccine for H1N1 and seasonal flu in 2009 – in both North America and internationally – has demonstrated just how many infrastructural weak-nesses there are.

At least as important as buttressing existing disease prevention systems, though, is the need to rethink how we conceive of public health. To imagine it as a robust system, one that can adapt to new situations and work *throughout people's lives* rather than the current notion of a heroic mechanism that sweeps in at critical moments to vanquish death and maintain the workforce, would constitute a major shift in policy goals and money allocations. This new and different type of long-term public health response likely would have more goals in common with the educational system or other institutions of civic infrastructure than with the military, making it a shift from the sorts of public programs that have historically received large amounts of funding in the United States, programs whose goals align with those of national security. We North Americans panicked over SARS and the permeability of our borders, and we panic over bioterrorism, to the surveillance of which our governments have given strong funding, but the US government, media, and mainstream population have been slow to worry about influenza. As the military prepares in peacetime for the possibility of wartime, it would make sense to make public health development a continuous, far-sighted endeavor that sees to everyday health concerns toward the end of also being prepared for outbreaks when they occur.

Disasters and disaster preparedness have received much attention in public health policy and the social sciences over recent years, especially as emerging epidemics have garnered increasing amounts of journalistic and public awareness. Most of this attention, however, has focused on a case-by-case basis or on financial liability, leaving all too little space for the most crucial question of how to produce public health and emergency systems that are always prepared and that focus on real prevention rather than just controlling scared populations after a disease threat materializes.

The ever-present possibility of an influenza pandemic presents a particularly thorny problem because we have been living with this potential for generations. We must expect to live with it for generations to come as well. Even ordinary influenza results in over 100,000 hospitalizations in the United States each year. Flu pandemics like the "Spanish" flu of 1918–1919, the "Asian" flu of 1957–1958 (which killed well over 1,000,000 people), the "Hong Kong" flu of 1968–1969 (which killed over 500,000 people), and this year's H1N1 are extraordinary in their transmissibility and adaptability (Snacken, Kendal, Haaheim, & Wood, 1999), but influenza viruses mutate constantly. Pandemic flu is always a possibility and invariably stretches even good public health systems to their limits. This means that preparing for pandemic flu is a good test for health systems to gauge their readiness for any potential large-scale emergency, whether caused by a disease agent or natural disaster, and *to integrate broad and robust prevention care with emergency planning.*

In this chapter, I will review the history of influenza pandemics since 1918 up to 2009, discuss the relationship between pandemic flu and seasonal flu, and then consider how public health and epidemiology have responded to these crises as opposed to the more integrated and active role that public health could play in preventing disastrous pandemics and the panic that surrounds them.

My two, closely tied, main points are as follows: (1) we must think ecologically and with a wide and historical view to understand influenza or the possibility of any airborne pandemic, and not only in terms of momentary panics or emergencies – unlike a major storm or earthquake. Flu pandemics occur over the space of many months and most of the globe and require much more than basic disaster response (which, in any case, is often inadequate even in the face of other natural disasters, such as the Indian Ocean tsunami of 2004). (2) The major boundaries that constitute a significant aspect of how most people think of infections and epidemics – national; ethnic, communal, and racial; interpersonal; and species – are all *permeable* and, in some cases regarding flu, functionally meaningless, such that their invocation can cause misinformation and harm.

Sociology's role in preventative public health and disaster preparedness may go beyond its contribution to understanding how different institutions can share power and develop compatible functions to work together. Sociology can, as Barbara Katz Rothman writes (see her introduction, 1998), offer a different set of priorities for public health as a large and complex mechanism that works toward reducing suffering and social inequities; it can offer a different vision of how we, the public, imagine an *ideal* health care system. Philosopher Barry Hoffmaster, in his introduction to the volume *Bioethics in Social Context*, advocates attention to the practical implications of every biomedical ideal, to the "fundamental matter of medical–moral responsibility" (2001, p. 4). It is crucial to remember, especially in the midst of responding to a population-level panic over an infectious disease outbreak, that the welfare of individuals is at the heart of why the population they comprise matters.

BACKGROUND: WHAT MAKES A PANDEMIC, AND WHEN IS FLU DEADLY?

The threat of pandemic influenza is a topic about which everyone now knows something. What each person knows, however, varies considerably throughout even small communities (such as a school district in New York City), let alone on a national or international scale. There is great variance, too, in estimating how much concern we should devote to this issue. Is panic reasonable? Or is the fear bamboozling us into forgetting the war in Iraq? Are the shelter-in-place directives (basically, food, water, and batteries to last two weeks, now applied to all potential disasters) fail-safe or absurd, and will there be enough flu vaccine to supply even the highest risk groups?

Mike Davis, in an article for *The Nation* in 2005, when the primary pandemic flu threat was avian influenza, H5N1, wrote:

Avian influenza is a viral asteroid on a collision course with humanity. Since the horrific autumn of 1918, when a novel influenza killed more than 2 percent of humanity in a few months, scientists have dreaded the reappearance of a wild flu strain totally new to the human immune system .... Governments have had ample warning, unlike the surprise of HIV/AIDS, that a new plague is coming. Indeed, Washington has had almost nine years to heed the advice of top influenza experts and mobilize the nation's resources to battle H5N1 in Asia and at home. The Bush Administration's failure to do so makes "homeland security" into a sick joke whose punch line may be a repetition of the 1918 catastrophe. (2005b, pp. 1–2)

A report published in November of 2006 by the Financial Services Roundtable's committee on "mega-disasters," making recommendations to the US Congress and to insurers, stated baldly:

No one is ready if the pandemic occurs within the next several years .... We must be better prepared. This report recommends a series of steps that the federal government should take, many in concert with governments of other countries, to reduce the threat to lives and the global economy. We believe a comprehensive plan would cost roughly $10 billion more than the $7 billion the U.S. Government has committed to spending already. This additional sum is less than 1/10th the amount the federal government has devoted to relief and recovery from Hurricane Katrina. Additionally, it is a tiny fraction of the more than $500 billion in lost output in the United States alone that a pandemic could cause. (2006, p. 8)

However, several months on from the original recorded outbreak of the H1N1 influenza virus in Mexico (this paper is being finalized in the autumn of 2009), it seems that pandemic flu has fallen short of the terrifying threat it seemed to promise. H1N1 has proven to be frightening and to be quicker moving, more virulent, and two to three times more likely to cause death than this year's seasonal flu, but, thankfully, it has not delivered the disaster of the major and deadly pandemic that many expected. Seasonal flu, meantime, continues to cause about 35,000 deaths per year in the United States and to cause widespread workplace shortages. What, then, distinguishes pandemic flu from the seasonal variety, and what makes influenza both so much a mundane part of everyone's life and a true disease threat? Pandemic flu is marked by its novelty (that it is caused by a strain not previously seen in humans), by its virulence, and by its ease of transmission. In the northern hemisphere in the fall of 2009, for example, pandemic H1N1 was outstripping all the seasonal flu strains with respect to its rate of spread and the likelihood that those who contracted the virus grew sick, often very sick.

The 1918–1919 influenza pandemic killed between 50 and 100 million people worldwide, but the figures are difficult to pin down because the ongoing war made record-keeping very difficult (Barry, 2005; Kolata, 1999). The 1918–1919 pandemic was widely referred to as the "Spanish influenza" because it was first reported in large numbers in Spain. Some contemporary theories attributed its origins to China (see "The Influenza Pandemic of 1918" at http://virus.stanford.edu/uda/), but it seems the first eruptions of influenza occurred on military bases in the American Midwest. A recent study conducted in London suggested the pandemic might actually have emerged in France, from the ecology of juxtaposed soldiers, gas, pigs, and fowl (Oxford et al., 2005). The longstanding association of certain diseases – particularly the flu – with nations, regions, or races (particularly Asians in the 20th century) is, I argue, part of why the United States and global public health bodies like the World Health Organization (WHO) were slow to respond to H5N1 virus in Hong Kong in 1997. Even since 2004, when H5N1 began to draw much international attention, there has been consistent debate about whether wealthier nations should rush resources to the source of an avian influenza epidemic – should that epidemic start in Asia or Africa – or wait until the virus reaches their borders.

In 1997, 18 people in Hong Kong were hospitalized with a strain of H5N1 avian influenza that was new in humans; 6 of these people died of the disease. Every human exposure in this case was linked to live bird markets, and the strain did not transmit easily among humans or extend beyond the initial outbreak (Davis, 2005a; Snacken et al., 1999). From 2003 to 2009, small outbreaks of H5N1 infection in humans emerged through much of Asia and beyond, extending to Bangladesh, Egypt, and Turkey. During this same period, H5N1 was found in wild, migrating birds throughout most of Africa and into the colder regions of North America.

Scientific and public anxiety about H5N1 grew, climaxing in 2005 and 2006, following the most worrying H5N1-related incident in 2004, when Pranee Thongchan contracted H5N1 virus from her daughter Sakuntala as she nursed the girl through the final hours of an acute infection in the Thai town of Kamphaeng Phet. Both mother and daughter died from H5N1 within a few days, and this remains the only confirmed instance of human-to-human transmission for this strain. In this case, it required many hours of intimate contact with large quantities of virus-laden bodily fluids, which meant the virus was still not easily transmissible. With this case, H5N1 became a matter of major international concern, as influenza experts like Robert Webster decried the fact that it had taken seven years to turn so much attention to it.

When the H1N1 outbreak was confirmed in Mexico in the spring of 2009, many flu researchers were shocked because attention had been focused on Asia for the past 12 years. By July, the WHO had declared a "phase six pandemic." Later in the summer, research showed that the strain behind the Mexican pandemic was extremely similar to one that had caused a small human outbreak in the American Midwest four years earlier, suggesting that this epidemic had been in the wings for some time (Garrett, 2009).

The discovery in 2006 that the 1918 pathogen was likely a mutated avian or swine flu contained some hope for future action. Assuming that it was the very unfamiliarity of the virus that killed so many infected with it, the 1918 virus, now genetically recreated from frozen tissue samples, could potentially lead to a vaccine that sufficiently resembled what a mutated H5N1 might look like. Such a vaccine might not be a perfect enough match to prevent sickness, but it might give the immune system enough familiarity with the antigen to reduce the number of deaths from the disease (Matthews, 2006; Leavitt, 2006). Having an imperfect-match vaccine stockpiled might curtail hospitalizations and deaths in the months it takes to produce a perfect-match vaccine, as we have seen with H1N1 vaccine production in 2009.

VACCINES, INTERNATIONAL BORDERS, AND INTERPERSONAL BARRIERS

The obstacles to smooth and effective population-level vaccination, however, are many. Influenza vaccines, which are generally still produced by infecting fertile chicken eggs with the virus and then harvesting antigens and killed viral particles, decompose rapidly and, even while potent, they quickly lose efficacy as the circulating strains mutate. For vaccine programs to be effective at the population level, to achieve what infectious disease specialists refer to as "herd immunity," a majority of the population (ideally, 60–70%) would need to be vaccinated. Even if enough vaccine could be produced, many people harbor suspicions about the possible side effects. In any case, it is difficult to produce enough vaccine because inoculation is not a profit-making branch of medicine and because vaccines need to be distributed inexpensively and are typically administered only once or twice (see, e.g., the World Health Assembly's 60.28 working paper, "Patent Issues related to Influenza Viruses and their Genes").

Medicine production is, certainly in the global North and, to a significant degree, throughout the world, a profit-making business. This affects vaccination programs both because vaccine production cannot be lucrative and because the greed and wealth of many pharmaceutical conglomerates make people, and some governments, suspicious of them. Regarding the former issue, the 1976 flu vaccine controversy in the United States offers a cautionary tale. After an outbreak of swine flu at Fort Dix military base in New Jersey, the US government began an active, government-led, and subsidized campaign to inoculate the nation's population against the strain. President Ford's vaccination was photographed for publicity, and Congress earmarked US$ 137 million for the program. Soon after vaccinations began, however, the plan dissolved amidst controversy. The pharmaceutical manufacturers charged with making the vaccines demanded indemnification against possible lawsuits, raising public doubts about the safety of the vaccine. Then, some cases of Guillain–Barre Syndrome developed in individuals who had received the swine flu vaccine. Although the number of cases was small (fewer than 50 such cases associated with all flu vaccinations between 1976 and 2006) and causality has never been determined, the co-occurrence confirmed the fears many people had, and the program ground to a halt (for an history of this event, see Sencer & Millar, 2006).

Regarding the latter issue, associating the United States with pharmaceutical conglomerates and with the UN has prompted some nations to suspect the United States and UN of colluding to actually spread influenza viruses in order to later reap profits from selling vaccines to those countries in which they had planted epidemics. In 2007, the Indonesian government refused to share any more flu virus samples found in the country with the WHO after the pharmaceutical company CSL produced a vaccine based on samples from Indonesia. "Jakarta argue[d] it has an intellectual property right to the country's flu strain and to designate who develops a vaccine and profits from it. It says it is willing to share samples with those who agree they will not use them for commercial [purposes]," Reuters reported (Perry, 2007), regardless of the fact that the virus had already been traveling across state borders in the bodies of migrating birds. While the idea of any nation "owning" a flu virus is illogical and dangerous, it is also supported by the market economy (again, see the World Health Assembly's 60.28 working paper, "Patent Issues related to Influenza Viruses and their Genes").

All too similar is the notion that wealthier nations would do better to hoard their antivirals or vaccine stockpiles and wait for the virus to come to them rather than to advance these to the first local epidemics. In Atlantic Storm, a 2005 tabletop exercise simulating an international smallpox attack, Madeleine Albright, acting as the US President, held the position that the

United States would not share its vaccine stockpiles with nations that had not supported the US-led war in Iraq (see UPMC Biosecurity Center, 2005). While the situation was hypothetical and the actors were performing, this thinking is in line with much US foreign policy at the time and, perhaps, with complicated and incoherent ways in which public health and security issues intersect in many people's minds.

Indeed, shoring up national borders to prevent the importation of infectious agents is standard practice but, in the case of airborne pandemic, very difficult to enforce effectively. As the death toll from India's H1N1 epidemic rose to 100 in the summer of 2009, airport security staff in India and other Asian countries brought out the thermal scanners used during the SARS scare seven years earlier to scan all disembarking passengers. The scanners had provided some use in containing SARS because that disease is marked by a rapid fever spike. With influenza infection, the fever might come more slowly, and the ill individual is infectious before the fever begins. The first few months of the H1N1 pandemic also saw travelers the world over prone to being tested and quarantined on the basis of their point of origin, with Mexicans under surveillance first and then New Yorkers. Here in New York City, the borough of Queens, where the first domestic outbreaks were concentrated around students returning from spring vacations in Mexico, became associated with H1N1.

Unsurprisingly, however, the H1N1 virus had traveled quickly beyond the highly organized Mexican quarantine and curfews and the immediate school closures in Queens, across the tourist isolation in Hong Kong (where authorities must have felt slightly bemused that the influenza pandemic long expected to originate in their city had arrived from elsewhere), and past the thermal scanners in Asian airports. Because influenza is airborne, because infected individuals are contagious before they show symptoms, and because H1N1 proved to be particularly transmissible, it is not surprising that all these measures might have slowed its spread but could not stop it. As this strain became a full global pandemic, its death toll rose as well, although the greatest concentration of fatal cases has remained in Mexico in the spring and in India in the summer, where they were likely exacerbated by poverty and co-infections.

As H1N1 has spread throughout the world, past international borders, interpersonal barriers have become a matter of ever-greater concern to most people. In the 1918 influenza pandemic, quarantines and face masks were used widely and often enforced strictly. Neither is likely to have been very effective, though. Again, because individuals with the flu are contagious before they show any symptoms, quarantines can, at best, only slow the spread of the virus. Once an individual is infected and ill, the fact that influenza replicates in mucus membranes means that face masks are not always practicable; the respiratory discharges, violent coughs, and difficulty breathing that are symptomatic of serious flu make it impossible to wear one. Even before one is ill, face masks are uncomfortable and usually too porous to block viral particles (Barry, 2005; Davis, 2005a). Vaccines suit the common contemporary mindset about disease in that they seem to promise quick, efficient, and total protection from the effects of pathogens. Where no vaccine is yet available, the search for equally efficient and complete protection from pathogens continues. Quarantines and face masks at least offer this symbolically. The 2009's ubiquitous directives to carry hand sanitizer, to wash hand for at least 15 s, to smother coughs, and to stay home when sick work toward similar security. Each of these directives is a good idea, but none can fully diminish the risk of contracting flu.

I do not mean to argue that it is wrong to reinforce international and interpersonal barriers to contain flu contagion. Of course we should, and studying the sociology of infectious disease has made me into an avid hand washer myself. However, unless an influenza outbreak is contained quickly, strategically, and completely at its source, it is naive to expect that the virus will respect national borders or the good hygiene of individuals. Airborne viruses, in particular, can pass from one person to another through a cough, even a smothered one, while they are waiting to go through customs or despite their very clean hands. These measures make sense, but they do more to reinforce individuals' need for some control and a feeling of security in the face of an epidemic than they actually enhance biosecurity. A critical aspect of our emphasis on these borders is, I argue, our reluctance to admit that we 21st-century humans remain a part of, and subject to, the natural world and, therefore, vulnerable to its diseases and predations just as it is to ours.

I move now to a discussion of the significance of species boundaries when considering the management of influenza viruses that can hop from one kind of animal to another.

SPECIES BOUNDARIES AND THE ROLE OF INDUSTRIALIZED MEAT FARMING

With respect to avian influenza, the WHO, the World Organization for Animal Health (OIE), and the UN's Food and Agriculture Association

(FAO) have given a great deal of attention to developing health policies for live bird markets (see FAO/OIE/WHO joint report, 2005). Live bird markets are a concern because birds from many different sources are kept in very tight proximity to each other and because they are kept in conditions that create extreme stress for them, which reduces their immunity. In industrial meat and egg farms in the United States, we see the same issue. Animals bought from many different auctions, coming from different regions, are kept in extremely overcrowded and highly stressed conditions. As well, as Jean Halley discusses in her work on cattle ranching, industrially farmed animals are bred to have abbreviated lives – they are essentially born to die (personal communication, July 29, 2009). This means that animals can contract viruses and then be sent to slaughter before the viral infection begins to show visible symptoms. Richard Rhodes, in his book on mad cow disease, discusses how this compressed birth-to-slaughter time-frame makes it practically impossible to know if beef cows are infected or not, especially if the infectious agent at issue is a slow virus like the one that causes mad cow disease (1998). This matter of diagnosis is exacerbated by the fact that most animals that are industrially farmed for slaughter exist in such inadequate conditions that many of them are sick all the time. Most companies compensate for this by feeding them large doses of antibiotics as a common course. Aside from the concern about creating population-level antibiotic resistance, this practice has the added downside of the false but common American perception that antibiotics can cure everything (see, e.g., Andremont & Tibon-Cornillot, 2006). They do not, certainly, provide any protection against viruses. So it was a reasonable – though not necessarily accurate – guess that the H1N1 virus may have been produced on an industrial pork farm in Mexico.

In a *Newsweek* article in 2009, Laurie Garrett wrote about the inaccuracies and uses of referring to H1N1 as swine flu:

A [wise] set of pig-related actions would turn to the strange ecology we have created to feed meat to our massive human population. It is a strange world wherein billions of animals are concentrated into tiny spaces, breeding stock is flown to production sites all over the world and poorly paid migrant workers are exposed to infected animals [who are, in turn, exposed to infected humans and to other livestock] …. Back in 1980 the per capita meat consumption in China was about 44 pounds a year; it now tops 110 pounds. In 1983 the world consumed 152 million tons of meat a year. By 1997 consumption was up to 233 million tons. The UN FAO estimates that by 2020 world consumption could top 386 million tons of pork, chicken, beef, and farmed fish. This is the ecology that, in the cases of pigs and chickens [and ducks], is breeding influenza. It is an ecology that promotes viral evolution.

Both with H5N1 and with H1N1, local and international authorities have often responded to outbreaks with culls of domestic and/or wild animals in the area, although this has sometimes been more a panicked, almost ritualistic purging than a strategic program to contain infection. The FAO and the OIE provide fairly clear and specific guidelines for animal culling, indicating when it is necessary and when it is not, how many animals should be killed and in what sort of a spatial range from the estimated point of infection, and how culling can be performed most humanely and hygienically. However, many of the birds, dogs, and domestic cats that were culled in Southeast Asia in 2005 and 2006 were simply buried alive and conscious. The welfare of the animals may or may not seem important to everyone in the face of a pandemic threat, but its context is that many of these animals were household pets and that much of this culling was excessive, ineffective, and conducted in an unplanned and haphazard manner, almost more for metaphoric purification than as epidemiological strategy. The World Bank and FAO specify that compensating people for their animals is important, both to prevent local economic collapse and to encourage people to surrender animals when a cull is called for. The FAO guidelines suggest compensation at a rate of about two-thirds the animal's market value, which is a significant depreciation for a family that relies on its animals for part or all of its livelihood, and this two-third compensation is not always feasible or achieved.

In a 2006 report on culling and compensation to eradicate H5N1 in Asia, the World Bank wrote:

> Payment of compensation to farmers whose animals are being culled enhances producer cooperation through better motivation to comply with the disease reporting and culling requirements of disease control packages. It reduces the time lag between an outbreak and containment actions, and hence diminishes the overall cost of control. To the extent that it reduces the virus load, it also reduces the risk of the virus mutating to become transmissible from human to human. Enhancing early reporting and complete culling of diseased or suspected birds is thus the first objective of compensation schemes. A second objective can be to reimburse losses of private citizens who have complied with a disease control process for the public good. This is compatible with the first objective ….

> While the imperative of disease containment drives compensation schemes, the reality of the severe impact of culling on very poor people cannot be ignored. (2006, p. iii)

Meanwhile, the OIE has produced a set of 10 principles for the killing of animals for disease control, which are included as part of its Terrestrial Animal Health Code. As they put it, these principles are "based on the premise that a decision to kill the animals has been made, and address the need to ensure the welfare of the animals until they are dead." Just as the

World Bank's principles are noteworthy for their focus on the economic needs of small farmers and other stakeholders in micro-markets, the OIE's principles are noteworthy for a repeated emphasis on the welfare of the animals to be culled. In 2009, these principles included:

- All personnel involved in the humane killing of animals should have the relevant skills and competencies. Competence may be gained through formal training and/or practical experience.
- Methods used should result in immediate death or immediate loss of consciousness lasting until death; when loss of consciousness is not immediate, induction of unconsciousness should not cause anxiety, pain, distress, or suffering in animals.
- There should be continuous monitoring of the procedures by the competent authorities to ensure they are consistently effective with regard to animal welfare, operator safety, and biosecurity (World Organisation for Animal Health, 2009, p. 1).

The issue of biosecurity during a cull is an essential one that is too easily overlooked. Biosecurity can be compromised in a number of ways. If management is poor, infected animals have greater motivation and better opportunities to escape. If those people involved in the cull are not competent and experienced, they run a higher risk of becoming infected themselves. Further, if culls are not properly controlled, a large gathering of spectators or informal participants increases the likelihood of contagion among the crowd. Again, while the welfare of the animals to be culled is usually a low priority in the panic surrounding culls, under the best circumstances, it *should* matter of its own accord. As well, it *should* matter for how deeply integrated it is with a number of other issues that are essential to effectively containing infection and reducing the epidemic risk.

It is the crisis situation, the rush to contain terror at a new disease contagion, that prompts hurried, haphazard culls. While the FAO and OIE do, as we have seen, have principles in place that should guide such measures, these principles are mere ideas until the far-sighted, collaborative, practical work is done to make them logistically deployable. Unless such practical plans exist, animal culls are more likely to cause harm than to contain influenza outbreaks. As domestic fowl and other animals were being culled in Turkey in 2005, for example, wild fowl carrying H5N1 were already migrating elsewhere. To return to Laurie Garrett's words, wise action would turn to ecology for its perspective, a viewpoint cognizant of how microbes, animals, and humans all function together and affect each other irrespective of the socially constructed borders (economic, national, and species) that fundamentally structure how most people conceive of the world but are meaningless on an animal or microbial level. For example, how does the ecology through which cheap meat is produced, killed, and distributed internationally produce new microbes and how does it increase the vulnerability of farmed animals and the workers at those farms, slaughterhouses, and warehouses? How do people and animals coexist and, in sharing space, also share the risk of influenza infection?

Jeffrey Bussolini, translating and interpreting Roberto Esposito's *Immunitas*, describes how Esposito draws on Rene Girard's *Violence and the Sacred* to draw a parallel between the contemporary hopes for vaccines and the ancient practice of eliminating plagues by designating a scapegoat which is "externalized" by driving it, with the burden of the plague, outside community boundaries. As Bussolini told me, Esposito writes that the medical condition consists of inoculating a limited amount of the disease just as, in rituals, a little bit of violence (the burdening and driving out) is injected into the social body to prevent greater violence (turmoil within the community). Girard draws a link between this ancient form of managing violence and the modern act of inoculation. This injection (the inoculation) is a repetition of the sacrifices (as in the scapegoat) and, "as in all types of sacrificial protection, naturally contains the possibility of a catastrophic inversion" (personal communication, April 11, 2009).

With vaccination programs, hygiene, quarantine, and animal culling, it is crucial to be strategic, to be precise, to be *practical*, and for institutions or states with different perspectives and areas of expertise to work together in order to respond effectively to a pandemic rather than letting panic and bad planning exacerbate existing inequities in the name of disaster response.

CONCLUSION

My concerns, then, are about the ebb and flow of public panic that flu news both responds to and generates. It is important to discern between "pandemic threat" and the constant threat of flu but to also understand that virulent and pandemic influenza is a possibility at almost any time. An emphasis on isolating specific pandemic threats only as they seem to emerge creates fits and starts of attention but very little consistent, systemic thought about prevention. There is a real need for a robust public health perspective – one that can be flexible enough to monitor flu activity all over the world by cooperating with respect to surveillance and treatment – and an ecological one – one that thinks in terms of systems and their interactions with each other. How do changes in global meat consumption affect the development of novel viruses? How should vaccines be distributed to have the most population effect worldwide? Perhaps most importantly, how can this public health perspective address income difference and the enhanced vulnerabilities of the poor?

In 2005, Paul Farmer wrote, "[Making] social and economic rights a reality is the key goal for health and human rights in the twenty-first century." Three years later, Sir Michael Marmot, Chair of the WHO's Commission on Social Determinants of Health, said, "We rely too much on medical interventions as a way of increasing life expectancy. A more effective way of increasing life expectancy and improving health would be ... to make health and health equity a marker for government performance" (WHO, 2008). It is fair and reasonable that we, as citizens, expect our governments to act responsibly and with foresight, to collaborate with other governments and with the private sector when necessary, and to dedicate sufficient funding and human expertise to developing preventative health systems that are practical, responsive, and functional and that are an integral aspect of everyday life as well as disaster preparedness.

ACKNOWLEDGMENTS

I am grateful to the following individuals for their comments, often offered in a workshop setting: Jeffrey Bussolini, Grace Cho, Rafael de la Dehesa, Jean Halley, Hosu Kim, Ron Nerio, Barbara Katz Rothman, Dan Skinner, and Neil Smith. I presented earlier versions of this chapter at the Rockefeller-funded seminar run by the Center for Place, Culture, and Politics at the CUNY Graduate Center and at the annual meeting of the Society for the Study of Symbolic Interaction.

REFERENCES

Andremont, A., & Tibon-Cornillot, M. (2006). *Le Triomphe des Bacteries, La Fin des Antibiotiques?* Paris: Max Milo.
Barry, J. (2005). *The great influenza: The epic story of the deadliest plague in history*. New York: Penguin.

Davis, M. (2005a). *Monster at our door: The global threat of avian flu*. New York: New Press.

Davis, M. (2005b). Avian flu: A state of unreadiness. *The Nation*, July 18.

Farmer, P. (2005). *Pathologies of power: Health, human rights, and the new war on the poor*. Berkeley: University of California Press.

Financial Services Roundtable. (2006, November). *Preparing for pandemic flu: A call to action*. Washington, DC: Financial Services Roundtable.

Food and Agriculture Association. (2005, July). *FAO/OIE/WHO consultation on avian influenza and human health: Risk reduction measuring in producing, marketing, and living with animals in Asia*. FAO, Kuala Lumpur.

Garrett, L. (2000). *Betrayal of trust: The collapse of global public health*. New York: Hyperion.

Garrett, L. (2009, 2 May). The path of a pandemic: How one virus spread from pigs and birds to humans around the globe. And why microbes like the H1N1 flu have become a growing threat. *Newsweek*, New York, viewed 28 July 2009. Available at http://www.newsweek.com/id/195692/page/1

Hoffmaster, B. (2001). Introduction. In: Hoffmaster (Ed.), *Bioethics in social context*. Philadelphia: Temple U Press.

Katz Rothman, B. (1998). *Genetic maps and human imaginations: The limits of science in understanding who we are*. New York: WW Norton and Co.

Kolata, G. (1999). *Flu: The story of the great influenza pandemic*. New York: Touchstone.

Leavitt, M. O. (2006, 13 November). *Pandemic planning update III*. US Department of Health and Human Services, Washington.

Matthews, J. T. (2006). Egg-based production of influenza vaccine: 30 years of commercial experience. *The Bridge*, *36*, 3. Viewed 10 October 2006. Available at http://www.nae.edu/Publications/TheBridge/Archives/V-36-3EngineeringandVaccineProductionforanInfluenzaPandemic/Egg-BasedProductionofInfluenzaVaccine30YearsofCommercialExperience.aspx

Oxford, J. S., Lambkin, R., Sefton, A., Daniels, R., Elliot, A., Brown, R., & Gill, D. (2005). A hypothesis: The conjunction of soldiers, gas, pigs, ducks, geese, and horses in northern France during the Great War provided the conditions for the emergence of the 'Spanish' influenza pandemic of 1918–1919. *Vaccine*, *23*(7), 940–945.

Perry, M. (2007). Indonesia ban risks WHO flu protection system. *Reuters*.

Rhodes, R. (1998). *Deadly feasts: Tracking the secrets of a terrifying new plague*. New York: Simon and Schuster.

Sencer, D. J., & Millar, J. D. (2006). Reflections on the 1976 swine flu vaccination program. *Emerging Infectious Diseases*, *12*(1), 29–33.

Snacken, R., Kendal, A., Haaheim, L., & Wood, J. (1999). The next influenza pandemic: Lessons from Hong Kong, 1997. *Emerging Infectious Diseases*, *5*(1), accessed in 1 October 2006, available at http://www.cdc.gov/ncidod/eid/vol5no2/snacken.htm

The World Bank. (2006). *Enhancing control of highly pathogenic avian influenza in developing countries through compensation: Issues and good practice, executive summary*. London: The World Bank.

UPMC Biosecurity Center. (2005). *Exercise illuminates transatlantic leaders' reactions to bioterror attack*. UPMC, Pittsburgh, viewed 15 October 2009. Available at http://www.upmc-biosecurity.org/website/center/newsroom/archive/2005-01-17_atlanticstorm.html

World Health Assembly. (2007). *Patent issues related to influenza viruses and vaccines*. Geneva: The World Health Organisation.

World Health Organisation (WHO). (2008). *Inequities are killing people on a grand scale, reports WHO's Commission.* The World Health Organisation, Geneva, viewed 1 September 2008. Available at http://www.who.int/mediacentre/news/releases/2008/pr29/en/index.html

World Organisation for Animal Health. (2009). *Killing of animals for disease control purposes.* Paris: OIE.

PART III
THE POLITICS OF RHETORIC AND CATEGORIZATION

THE POETICS OF AMERICAN CIRCUMCISION ON THE MARGINS OF MEDICAL NECESSITY

Daniel Skinner

ABSTRACT

Purpose – *This chapter sketches the major historical shifts in American circumcision discourse and examines the sociopolitics of those shifts.*

Methodology/approach – *The chapter centers on a critical analysis of competing narratives and knowledge claims about circumcision. It re-examines these narratives and claims, most of which are packaged in a rhetoric of health, specifically for their political valence.*

Findings – *The medical necessity of circumcision in the United States cannot be ascertained without attending to the disciplinary systems designed to produce and maintain religious, sexual and other cultural norms.*

Contribution to the field – *The chapter provides a clear and focused synthesis of many different literatures and contentions about circumcision that have yet to be brought together into a single narrative accessible for students and scholars of the medical humanities and medical politics.*

Understanding Emerging Epidemics: Social and Political Approaches
Advances in Medical Sociology, Volume 11, 145–163
Copyright © 2010 by Emerald Group Publishing Limited
All rights of reproduction in any form reserved
ISSN: 1057-6290/doi:10.1108/S1057-6290(2010)0000011012

INTRODUCTION

What justifications or perceived dangers underpin the story of male circumcision? How are the very terms of the debate over routine circumcision set, maintained and challenged? This chapter attempts to answer these questions by examining the rhetorical structures that have made circumcision a common procedure and object of faith in the United States, legitimizing and situating circumcision as a necessary and normal 'procedure'. In this chapter I sketch the major historical shifts in American circumcision discourse and examine the sociopolitics of those shifts. In taking this approach I seek to better understand the social forces that shape American circumcision discourse.

HISTORICAL DEVELOPMENT FROM ABRAHAM TO AMERICA

A series of comprehensive histories of circumcision have been published in the last few years (Glick, 2005; Gollaher, 2000). Despite differences in the way these histories narrate the story of circumcision, and their different emphases of circumcision's religious, medical and aesthetic justifications, taken together they make clear that American circumcision is an extraordinarily complex cultural phenomena. Yet, it is also clear that the depth of the surgery's social value has only begun to be recognized more widely, perhaps because it intersects with a complex of sociopolitical, including psychological, discourse. Understanding the relationships between these levels of discourse can help us understand what, if any, political questions circumcision intersects.

Though anthropologists have uncovered earlier accounts of Egyptian circumcision rituals (Gollaher, 2000), most studies point to circumcision's origins in Judaism, in the so-called 'Abrahamic covenant' (Van Ryzin, 2000). Here, according to Biblical accounts, circumcision constitutes the outward mark of the Jew and sign of membership in the community. Yet, the reason for this circumcision, beyond its cultural or symbolic value, is unclear. Gilman (1997) points to the merging of health and beauty that marks the history of circumcision, with Jews cast aside by the ancient Greeks, for whom beauty was found in the unaltered body. According to Gilman (1997), some attempted to 'pass' as gentiles, using weights and other strategies to stretch what remained of their foreskins. Such attempts to obscure one's circumcision were aided by the fact that these ritual circumcisions were far less complete than contemporary operations that remove a larger percentage of the foreskin. By the late 19th century, some German Jews would seek decircumcision surgery to restore them. These efforts underscore the indisociability of anti-semitism and other social forces such as hygiene, with the nation understood as a larger 'body'. One need only remember the centrality of dirt and vermin to Hitlerian rhetoric to see the connection (Burke, 1964). But social perspectives also shape cultural aesthetics more generally, both laterally within extant populations and across time, in family lineages.

While circumcision's centrality to Judaism is contested (Gollaher, 2000; Judd, 2007), we need not reconcile competing interpretations to write the story of American circumcision. The relatively small Jewish population in the United States does not help explain why, by 1965, about 85% – the precise opposite of global levels – of American boys would be routinely circumcised (Laumann, Masi, & Zuckerman, 1997). (If anything, one might expect anti-Semitism to provide friction *against* routine circumcision.) Though levels have declined since 1965, at 56% in 2005, circumcision was still the 'third most common inpatient surgery performed in the U.S.', though levels vary greatly across the various regions of the United States (Merrill, Nagamine, & Steiner, 2008). These differences suggest that circumcision intersects not merely with the medical, hygienic and aesthetic arguments with which it is commonly associated, but that these categories are themselves cultured. Circumcision politics impact different populations in different ways, as the surgery carries with it a rich set of cultural significations.

For example, Merrill et al. (2008) speculate that these regional differences (74.9% in Midwest, 64.5% in Northeast and 30.1% in West) stem at least in part from different ethnic associations with circumcision. As the US Hispanic population rises, it is likely that circumcisions will become increasingly rare because circumcision is not common in most Hispanic cultures. Similarly, as new studies (Bloemenkamp & Farley, 2000; Weiss, Quigley, & Hayes, 2000) find new uses for circumcision as a preventive measure for sexually transmitted disease (STD) transmission, it is also possible that circumcision will become increasingly associated with at risk populations, such as gay men and African Americans, both of whom are currently experiencing a resurgence of HIV/AIDS infections and are being targeted by health authorities as possible candidates for circumcision (McNeil, 2007). As the United States begins to discuss the development of a national health care system, all costs – and especially those lacking medical justification – will likely be called into question. Each of these cases points to the possibility that circumcision politics are changing in the United States.

A POLITICAL TOPOGRAPHY OF
AMERICAN CIRCUMCISION

American circumcision debates can be grouped into two main (though often overlapping) categories. On the one hand are questions concerning the medical necessity of routinely – that is, in the absence of any medical complications – removing the foreskin. Some groups argue that routine neonatal circumcision is never medically necessary since clinical problems with a baby's foreskin tend to arise days, weeks or months after birth; phimosis – or a foreskin that does not retract – can only be diagnosed when the foreskin does not retract as babies grow, a process that takes anywhere from six months to two years (Dewan, Tieu, & Chieng, 1996). On the other hand, critics question the ethics of operating – again, routinely – on babies who cannot be consulted and who experience high levels of pain during the operation, pain that some (Goldman, 1997; Boyle, Goldman, Svoboda, & Fernandez, 2002) say may cause life-long trauma and even violent tendencies. The ethical and medical arguments (but also their many intersections) collide with religious, sociocultural, sexual and aesthetic arguments.

With respect to beauty, the contemporary United States has reached the precisely opposite position from earlier (especially the Greek) histories, and many uncircumcised American men fear that their partners will be repulsed by their penises (two television shows, *Nip/Tuck* and *Sex and the City*, equated the intact penis with Shar-Peis). Studies suggest that there is good reason to believe this, as many Americans have internalized stereotypes of the uncircumcised penis as unhealthy, unclean and unattractive (Bonner, 2000). Could this American aesthetic be enough to account for the small difference between circumcised and uncircumcised men of STD transmission, with uncircumcised men being more self-conscious of the way their bodies will be viewed by new partners? These aesthetics, of course, change with other cultural indicators. For example, both of these television programs focus on upper class Whites; Hispanic Americans are far less likely to circumcise their children (which probably accounts for the relatively low percentages of circumcised boys in the American West (Merrill et al., 2008)). Still, the point remains that in American popular culture, the circumcised penis has become both sexually and aesthetically normalized. Of those Americans who are not circumcised at birth, some chose to be circumcised at some point in their early sexual lives, often at the encouragement of their partners (Bell, 2005), but most often to deal with medical problems such as phimosis.

Yet, how circumcision became associated with medical discourses seems a slightly different matter, and one that requires attention to the logic and politics of medicalization itself. It is now well known that the medicalization of childbirth was integral to the institutionalization and legitimation of medicine in America. As Wertz and Wertz (1977) note, 'Medicine in America may have had minimal scientific authority, but it was beginning to develop social and processional organization and leadership; unorganized midwives were an easy competitive target for medicine'. These efforts to medicalize childbirth were integral to the founding of both the American Medical Association (AMA) and American Academy of Pediatrics (AAP), which raises the question: did childbirth need to be medicalized, or did the new (male-dominated) institutions prey upon easy targets to legitimize themselves?

Without resolving this question here, I want only to note that the story of circumcision, too, is bound up with the professionalization of medicine in post-Civil War, Victorian America. Around the same time that midwifery was marginalized, the war on masturbation had become an American obsession, which critics linked to the sensitive nerve endings of the foreskin (much in the same way advocates of clitoridectomies understand female masturbation). Yet, at this point, the foreskin also began to be subsumed by volumes of medical and social mythology. The Victorian use of circumcision as an effort to curb masturbation faded to the background and was largely replaced, at least explicitly, by medical justifications and scientific reasoning. Lewis Sayre, a founding member of the AMA (and eventual president), began to experiment with circumcision as a possible means for helping patients with a wide range of afflictions, including 'malnutrition', 'derangement of the digestive organs', chorea, convulsions, hysteria and other nervous disorders (Boyd, 1998, p. 330). Sayre's experiments contributed to not only the medicalization of circumcision (Boyd, 1998), but also the legitimization of the fledgling AMA.

Today, the medical benefits of circumcision are still being studied and considered. An AMA study (2000) has concluded that circumcision decreases the incidence of urinary tract infections in newborns, as well as penile cancer in adults. It also indicated that circumcised men were slightly less likely to contract HIV and other STDs. Yet, the study also notes that all of these findings are mitigated by other factors, such as the extremely low total incidences of penile cancer in the United States and the fact that the number of a man's sexual partners correlates more closely with STDs and penile cancer than rates of circumcision (Van Ryzin, 2000). In general, circumcision's potential benefits concern young adults and adults, and are almost always correlated with other indexes of health, such as hygiene and social behavior (Spach, Stapleton, & Stamm, 1992).

The AAP's (1999) rejection of routine neonatal circumcision also weighed potential benefits with the problems associated with subjecting babies to routine surgery at a very fragile stage of life and other complications. Yet, from the perspective of social discourse, it is precisely the absence of danger and controversy – since circumcision has come to be seen as rote – that makes circumcision interesting. If so many of circumcision's potential benefits are correlated with social behaviors and socioeconomic indicators (which one would expect to bear on social hygiene), then why would a rich nation such as the United States deploy such strong rhetorics of cleanliness and disease to support a practice that as Boyle et al. (2002, p. 330) note, 'no national medical association anywhere in the world that has studied the issue recommends …'? (See also AAP, 1989, 1999.) Not only is routine circumcision not recommended, but Boyle et al. suggest, aside from ethical considerations (cf. Denniston, 1996; Fadel, 2003; Mukherjea, 2008), the surgery's positive social benefits for an extremely small subset may outweigh its negative effects on the larger population.

Whatever the medical judgments, however, Bell (2005) notes a crucial sociopolitical phenomenon: 'The biomedical debates about male circumcision in the United States do not seem to have infiltrated public attitudes toward the practice to any significant degree'. This suggests the presence of a medical discourse not informed or driven by the judgments of medical experts, a non-medical medical discourse or what Van Ryzin (2000, p. 24A) calls 'perceived medical reasons'. Such divides suggest that attempts to generate serious discussion about epidemics and disease must grapple with broader social understandings and projections about disease that are encumbered by social metaphors, body politics and various levels of psychological interference (see, e.g. Laqueur, 1990; Pitts, 2003).

The different perspectives and data sets here indicate why I have framed American circumcision as a web of sometimes competing, sometimes reinforcing discourses. Most studies of male circumcision as a sociopolitical phenomena, including Glick's and Gollaher's, do not resolve the tensions inherent in circumcision politics because there are so many levels of culture at play, many of which cannot be organized into clear causal sequences.

We cannot simply say that conceptions of cleanliness lead to perceptions of medical necessity; hygiene does not constitute, in and of itself, grounds for declaration of medical necessity. Similarly, one cannot ascertain whether cleanliness is a response to perceptions of hygiene, whether associations of disease are results of moral prohibitions and rejections of or the management of pleasure, or whether routine circumcision is, at least in part, a simple attempt to maintain an aesthetic order, a perpetuation of predominant appearance of American penises, as, for example, in father–son relations. Religious rituals and medical discourses, too, cannot be so easily dissociated, especially when we consider the possibility, as Glick (2005) has argued, that religious ritual may evolve into a medical practice that may itself become ritualized. Similarly, aesthetic orders do not, in themselves, correlate to hygiene any more than morality is necessarily linked to cleanliness. These connections constitute a tight network of knowledge that makes these various discourses impossible to disentangle. It is clear, however, that considerations of how meanings are produced and related to social questions must be part of the study, of not only circumcision, but also medical practices generally. All diseases, and not just epidemics, tend to acquire meanings (Treichler, 1987; Sontag, 1990; Weiss, 1997). A medical and epidemiological politics must work with and through those meanings.

SYNERGIES AND TENSIONS: RELIGION, MEDICINE AND SEXUAL POLITICS

Arguments about circumcision are so closely related, not only to the belief that foreskins harbor dirt and disease, but also that the sensitivity of the foreskin increases pleasure and that the transmission of STDs is as much part of the story of circumcision as is the regulation of masturbation and sexual pleasure (Gollaher, 2000; Glick, 2005; Mukherjea, 2008, p. 232). This suggests that a politics of the metaphor, and a critique of those metaphors, must be part of a politics of circumcision. Its meaning constituted through its metaphors, masturbation is not prone to uncleanliness, but is understood as fundamentally unclean, where specters of dirt become actual. Circumcised penises are understood as part of the broader American pursuit of cleanliness that Bushman and Bushman (1988) and Hoy (1995) have detailed, within an aesthetic order that economizes health as well as beauty. These clustered metaphors are powerful because they are capable of subsuming many different questions into one discursive field. These intertwined discourses make appeals to the scientific or medical justifications for circumcision problematic because, in these metaphors, a purely 'medical' knowledge is elusive.

Aside from potential benefits, some studies have found that circumcision may cause a series of complications and illnesses, including meningitis (Scurlock & Pemberton, 1977) and, more often, urinary tract (Goldman, Barr, Bistritzer, & Aladjem, 1996) and 'staph' infections (Nguyen, Bancroft, Mascola, Guevara, & Yasuda, 2007). Complications, though relatively rare in the United States, also include the disfiguration of the penis itself as a result of incorrect cutting (Bonner, 2000). In some countries, the same substandards of hygiene that lead some to argue in support of routine circumcision may exacerbate potential harms stemming from it. These complications indicate that the establishment of routine surgeries must be accompanied by considerations of routine complications: from mistakes; from exposing the body to airborne germs; or from systemic problems with health care infrastructure, protocol and political economy (Bonner, 2000, pp. 147–148).

Even when done 'correctly' and without 'complication', circumcision – as with all surgeries – has negative effects. The physical problems associated with circumcision differ, of course, depending on the conditions under which the surgery is carried out. As Gollaher (2000) and others (Gesundheit et al., 2000) have noted, the circumcision ritual of *Metzizah b'peh*, practiced in some Hasidic communities, was believed to have been the cause of an occasional outbreak of neonatal herpes in New York in 1988, 1998 and again in 2005 (Newman, 2005). In this ritual, the *mohel* (circumciser) affixes his mouth to the baby's penis after circumcising in order to stop bleeding and purify the wound. While the case of *Metzizah b'peh* is specific to a small number of orthodox sects, it does indicate a fundamental tension at the center of circumcision discourse. Not only are practices like circumcision considered by critics to be (ethical as well as sexual, psycho- and physiological) epidemics themselves, but they can, like all invasive procedures, by dint of exposing the body to germs and other related effects, produce disease themselves.

To opponents of routine neonatal circumcision, the epidemic associated with genital cutting is not that which it purports to curb, but that which it causes. Studies critical of circumcision's effects deploy not only the languages of trauma (AAP, 1999; Boyle et al., 2002), but also long-term trauma, with effects similar to those found in victims of PTSD, including suicidal gestures (Anand & Scalzo, 2000). Traditionally, circumcisions are performed without anesthesia (Lander, Brady-Fryer, Metcalfe, Nazarali, &

Muttitt, 1997), leading some (Rhinehart, 1999) to suggest that circumcision has long functioned as an early encounter with violence. These critics suggest that *routine* circumcision may cause *routine* harm (Boyle et al., 2002). Still others indicate that routine circumcision may create populations prone to exacerbate social dangers, such as a study by Laumann et al. (1997) that found (contrary to the 2000 AMA study) that circumcised men may be statistically more *likely* to acquire and transmit STDs.

A series of anesthetic techniques have been normalized in recent years and post-neonatal circumcisions are generally performed under general anesthesia (Bonner, 2000). Other studies (Boyle et al., 2002) consider the possibility that the psychological effects of circumcision may be similar to those stemming from child abuse and rape. Citing a series of studies based on testimonies of circumcised men, Boyle et al. (2002, p. 333) argue that 'Some men circumcised in infancy or childhood without their consent have described their present feelings in the language of violation, torture, mutilation and sexual assault'. Despite variations in psychological evidence, most anti-circumcision groups agree that it is unethical to perform a medically unnecessary surgery on unwilling babies lacking the capacity for consultation or decision. Many associations between circumcision and trauma stem from the vulnerability of babies to a painful surgery.

Because circumcision is not merely a form of body alteration but a form of specifically *genital* cutting, each of these potential effects finds correlates in the politics of male sexuality. Freud understood circumcision not only as a mark of the Jew, but also as inherently bound up with Jewish sexuality. The intertwinedness of genital cutting with sexuality and gender suggests that the question of male genital cutting must be addressed within the context of gender politics more generally. This is not only due to circumcision's roots in anti-masturbation campaigns, but also because its primary social effects *are* sexual, whether they bear on pleasure, performance, aesthetics and social approval, or a trauma that leads to effects from melancholy to aggression.

Even if routine circumcision is 'useful as a preventative to masturbation', as J.M. McGree argued way back in 1882 (Gollaher, 2000, p. 85), then this effort at sexual regulation reinforces a central claim of the anti-circumcision movement that the reduction of pleasure is not a side effect of circumcision, part of its very purpose. The Jewish philosopher Moses Maimonides explicitly indicated that decreased sexual gratification was a key goal of circumcision (Maimonides & Friedländer, 1956, p. 378). Boyle et al. (2002, p. 334) note 'an inevitable reduction in sexual sensation experienced by circumcised males' by the simple fact that the surgery removes thousands of sensitive nerve endings. The Victorian prohibition on masturbation and the use of circumcision to combat it provide fodder for equating male circumcision with so-called 'female circumcision' or genital mutilation (FGM), as both are cast in terms of the management of economies of pleasure.

Feminist theorists have successfully foregrounded women's bodies in debates over reproductive rights and health crises such as breast cancer, while men have been addressed primarily in terms of aggressive tendencies and sexual violence, as either lacking an understanding of the embodied reality of women's experience or perpetrating acts of violence against them. Circumcision politics are unique in their concern with men's bodies, rivaled only in contemporary America by discussions about erectile dysfunction. In addressing circumcision, men's bodies are foregrounded, bringing with them a series of arguments familiar to students of the feminist movements: trauma in the service of gender norms, the ethics of living in a body that is not in one's control, subject to violation and the sense of loss stemming from the denial of sexual pleasure. Circumcision provokes questions about not only sexual politics, then, but also the violence wrought in pursuit of the maintenance of gender norms, where surgery functions as a means by which those norms are replicated. The social consequences of routine neonatal circumcision must be located within a politics of cutting non-volitional subjects more broadly (Fausto-Sterling, 2000).

In this sense, considerations of male genital cutting could be useful for throwing light on genital manipulation more generally, moving debates over those manipulations from the margins to the center of contemporary discussions of sexual health, as well as the use and abuse of 'medical necessity' determinations. In other words, the discursive intersections of circumcision debates could be redeployed to open those discourses for political engagement. Because of the historical male domination of the medical industry, circumcision is one of the few examples of a forced modification of men's bodies, which makes it useful for thinking about the ethics and sociopolitics of medical economies – from birth control to forced sterilization to castration to clitoridectomy to hymenoplasty.

Bell (2005) notes that while the mutilation of female genitalia has evoked a widespread response because it is understood as a violent act perpetrated as a form of gendered violence, the cutting of the penis has not been framed similarly, largely because the foreskin has been treated as 'extra skin', rather than part of the penis itself. Since men's bodies are subject to a different gender and sexual politics, male circumcision is not allowed to enter into the very order of discourse that could allow us to think critically about it. The question is: how can we think about men's and women's bodies in such a way that we can think about the sociopolitics of genital cutting without paving over the important differences in the politics of American gender? On the one hand, we surely do not want to simply equate male circumcision with clitoridectomy; on the other, to understand circumcision as an ethical matter within a public health crisis – in terms of the justifications both for and against circumcision – how shall we conceptualize the problem but by drawing on those politics that have been able to capture public attention?

The sociopolitics of circumcision cannot be dissociated from what Faludi (1999) has called 'the betrayal of the American man' and can be read as a symptom of the immature state of American gender politics. According to Bell (2005), 'This connection between circumcision and male sexuality is most evident in popular perceptions that circumcised men "last" longer during sexual intercourse'. In this case, circumcision is bound up with what has been advertised as a medicalized epidemic in male sexuality, of dysfunction. Some men identify their circumcised penises as a cause of sexual dysfunction, with some studies suggesting that circumcision reduces penile sensation by as much as 90% (Van Ryzin, 2000).

Considering their visibility, we can understand why circumcision debates, in so far as they attract any widespread attention, would quickly become associated with the burgeoning industry of remedies for erectile dysfunction. For precisely the same reason, the discourses called upon by some anti-circumcision groups (such as the National Organization of Circumcision Information Resource Centers, or NOCIRC) also reinforce problematic gender stereotypes – as when dysfunction (in arousal or 'staying power') becomes a key argument about circumcision's ethicality. Such arguments engender a politics of resentment that simultaneously reinforce the very norms that might foreclose opportunities to think about gender in relation to body modification and the medicalization of male sexuality.

For our purposes in thinking about circumcision discourse in relation to epidemics, we need not resolve these tensions between medicine, religion and sexuality. We need only notice the merging of discourses and raise a skeptical eye toward medical arguments so intimately related with sexual and gender norms. If surgery is understood as a cause of a widespread dysfunctionality, then surgery may also be prescribed as the cure. Either way, the various discursive fields cannot be altered if circumcision is not understood – diagnosed? – in its rich cultural complexity.

Bell (2005), who reviewed a series of circumcision web boards, argues that women reporting increased pleasure with their circumcised partners constitute an important source of pro-circumcision rhetoric. Her argument is worth quoting at length:

> Importantly, these anecdotes speak to the role that sexual competence plays in constructions of contemporary masculinity, as many men clearly believe that any loss of sensitivity that accompanies circumcision is compensated by their enhanced sexual performance. Indeed, what is interesting here is how irrelevant the issue of reduced sensation is for both the men who have this operation and their sexual partners. This poses a striking contrast to the dominant discourses surrounding female genital cutting, where the idea of a woman undergoing genital cutting to enhance her partner's sexual pleasure (while concomitantly reducing her own level of sensation) strikes most observers as "barbaric" and misogynistic. The differing reaction these operations evoke is hardly surprising in light of the assumptions regarding instinctive, active male sexuality and fragile, passive female sexuality ....

To properly situate male circumcision in a larger framework of American health discourse, including sexual health, a number of new perspectives need to be opened. The first concerns the way the body is conceptualized. Bell (2005) argues that female bodies are understood through male bodies, with the clitoris understood as the female equivalent of the penis. While the castration metaphor may be useful politically for emphasizing the seriousness of FGM, these metaphors only open doors to cycles of competitive victimization. Were male and female bodies understood on their own terms, and not metaphored through one another, these comparisons would not control social understandings of genital cutting (the expression 'genital cutting' is of course itself strategic in its gender neutrality). The history of this view is deposited in the very word circumcision, which suggests that the organ is being 'cut around', rather than seeing the foreskin as part of the organ. Reframing circumcision as cuttings 'of' – rather than cuts 'around' supposedly more central parts – ascribes a similar logic to men's and women's bodies without closing spaces for different modes of gender analysis. This approach does not subsume the bodies of different individuals under one epistemic umbrella.

Our understanding of circumcision can benefit from recent debates over the ethics of operating on intersexed babies (babies born with gender indeterminant genitalia). Recent studies (Dreifus, 2005) have suggested that the psychological effects of operating on intersexed babies may be greater than leaving them intact until they grow to an age at which they can decide what – if anything – to do. Others (see Weil, 2006) have emphasized the ethicality of this approach, advocating gender self-determination. Blizzard (2002, p. 619) notes that though 'In most instances of an intersex problem, a *medical emergency* is not present but a *mental and/or social emergency* very likely is' (emphasis original). At issue here is a balancing of the rights of parents to make these determinations for their children, weighing the ethics of non-volitional surgery with the potential struggles an intersexed person (and their parents) may endure (Weil, 2006).

As with intact foreskins, there are surely cases where intersexuality poses a danger to newborns, but these are the exceptions, not the rule. In this sense, it is precisely in and with the 'exceptions' that the politics and ethics of circumcision is both most pronounced and clearly articulated. The politics of intersexuality suggests a question for routine circumcision politics: what should be the relationship between the medical establishment and the management of social, and especially sexual, norms?

POLICY CONSIDERATIONS OF CIRCUMCISION

As one would expect, the future of American circumcision is constrained by the policies, practices and traditions of the past. Bollinger (2007) argues that the history of routine neonatal circumcision in the United States has left the United States today with a 'penis-care information gap', where American doctors and parents do not know how to care for intact penises, which could produce precisely the same epidemiological effects as those who assume that intact penises are dirty fear. This 'gap', according to Bollinger (2007, p. 205), puts the intact boy 'at risk for losing his foreskin to the scalpel due to improper care of the foreskin'. As health insurance coverage of the surgery wanes (Bollinger, 2007, p. 207), and fewer Americans opt for a circumcision that they will have to pay for, Americans will need to learn about foreskin maintenance if declining circumcision rates are not to produce increased instances of STDs, penile cancer and other related afflictions.

There is also an important psychological dimension to these histories that policy planners must consider. Boyle et al. (2002) note that many men are incapable of thinking critically about circumcision because they do not want to consider the possibility that they, too, may have been violated (Goldman, 1998; Boyle et al., 2002). This underscores the possibility that the psychological effects and identifications stemming from a culture of circumcision may produce a resistance to change. Here, circumcision's injurious effects are bound up in a gender politics, constrained by norms whereby American men refuse to see themselves as vulnerable, ultimately resulting in an unwillingness to be tested and checked by doctors (Rabin, 2006).

Boyle et al. note that parents are bound in these discursive webs as well. Parents who have circumcised their children may be resistant to the idea that they might have done so wrongly or unnecessarily while new parents may choose to circumcise to avoid clashing with the narratives and histories that sustained them; in short, 'beliefs may be adopted to conform with one's decision to circumcise' (Boyle et al., 2002, p. 337), and not the reverse. Still others (Gilman, 1997) have suggested that the 'child abuse' experienced by circumcised children may make them abusers themselves: 'child abuse turns abused children into child abusers; they then circumcise their own children, who go on in the same vicious circle'. Though many people will surely question these associations, the questions raise the possibility that attachments to cultural patterns may replicate and repeat the trauma and bodily dangers associated with circumcision, using a vague sense of medical legitimacy as justification.

In recent years circumcision has received renewed attention with regard to the HIV/AIDS crisis, with studies suggesting that routine circumcision does, in some cases and contexts, reduce transmission (Marx, 1989; AMA, 2000; Bloemenkamp & Farley, 2000; Weiss et al., 2000). Most HIV/AIDS circumcision discussions have centered on Africa, but the City of New York has recently considered encouraging circumcision in high-risk populations as well (McNeil, 2007). Yet discussions about circumcision in Africa suggest the need to apply the critical lens that Americans usually reserve for those 'others' to the United States itself. The critique 'point[s] to the hypocrisy in decrying only those surgeries that are performed in non-Western contexts' (see Boyd, 1998; Gollaher, 2000), such as FGM, but also the ethicality of maintaining surgical customs for cultural – not medical or scientific – reasons. Similarly, is the mostly 'Western' scientific data immune to the aestheticization of hygiene, or the role that racism often plays in conceptualizing African bodies as sites of neocolonial intervention?

While the question of circumcision in Africa is beyond the scope of this chapter, a similar contrast between the HIV/AIDS crises in the United States and Africa does shed light on circumcision in America. The New York case, in fact, has been compared to the African case, as when Dr. Thomas R. Frieden, Commissioner of Health in New York City, said that 'In some subpopulations, you have 10 to 20 percent prevalence rates, just as they do in parts of Africa' (McNeil, 2007). These 'subpopulations', it turns out, are two traditionally marginalized groups: Black men and gay men. Far from framing HIV/AIDS in ways that could be useful for combating it, equating these people with 'Africa' seems to foreclose understanding of the HIV/AIDS crisis in these communities. In part, this is because the analogy does not hold up; not only are socio-economic and hygienic conditions significantly worse in 'Africa' than they are in the United States – which is the primary point of the AAP (1999) rejection of routine neonatal circumcision – but also the US government has resources at its disposal that less wealthy countries do not.

A politics of American circumcision must be attentive to the sociocultural positions of targeted populations. One cannot ignore the fact that this concession to palliative surgery would arrive in the form of the irreversible modification of bodies that conjures the more sordid moments in the history of American medicine, such as forced sterilization (Davis, 1983; Reilly, 1991). This reduction by analogy, of 'Africa' to the United States, only serves to erase the particular sociopolitical conditions and histories of these groups and these epidemics, which constitute the very grounds on which a sociopolitical response to epidemics must take place. Given that American circumcision's early history is bound up with the management of economies of pleasure, is it a coincidence that the two groups being targeted for circumcision have historically been branded promiscuous, sexualized in the context of a host of deviances? The ethics of the contemporary politics of HIV/AIDS cannot be dissociated from its history; what are the ethical implications of following historical silences (White, 2004) with routine surgeries?

Given the depth of these cultural intersections, it is possible that the defunding of circumcision by HMOs and Medicare may provide the best possibility for a critical reconsideration whether or not to circumcise, as occurred in the United Kingdom when, in the 1950s, the National Health Service (NHS) stopped paying for circumcision, based largely on an influential study published by Gairdner (1949). As with many treatments and surgeries in the United States, the patchwork health care system has enabled the United States to avoid serious debates over the wisdom and necessity, but also ethics, of certain medical practices. Before we can consider circumcision in the United States as a singular phenomenon – not to mention epidemic – we must make sense of the ways in which medicine itself is decentralized, regionalized and – in the case of determining whether practices are necessary, elective or cosmetic – privatized. If the costs of routine circumcision were socialized, then a broad social debate and decision about circumcision would seem to be necessary (as occurred, e.g. in the United Kingdom (Gollaher, 2000, p. 114), and Canada (Charles, Lomas, Giacomini, Bhatia, & Vincent, 1997)). Both cases, motivated by a cost–benefit analysis that forced them to re-evaluate their understanding of medical necessity, ultimately came to regard circumcision as a cosmetic surgery. In both cases, circumcisions are paid for by parents.

CONCLUSION

Despite its unique place in the culture order, circumcision opens pathways for thinking through the broader sociopolitics of epidemics more generally. Even a cursory consideration of the question of medical necessity and circumcision foregrounds the relationship between perceived crises and culturally refracted concepts such as cleanliness, moral and physical hygiene, and the gendered politics of sexual behavior. As they constitute the field of cultural knowledge that informs the sociopolitical conditions that provide the context for circumcision, these social forces determine where the line between social engagements end and surgery begins.

I have suggested that in order to understand the political fault lines of circumcision discourse, as well as the ethical considerations that must be part of engagements with those lines, we must attend to the complicated network of meanings that accompany circumcision. Such an analysis, however, needs to be as multi-faceted and layered as medical discourse itself, where meanings are constructed relationally and over time, and within specific political contexts. As I have suggested, medical discourse is constituted through and by a gender politics, just as conceptions of health and cleanliness that drive conceptions of the medical are refracted through that politics. Just as importantly, circumcision's historical transmission has been fueled by traditions that make it difficult to distinguish medical, hygienic and sexual knowledge from habit and culture. This suggests that the associations between circumcision and disease that drive political interventions and policy initiatives require careful ethical, as well as critical, political consideration.

REFERENCES

American Academy of Pediatrics. (1999). Circumcision policy statement. *Pediatrics, 103*, 686–693.
American Academy of Pediatrics Task Force on Circumcision. (1989). Report of the Task Force on Circumcision. *Pediatrics, 84*, 388–391.
American Medical Association. (2000). Report 10 of the Council on Scientific Affairs. Available at http://www.ama-assn.org/ama/pub/category/13585.html
Anand, K. J., & Scalzo, F. M. (2000). Can adverse neonatal experiences alter brain development and subsequent behavior? *Biology of the Neonate, 2*, 69–82.
Bell, K. (2005). Genital cutting and Western discourses on sexuality. *Medical Anthropology Quarterly, 19*, 125–148.

Blizzard, R. M. (2002). Intersex issues: A series of continuing conundrums. *Pediatrics, 110*, 616–621.

Bloemenkamp, K., & Farley, T. M. M. (2000). *HIV and male circumcision*. Geneva, Switzerland: World Health Organization.

Bollinger, D. (2007). The penis-care information gap: Preventing improper care of intact boys. *Thymos: Journal of Boyhood Studies, 1*, 205–219.

Bonner, K. (2000). Male circumcision as an HIV control strategy: Not a 'natural condom'. *Reproductive Health Matters, 18*, 143–155.

Boyd, B. R. (1998). *Circumcision exposed: Rethinking a medical and cultural tradition*. Freedom, CA: The Crossing Press.

Boyle, G. J., Goldman, R., Svoboda, J. S., & Fernandez, E. (2002). Male circumcision: Pain, trauma and psychosexual sequelae. *Journal of Health Psychology, 7*, 329–343.

Burke, K. (1964). *Terms for order*. Bloomington: Indiana University Press.

Bushman, R. L., & Bushman, C. L. (1988). The early history of cleanliness in America. *The Journal of American History, 4*, 1213–1238.

Charles, C., Lomas, J., Giacomini, M., Bhatia, V., & Vincent, V. A. (1997). Medical necessity in Canadian health policy: Four meanings and … a funeral? *The Milbank Quarterly, 75*, 365–394.

Davis, A. Y. (1983). *Women, race & class*. New York: Vintage Books.

Denniston, G. (1996). Circumcision and the code of ethics. *Humane Health Care International, 12*, 78–80.

Dewan, P., Tieu, H., & Chieng, B. (1996). Phimosis: Is circumcision necessary? *Journal of Paediatrics and Child Health, 32*, 285–289.

Dreifus, C. (2005). Declaring with clarity, when gender is ambiguous. *The New York Times*.

Fadel, P. (2003). Respect for bodily integrity: A Catholic perspective on circumcision in Catholic hospitals. *The American Journal of Bioethics, 3*, 23–25.

Faludi, S. (1999). *Stiffed: The betrayal of the American man*. New York: HarperCollins Publishers.

Fausto-Sterling, A. (2000). *Sexing the body: Gender politics and the construction of sexuality*. New York: Basic Books.

Gairdner, D. (1949). The fate of the foreskin. *British Medical Journal, 2*, 1433–1437.

Gesundheit, B., Grisaru-Soen, G., Greenberg, D., Levtzion-Korach, O., Malkin, D., Petric, M., Koren, G., Tendler, M. D., Ben-Zeev, B., Vardi, A., Dagan, R., & Engelhard, D. (2000). Neonatal genital herpes simplex virus type 1 Infection after Jewish ritual circumcision: Modern medicine and religious tradition. *Pediatrics, 114*, e163–e259.

Gilman, S. L. (1997). Decircumcision: The first aesthetic surgery. *Modern Judaism, 17*, 201–210.

Glick, L. B. (2005). *Marked in your flesh: Circumcision from ancient Judea to modern America*. Oxford/New York: Oxford University Press.

Goldman, M., Barr, J., Bistritzer, T., & Aladjem, M. (1996). Urinary tract infection following ritual Jewish circumcision. *Israel Journal of Medical Sciences, 32*, 1098–1102.

Goldman, R. (1997). *Circumcision: The hidden trauma*. Boston, MA: Vanguard.

Goldman, R. (1998). *Questioning circumcision: A Jewish perspective*. Boston, MA: Vanguard.

Gollaher, D. (2000). *Circumcision: A history of the world's most controversial surgery*. New York: Basic Books.

Hoy, S. (1995). *Chasing dirt: The American pursuit of cleanliness*. New York: Oxford University Press.

162   DANIEL SKINNER

Judd, R. (2007). *Contested rituals: Circumcision, kosher butchering, and Jewish political life in Germany, 1843–1933.* Ithaca: Cornell University Press.

Lander, J., Brady-Fryer, B., Metcalfe, J., Nazarali, S., & Muttitt, S. (1997). Comparison of ring block, dorsal penile nerve block, and topical anesthesia for neonatal circumcision: A randomized controlled trial. *Journal of the American Medical Association, 278,* 2157–2162.

Laqueur, T. (1990). *Making sex: Body and gender from the Greeks to Freud.* Cambridge: Harvard University Press.

Laumann, E. O., Masi, C. M., & Zuckerman, E. W. (1997). Circumcision in the United States: Prevalence, prophylactic effects, and sexual practice. *Journal of the American Medical Association, 277,* 1052–1057.

Maimonides, M., & Friedländer, M. (1956). *The guide for the perplexed.* New York: Dover Publications.

Marx, J. L. (1989). Circumcision may protect against the AIDS virus. *Science, 4917,* 470–471.

Mcneil, D. G. (2007). New York City plans to promote circumcision to reduce spread of AIDS. *The New York Times.*

Merrill, C. T., Nagamine, M., & Steiner, C. (2008). Circumcisions performed in US community hospitals, 2005. *Healthcare Cost and Utilization Project, statistical brief #45.*

Mukherjea, A. (2008). Cutting risk: The ethics of male circumcision, HIV prevention, and wellness. *Advances in Medical Sociology, 9,* 225–243.

Newman, A. (2005). City questions circumcision ritual after baby dies. *The New York Times.*

Nguyen, D. M., Bancroft, L., Mascola, R., Guevara, R., & Yasuda, L. (2007). Risk factors for neonatal methicillin-resistant *Staphylococcus aureus* infection in a well-infant nursery. *Infection Control and Hospital Epidemiology, 28,* 406–411.

Pitts, V. (2003). *In the flesh: The cultural politics of body modification.* New York: Palgrave Macmillan.

Rabin, R. (2006). Health disparities persist for men, and doctors ask why. *The New York Times,* New York.

Reilly, P. (1991). *The surgical solution: A history of involuntary sterilization in the United States.* Baltimore: Johns Hopkins University Press.

Rhinehart, J. (1999). Neonatal circumcision reconsidered. *Transactional Analysis Journal, 29*(3), 215–221.

Scurlock, J., & Pemberton, P. J. (1977). Neonatal meningitis and circumcision. *Medical Journal of Australia, 1,* 332–334.

Sontag, S. (1990). *Illness as metaphor; AIDS and its metaphors.* New York: Doubleday.

Spach, D. H., Stapleton, A. E., & Stamm, W. E. (1992). Lack of circumcision increases the risk of urinary tract infection in young men. *Journal of the American Medical Association, 267,* 679–681.

Treichler, P. A. (1987). AIDS, homophobia, and biomedical discourse: An epidemic of signification. *AIDS: Cultural Analysis/Cultural Activism, 43,* 31–70.

Van Ryzin, L. (2000). The circumcision debate. *The American Journal of Nursing, 100,* 24A–24B.

Weil, E. (2006). What if it's (sort of) a boy and (sort of) a girl? *The New York Times Magazine.*

Weiss, H. A., Quigley, M. A., & Hayes, R. J. (2000). Male circumcision and risk of HIV infection in sub-Saharan Africa: A systematic review and meta-analysis. *AIDS, 15,* 2361–2370.

Weiss, M. (1997). Signifying the pandemics: Metaphors of AIDS, cancer, and heart disease. *Medical Anthropology Quarterly, 11,* 456–476.

Wertz, R. W., & Wertz, D. C. (1977). *Lying-in: A history of childbirth in America.* New York: Free Press.

White, A. (2004). Reagan's AIDS legacy: Silence equals death. *San Francisco Chronicle,* June 8.

OF REBELS, CONFORMISTS, AND INNOVATORS: APPLYING MERTON'S TYPOLOGY TO EXPLORE AN EFFECTIVE HOME CARE POLICY FOR THE EMERGING ALZHEIMER'S EPIDEMIC

William D. Cabin

ABSTRACT

Purpose – *To explore how home care social worker perceptions of their organizations' dominant goals and means affect direct service home care professionals' care delivery and meeting of patient needs for persons with Alzheimer's disease.*

Methodology/approach – *The study used a convenience sample of 34 home care social workers in the New York City metropolitan area and an extensive literature review.*

Findings – *The study found that literature indicates a dissonance between effective, evidence-based research psychosocial Alzheimer's disease*

Understanding Emerging Epidemics: Social and Political Approaches
Advances in Medical Sociology, Volume 11, 165–181
Copyright © 2010 by Emerald Group Publishing Limited
All rights of reproduction in any form reserved
ISSN: 1057-6290/doi:10.1108/S1057-6290(2010)0000011013

interventions and Medicare home health policy which does not cover their use. Furthermore, interviews indicated home care social workers' different strategies to cope with organization demands, which affect their perceptions and care delivered to patients. The coping strategies are characterized using a modified version of Merton's (1957) adaptation model – conformist, innovator, and rebel.

Contribution to the field – *The study is the first to use the voice of home care social workers to explore how perceptions of organizational dominant goals and means affect direct service home care professionals' care delivery and meeting of patient needs. The study asserts the need for a home care-based policy model drawing on the Hospice Medicare Benefit (HMB) to address Alzheimer's disease more cost-effectively with a more positive quality of life manner, thus limiting the adverse consequences of the evolving epidemic.*

INTRODUCTION

In the United States, the $13 billion annual Medicare home health benefit is based on a medical model, providing limited medical and virtually no psychosocial care to this largely home- and community-based population. This chapter presents research using a convenience sample of 34 home care social workers in the New York City metropolitan area and an extensive literature review. The interviews were conducted from August 2006 to October 2007.

The chapter asserts that literature indicates a dissonance between effective, evidence-based research on psychosocial interventions and Medicare home health policy which does not cover their use. Further, interviews indicate home care social workers' different strategies to cope with organization demands affect their perceptions and care delivered to patients. The coping strategies which emerged are characterized using a modified version of Merton's (1957) adaptation model: *conformist, innovator, and rebel.* Merton hypothesized that individuals cope differently with societal expectations based on whether they accepted or rejected society's dominant goals (i.e., wealth accumulation) and means for obtaining success (i.e., education, work, and marriage). The conformist accepts both the dominant goals and means; the innovator accepts the goals, but creates alternative means; and the rebel rejects both the goals and means. I present interview results and evidence-based literature for the need for a home care-based policy model drawing on the HMB to address Alzheimer's disease more cost-effectively with a more positive quality of life manner, thus limiting the adverse consequences of the evolving epidemic.

ESTABLISHING CONTEXT: THE EVOLVING ALZHEIMER'S DISEASE EPIDEMIC

Alzheimer's disease is a major and increasing cause of illness and death in the United States, imposing significant social, economic, and psychological burdens on patients and their caregivers. Alzheimer's disease progresses with the aging process. Symptoms include a gradual and steady decline in being oriented, a decrease in memory and ability to participate in everyday activities, and personality changes. In the twentieth century, Alzheimer's disease became the most frequently identified type of dementia in the United States and Western society (Cohen, 1998; Whitehouse, 2001). Over 5 million Americans were estimated to have Alzheimer's disease in 2007, including 4.9 million over age 65 years and between 200,000 and 500,000 under age 65 years with early onset Alzheimer's disease and other dementias (Alzheimer's Association, 2007a, 2007b). The Alzheimer's Association (2006) estimates 4.5 million Americans, mostly over age 65 years old, had the disease in 2006 and 16 million are projected to have the disease by 2050.

Alzheimer's disease is the fourth leading cause of death for Americans aged 65 years and older exceeded only by cardiovascular disease, cerebro-vascular disease, and cancer. It is the third most costly disease in the United States with an estimated annual cost of $100 billion (Centers for Disease Control and Prevention, 2006; McConnell, 2004; Rice et al., 2001; Sadick & Wilcock, 2003). Worldwide, Alzheimer's disease is considered an epidemic by the World Health Organization (WHO), which estimates 18 million persons currently having the disease and a projected 34 million worldwide by 2025 (World Health Organization, 2008). Most of the increased worldwide spread of Alzheimer's is expected from worldwide aging in both developed countries which dominate the current statistics and developing countries, particularly in Southeast Asia (World Health Organization, 2008).

Alzheimer's disease is frustrating and burdensome because there is no known effective medical or pharmacological cure or treatment. Despite significant medical research on Alzheimer's disease (Albert, 2001; Santaguida et al., 2004; Stall & Firth, 2001), studies indicate no medical cure (Gauthier, 2002; Whitehouse, 2001) and little effective medical and pharmacological treatment (Dementia, 2003; Evans & Harris, 2004; Petersen, 2004; Santaguida et al., 2004). However, some significant research indicates that non-pharmacological interventions are effective at improving patient and caregiver symptom management and quality of life (Cohen-Mansfield, 2001; Mittelman, 2004; Rosack, 2006; Schulz et al., 2003; Small et al., 1997).

Managing the symptoms of Alzheimer's imposes significant patient and caregiver burdens. Alzheimer's disease patients display a combination of cognitive, behavioral, and functional symptoms. The symptoms vary by individual disease stage and over time (Small et al., 1997). Cognitive symptoms include memory impairment, speech and language comprehension problems, and impaired judgment. Behavioral symptoms may include personality changes, irritability, anxiety, depression, delusions, hallucinations, aggression, and wandering. Functional symptoms include difficulty with eating, dressing, bathing, getting to the toilet, walking, grooming, getting in/out of bed, meal preparation, shopping, moving within and outside the house, money management, and using the telephone or computer.

Caregiver burden also is a major issue for caregivers of persons with Alzheimer's disease and other chronic conditions, including multiple sclerosis, Parkinson's disease, diabetes, depression, and cardiovascular, heart, and respiratory diseases, among others (Dartmouth Atlas Project, 2006; Kennet, Burgio, & Schulz, 2000; Levine, 2000, 2003; Levine & Murray, 2004; O'Brien, 2004; Robert Wood Johnson Foundation, 1996, 2001). An estimated 70% of Alzheimer's patients live at home. Approximately 75% of this care is provided by family members and significant others, with the remainder provided by government or private care providers (McConnell & Riggs, 1999). Most caregivers report increased financial burden from supporting the household and paying out-of-pocket health care costs, estimated nationally at $15,000 and 18,000 a year. Caregivers' informal care reflects the dominance of personal and family responsibility in Alzheimer's care, as with much American health care. Employers, government, and private insurers provide limited coverage to assist patients and caregivers dealing with the burdens of home-based care (Fried, 2004; Levine, 2000, 2003; Levine & Murray, 2004; McConnell, 2004; McConnell & Riggs, 1999; MetLife Foundation, 2006; Morrow-Howell, Tang, Kim, Lee, & Sherraden, 2005; Society for Human Resource Management, 2003; Robert Wood Johnson Foundation, 1996, 2001).

Caregivers often experience increased stress, depression, substance abuse, loss of sleep, health and mental health problems, and increased personal isolation (National Alliance for Caregiving, 2004; Sadick & Wilcock, 2003).

Although caregiver burnout may necessitate the patient's placement in an institution, placement does not alleviate caregiver burden because of an ongoing sense of responsibility, loss, and guilt (McConnell & Riggs, 1999; Mittelman, Roth, Haley, & Zarit, 2004b; Schulz et al., 2004).

Non-pharmacological and social interventions have varying effectiveness in improving patient and caregiver quality of life and symptom management (Cohen-Mansfield, 2001; Schulz et al., 2003; Sloane et al., 2002). Social networks, support groups, counseling services, and environmental assessment, modification, and skills-building interventions generate the most evidence of positive outcomes, though there is some evidence of benefits from recreational therapies, respite care, and other therapies (Bennett, Schneider, Tang, Arnold, & Wilson, 2006; Cohen-Mansfield, 2001, 2004; Gitlin, Liebman, & Winter, 2003b; Gitlin et al., 2003a; Gitlin et al., 2003b; Mittelman, 2002, 2004; Mittelman et al., 1993, 1995; Schulz et al., 2003). Some research supports the assertion that psychosocial and non-pharmacological interventions may reduce costs of medically based home, community, or institutional care (Abt Associates, 1998; Brumley, Enguidanos, & Cherin, 2003; Chappell, Havens, Hollander, Miller, & McWilliam, 2004; Gage et al., 2000; Leon, Cheng, & Neumann, 1998; Newcomer, Miller, Clay, & Fox, 1999; Watt, Browne, Gafni, Roberts, & Byrne, 1999). These interventions will not be discussed in detail in this chapter. Their significance is that research indicates they are effective, yet they are not covered by Medicare home health policy.

ESTABLISHING CONTEXT: MEDICARE HOME HEALTH POLICY

Despite empirical support for the benefits of home- and community-based social services and an estimated 16% annual profit margin, the Medicare home health program does not cover such interventions (Fried, 2004; McConnell & Riggs, 1999; Medicare Payment Advisory Commission, 2006a, 2006b). The Medicare home health benefit is the government's primary home care benefit, covering nearly 3 million Medicare recipients annually (National Association for Home Care and Hospice, 2006; National Center for Health Statistics, 2006). Medicare currently spends $13 billion annually for home health care services (Kaiser Family Foundation, 2007; National Center for Health Statistics, 2006; Medicare Payment Advisory Commission, 2005).

Medicare home health is based on an acute care medical model, which requires eligible patients be: homebound; in need of skilled, part-time, or intermittent skilled nursing care or physical therapy; and suffering from a condition with a finite and definite end point, all as prescribed by a physician-certified plan of care (Health Care Financing Administration, 1999). If the requirements are met, the patient may receive additional skilled nursing, physical therapy, speech therapy, occupational therapy, home health aides, or social work services. Physical therapy and skilled nursing represent an estimated 72% of national home health visits (Medicare Payment Advisory Commission, 2003, 2004a). Social work historically represents only 1–2% of all national Medicare home health visits (Medicare Payment Advisory Commission, 2003, 2004a, 2004b). Consequently, many persons with Alzheimer's disease do not qualify for Medicare home health because they are not homebound, do not require skilled nursing or physical therapy, or their condition is viewed as chronic, without a finite and definite end point (*Duggan et al. v. Bowen*, 1988; Fried, 2004).

THE STUDY

This chapter emerged from a convenience sample of 34 home care social workers. The interviews occurred from August 2006 to October 2007 in the New York City metropolitan area. The study's goal was to explore factors influencing the decision-making process of home care social workers regarding Alzheimer's disease patients. The study paralleled an earlier pilot test of home care nurses (Cabin, 2007). Both studies were prompted by a literature review indicating a dissonance between the need for psychosocial care by Alzheimer's disease home care patients, statistically significant evidence of effective psychosocial interventions to improve patient and caregiver outcomes, and government home care policy which does not cover such interventions (Cabin, 2006a, 2006b). The study results may apply to other chronic conditions amenable to home care but also not currently covered by Medicare home health. Some examples are multiple sclerosis, Parkinson's disease, chronic diabetes, and persons with severe and persistent mental health conditions.

MERTON'S TYPOLOGY OF INDIVIDUAL ADAPTATION

In reviewing interview transcripts for common themes, it became apparent that Merton's five-mode typology of individual adaptation to cultural goals and institutional means might provide a useful analytic framework (1957). Merton's typology conceptually appeared applicable to individual coping strategies and organizational goals. Merton's first type was the conformist who accepted goals and their institutionalized means of achievement. Second was the innovator who accepted the goals, but devised different means of achievement. Third was the ritualist who scaled down or modified goals to increase likelihood of achievement while accepting the institutional means of achievement. Fourth was the retreatist who retreated virtually into their own world, creating different goals and means of achievement. Fifth was the rebel who viewed the goals as either totally or partially illegitimate and used a combination of existing institutional means and new means to achieve their goals.

Merton's typology enabled insight into how the social worker's perceptions of the legitimacy of their organization's goals and means of care affected the nature and extent to which they addressed patient and caregiver needs. Three modes of adaptation emerged among the 34 social workers. One was *the conformist*, who adhered almost mechanically and rigidly to the organization's policy and procedures, regardless of perceived patient need. At the other extreme was *the rebel* who modified or replaced organizational requirements with their personal and professional care standards when they believed the organizational goals frustrated fulfillment of patient need. In the middle was *the innovator* who adhered to corporate policy and procedure, but tried to create flexibility to meet more patient needs than would be met under the conformist's strict interpretation. Most of the social workers fit one dominant type, though some expressed views which ranged between *conformist* and *innovator* or *innovator* and *rebel*. However, overall most (19) were *conformists*, some (13) were *innovators*, and few (2) were *rebels*. Regardless of their dominant coping strategy, all the social workers expressed frustration and discussed significant unmet patient needs.

THE CONFORMIST

The conformist is the ultimate organization person, taking the agency's corporate care guidelines as gospel, regardless of patient need. Corporate guidelines typically focus around on the *Medicare Home Health Agency Manual* coverage guidelines (Health Care Financing Administration, 1999) and Medicare home health prospective payment system (PPS) which was implemented nationally on October 1, 2000. PPS is a managed care model which bases individual patient care on assessed categories of care.

Medicare pays a flat rate for each category, thus allowing the home health agencies to make profit if they keep their volume of care and costs below the payment rate. Thus, PPS creates a profit motive which may influence the nature and extent of patient care, regardless of patient need.

More specifically, PPS intensified the link between fiscal requirements, practice, and care delivery by linking reimbursement to a mandatory national home health assessment instrument. The 70-item instrument is the Outcome and Assessment Information Set (OASIS), which is used for reimbursement and outcome measures (Medicare Payment Advisory Commission, 2003, 2004a). An OASIS form is used for each patient's initial admission to a 60-day care episode, renewal for subsequent 60-day episode, transfer, and discharge. Twenty-three of the OASIS items are used to score the patient into 1 of the 153 Home Health Resource Groups (HHRGs), which are the basis for agency reimbursement during the 60-day period.

With the advent of OASIS and PPS, home health agencies are allowed to operate on a risk basis, keeping Medicare revenues exceeding cost while absorbing losses. As a result, there has been increased focus on limiting visits per episode to ensure costs are less than the HHRG payment (Medicare Payment Advisory Commission, 2003, 2004a, 2005). The decision on the nature and extent of care is made by a nurse who prepares a plan of care, subject to physician certification. The extent of social work involvement is determined by the nurse.

I just do what I'm told. It's no different than ever. Social work is not viewed as important. It's all about the wound, or the hip, the diabetes, the urinary problem. It's about medical issues. The people part is irrelevant. So, if I get a referral, I just do what little I can and block out the patient's needs. (Social worker AC)

Home care is not a long-term benefit. It's not for chronic patients. It doesn't matter that most of our patients are chronic. That's the way it is. The nurses and [physical] therapists treat the medical problems and I do a social work visit, if they ask me to. That's the playbook and there's no point in deviating. (Social worker SL)

I wish there was more I could do, but I can't. I feel it would be illegal. There are so many unmet needs, even with patients who have a lot of support at home. They [the patients and caregivers] really could benefit from more support. I just don't understand why Medicare won't pay for [individual and family] counseling, support groups, more social work, and other therapies, like art and music therapy. I think this would help many patients and allow some caregivers to care for longer periods with less stress. It would save money for everyone, but it's not allowed. I think of it as my fantasy world, but I can't let intrude on reality. I just make the visits the nurse includes in the care plan. That's it. (Social worker GA)

THE INNOVATOR

Despite the focus on acute care and PPS, there are some social workers who attempt to find flexibility in the corporate guidelines.

There's always room for more than meets the eye. You have to be a bit assertive with the nurses, but not too pushy. I talk to them informally and usually always they'll refer me an assessment visit. Some even let me come on their initial assessment. I find I can identify and communicate the patient needs better with the nurses. I usually get more social work visits from them, which is the whole point. If I do not get in early and politely to the nurses, then the patients get less. (Social worker LS)

It's simple. If you really read and know the regulations you know there is a lot of gray area. Some people just won't take the time. I do. It helps me advocate for the patient. They all have social work needs. The nurses know I know the regs so they trust me. Other social workers don't, so their patients get less. It's not because their patients do not have needs. It is because they take the easy way out. They do not take the time to become knowledgeable and advocate for their patients. I try talking about it in our [social work] supervisory meetings and in [interdisciplinary] team meetings, but we can't Those meetings are all business – quick case reviews and back to the field to do visits. It's more productive to approach the nurses one-on-one. (Social worker RG)

I know our [home health] patients would be better off if they had home modifications. Most have some level of dementia and mobility problems. So I convinced the quality assurance person to let me give an in-service on the value of a home environmental assessment by a nurse, PT [physical therapist], or social worker. I used material from another agency. It went over really well. The QA [quality assurance] person liked it so much she did a three-month pilot of a mandatory home environmental assessment protocol. She used social workers because she felt we could learn it and we cost less [than nurses and PTs]. She found it reduced the number and severity of falls which reduced our per Episode cost and length of stay. I wish they'd use us [social workers] more. (Social worker EH)

THE REBEL

Social work has a long history of advocating for social justice (Mullaly, 1997; Reisch & Andrews, 2002). There are some home care social workers who heed the call.

I became a social worker to help people. I never expect the system to be fair. If it was fair, there'd be no need for social workers. I go to work every day ready to fight for my client. I constantly meet and call nurses and therapists. I push them for social work referrals. Once I get them I do what is needed. I don't care if they ordered only two visits. If I feel four or five or more are necessary, then I do it and explain after. The nurses usually don't have a problem. They know there's more need for social work. (Social worker CA)

I think [Saul] Alinsky [the famous Chicago-born community organizer] when I do home care. The end justifies the means. I am here to help people so I find a way to do it. I get at least two-to-three times as many social work visits for my patients than others, even now with PPS. And my patients are no different than most. I just think I'm not as intimidated. It's not that other social workers don't care. They do, but they are worried about the rules, keeping their job, their evals, you now. I don't. I can always do social work somewhere. I shadow the nurses and [physical] therapists. I get them to let me do a lot of co-visits. They don't need to put that in the care plan so I get to give more visits and they don't get in trouble for violating rules or visit volume requirements. And I do free visits. I just go out on my own after regular hours and do visits. (Social worker BI)

Sometimes I wonder about politicians. Maybe they need to have a loved one with a chronic condition, or themselves, who wants to stay home. They think they'd get all this supportive care with counseling, resource management, family planning and support groups. That's hospice; not home care. Most times I stick to the plan. Every so often I just get fed up. It happened last week. Here is this poor dual eligible [a patient covered by Medicare and Medicaid] who with dementia who constantly gets discharged and readmitted. He's always falling. They [the nurse managing the case] would not make a social work referral. The home was not adapted in any way to the patient's mobility limitations. I identified what had to be done, talked to the family, and had my husband, who's in construction, do it [the modifications] for free. (Social worker KF)

LOOKING TO HOSPICE FOR GUIDANCE

The Medicare Hospice Benefit provides a stark contrast to Medicare home health. It was designed to deal with the Medicare problem of high cost institutionalized, low quality of life end-of-life care. The contrast can be viewed from the Merton typology. The development of Medicare hospice created a different set of appropriate goals and means for social workers, as well as nurses, physical, speech, and occupational therapists, volunteers, and spiritual care providers. Home care's goal is limited treatment for acute physical problems achieved by means of limited nursing, home health aide, social work, and physical, speech, and occupational therapy visits to address only patient (not caregiver) physical health problems. In contrast, hospice's goal is to replace treatment with a goal of maintaining and improving quality of life for patients with chronic conditions and their caregivers. The means to achieve the hospice goal is a focus on pain management and psychosocial care. As a result, hospice involves significant greater use of social work, mandated use of volunteers and spiritual care providers, and use of other therapies (i.e., reminiscence, music, art, and pet) as a means to maintain, if not improve, patient and caregiver quality of life.

In contrast to the home health medical model, the Medicare Hospice Benefit provides primarily home-based end-of-life care based on the *palliative care treatment model*, demonstrating cost reduction and improvements in patient and caregiver symptom management. Palliative care assumes that treatment is not curative and focuses treatment on patient, caregiver, and family psychosocial and spiritual needs, symptom management, and quality of life (World Health Organization, 2004; Forbes, 2002; National Hospice and Palliative Care Organization, 2004a).

The HMB was legislated in 1982. Patients must have an initial and ongoing physician-certified prognosis of six months or less to live and care is managed through a physician-led interdisciplinary team. Hospice patients relinquish all other Medicare coverage and the pursuit of curative, medical care. Hospice care includes physician involvement and direct medical care by nurses and physicians within the context of palliative care. Medicare-required services include respite care, pastoral care, and volunteer services as well as the six Medicare home health services, though art, music, massage, aroma, pet, and a variety of other palliative care therapies often are provided (Center for Medicare Education, 2001).

The Centers for Medicare and Medicaid Services (2006), unlike for home care, also has a specific set of national guidelines recognizing at least one major chronic disease category, Alzheimer's disease and related disorders, as a basis for HMB-covered terminal care. As a result, Alzheimer's disease and related disorders is the second highest non-cancer primary diagnosis for the HMB, representing 8.3% of all HMB primary diagnoses in 2002 (National Hospice and Palliative Care Organization, 2003b).

The HMB was based on results from a 28-site demonstration project indicating simultaneous improvement of patient and caregiver symptom management and quality of life and reduced Medicare end-of-life care expenditures (Gage et al., 2000; Mor & Kidder, 1985). The benefit uses a managed care, risk-sharing model focusing on simultaneous cost reduction while improving quality of life (Luft & Greenlick, 1996). Studies indicate that the HMB significantly reduces government expenditures (National Hospice and Palliative Care Organization, 2003a, 2003b; Pyenson, Connor, Fitch, & Kinzbrunner, 2004) and improves quality of life (National Hospice and Palliative Care Organization, 2004b, 2004c). There also is evidence that enhanced home-based hospice programs may save private insurers costs and improve patient and caregiver outcomes (Brumley et al., 2003; Brumley & Hillary, 2002; Gage et al., 2000).

MAKING PSYCHOSOCIAL CARE A CORE
ELEMENT OF HOME HEALTH CARE

The success of the HMB indicates that a different goal and means in policy can positively impact the decisions of social workers, and other providers, about the nature and extent of care for patients and their caregivers. The result is a focus on meeting patient and caregiver needs.

The Medicare hospice benefit presents prima facie evidence that making palliative care a core element can improve both patient and caregiver quality of life and reduce costs to patients, families, and the government, particularly for persons with Alzheimer's disease. There also are statistically significant research findings of psychosocial interventions which provide evidence of improved quality of life, and some evidence of cost savings, for community-dwelling elderly and their caregivers. The tested interventions include family and individual counseling (Mittelman, 2004; Mittelman, Epstein, & Pierzchala, 2003; Mittelman et al., 2004a; Mittelman et al., 2004b), support groups (Bennett et al., 2006; Kennet et al., 2000), and home-based environment assessments and skills-building programs for caregivers and patients (Gitlin, 2003; Gitlin et al., 2006).

Despite such evidence, neither the government nor private foundations have sponsored studies testing a palliative care-based Medicare home health component for persons with Alzheimer's disease and their caregivers. Pilot studies might use randomized controlled trials or other designs to test the quality of life and cost outcomes of specific new services. These might include support groups and individual and family counseling, using existing evidence-based protocols. Similar studies could be conducted using social work and occupational therapy-based environmental assessment, home modification, and environmental skills-building programs. Another option might be testing one or more new benefit design(s) for persons at high risk or falls or other high-risk characteristics associated with Alzheimer's disease.

Such a care model will not decrease the Alzheimer's disease epidemic; that remains a task of medical research. However, a home health palliative care component in addition to traditional acute medical care appears effective in reducing the physical, mental, and financial burdens of the disease while improving quality of life.

REFERENCES

Abt Associates, Inc. (1998). Evaluation of the program of all-inclusive care for the elderly (PACE) demonstration: The impact of PACE on participant outcomes, Final Report,

July. Retrieved on June 28, 2004, from http://www.cms.hhs.gov/researchers/demos/PACE.asp

Albert, S. M. (2001). Alzheimer's disease: Clinical. In: G. L. Maddox (Editor-in-Chief), *The Encyclopedia of aging: A comprehensive resource in gerontology and geriatrics.* (3rd ed., pp. 62–63). New York: Springer Publishing Company.

Alzheimer's Association. (2006). Fact sheet: Medicare home health benefit for caregiver training in 16 states. Retrieved on July 14, 2006, from http://www.alz.org

Alzheimer's Association. (2007a). Alzheimer's disease prevalence rates rise to more than five million in the United States. Retrieved on March 20, 2007, from http://www.alz.org/news_and_events_rates_rise_asp

Alzheimer's Association. (2007b). Alzheimer's disease facts and figures, 2007. Retrieved on March 20, 2007, from: http://www.alz.org

Bennett, D. A., Schneider, J. A., Tang, Y., Arnold, S. E., & Wilson, R. W. (2006). *The effect of social networks on the relation between Alzheimer's disease pathology and level of cognitive function in old people: A longitudinal cohort study.* Retrieved on June 27, 2006 from http://neurology.thelancet.com

Brumley, R. D., Enguidanos, S., & Cherin, D. A. (2003). Effectiveness of a home-based palliative care program for end-of-life. *Journal of Palliative Medicine, 6*(5), 714–715.

Brumley, R. D., & Hillary, K. (2002). *The TriCentral palliative care program toolkit.* San Francisco, CA: Kaiser Permanente.

Cabin, W. D. (2006a). *The phantoms of home care: Home care nurses' care decisions for Medicare home health Alzheimer's disease patients.* Unpublished paper, July 14, 2006. Hunter College School of Social Welfare, New York.

Cabin, W. D. (2006b). *Medicare fiscal requirements' impact on home care nurse care decisions for Alzheimer's disease patients.* Unpublished paper, May 27, 2006. Hunter College School of Social Welfare, New York.

Cabin, W. D. (2007). The phantoms of home care: Home care nurses' care decisions for Medicare home health Alzheimer's disease patients. *Home Health Care Management & Practice, 19*(3), 174–183.

Center for Medicare Education. (2001). *The Medicare hospice benefit* (Vol. 2, No. 9). Issue Brief. Washington, DC: Center for Medicare Education.

Centers for Disease Control and Prevention. (2006). Deaths: Final data for 2003. *National Vital Statistics Report, 54*(13), 1–2.

Centers for Medicare and Medicaid Services. (2006). *LCD for hospice Alzheimer's disease & related disorders (L16343).* Retrieved on July 15, 2006 from http://www.cms.hhs.gov/mcd.viewlcd.asp?lcd_id = 16343&lcd_version = 13&basket = lcd%3

Chappell, N., Havens, B., Hollander, M., Miller, J., & McWilliam, C. (2004). Comparative costs of home care and residential care. *The Gerontologist, 44*(3), 389–400.

Cohen, L. (1998). *No aging in India: Alzheimer's, the bad family, and other modern things.* Berkeley, CA: University of California Press.

Cohen-Mansfield, J. (2001). Nonpharmacologic interventions for inappropriate behaviors in dementia. *American Journal of Geriatric Psychiatry, 9*(4), 361–381.

Cohen-Mansfield, J. (2004). Advances in Alzheimer's disease research: Implications for family caregiving. Retrieved on December 16, 2004, from http://rci.gsw.edu/expanel_alz.htm

Dartmouth Atlas Project. (2006). *The care of patients with severe chronic illness: A report on the Medicare program by the Dartmouth Atlas Project.* Retrieved on July 25, 2006 from www.dartmouthatlas.org

Dementia. Retrieved on October 9, 2003, from http://www.geriatricsatyourfingertips.org

Evans, T., & Harris, J. (2004). Street-level bureaucracy, social work, and the (exaggerated) death of discretion. *British Journal of Social Work, 34*(6), 871–895.

Forbes, S. A. (2002). Palliative care. In: D. J. Ekerdt (Editor-in-Chief), *Encyclopedia of aging* (Vol. 3, pp. 1036–1038). New York: Macmillan.

Fried, L. (2004). *Medicare for people with Alzheimer's disease* (Issue brief, vol. 5, No. 8). Washington, DC: Center for Medicare Education.

Gage, B., Miller, S., Coppola, K., Harvell, J., Laliberte, L., Mor, V., & Teno, J. (2000, March). *Important questions for hospice in the next century*. Retrieved on June 28, 2004 from http://aspe.hhs.gov/daltcp/reports/impques.htm

Gauthier, S. (2002). Alzheimer's disease. In: D. J. Ekerdt (Editor-in-Chief), *Encyclopedia of aging* (Vol. 1, pp. 52–56). New York: Macmillan.

Gitlin, L. (2003). Conducting research on home environments: Lessons learned and new directions. *The Gerontologist, 43*(5), 628–637.

Gitlin, L., Burgio, L., Mahoney, D., Burns, R., Zhang, S., Schulz, R., Belle, S., Czaja, S., Gallagher-Thompson, D., Hauk, W., & Ory, M. (2003a). Effect of multicomponent interventions on caregiver burden and depression: The REACH multisite initiative at six-month follow-up. *Psychology and Aging, 18*(3), 361–374.

Gitlin, L., Liebman, J., & Winter, L. (2003b). Are environmental interventions effective in the management of Alzheimer's disease and related disorders? A synthesis of the evidence. *Alzheimer's Care Quarterly, 4*(2), 85–107.

Gitlin, L. N., Winter, L., Dennis, M. P., Corcoran, M., Schinfeld, S., & Hauck, W. W. (2006). A randomized trial of a multicomponent home intervention to reduce f unctional difficulties in older adults. *Journal of the American Geriatrics Society, 54*(5), 809–816.

Health Care Financing Administration. (1999). *Medicare home health agency manual* (HCFA Publication No. 11). Washington, DC: US Government Printing Office.

Kaiser Family Foundation. (2007). *Medicaid home health participants, 1999–2003*. Retrieved on May 25, 2007 from http://www.statehealthfacts.org.

Kennet, J., Burgio, L., & Schulz, R. (2000). Interventions for in-home caregivers: A review of research 1990 to present. In: R. Schulz (Ed.), *Handbook on dementia caregiving: Evidence-based interventions for family caregivers* (pp. 61–125). New York: Springer Publishing Company.

Leon, J., Cheng, C.-K., & Neumann, P. J. (1998). Alzheimer's disease care: Costs and potential savings. *Health Affairs, 17*(6), 206–216.

Levine, C. (2000). The many worlds of family caregivers. In: C. Levine (Ed.), *Always on call: When illness turns families into caregivers* (pp. 1–17). New York: United Hospital Fund of New York.

Levine, C. (2003). *Making room for family caregivers: Seven innovative hospitals programs*. New York: United Hospital Fund.

Levine, C., & Murray, T. (Eds). (2004). *The cultures of caregiving: Conflict and common ground among families, health professionals, and policy makers*. Baltimore: Johns Hopkins University Press.

Luft, H. S., & Greenlick, M. S. (1996). The contribution of group-and-staff HMOs to American medicine. *The Milbank Quarterly, 74*, 445–467.

McConnell, S. (2004). Testimony of Stephen McConnell to the U. S. Senate Committee on Aging, April 27. Retrieved on December 5, 2004, from http://www.alz.org/advocacy/ wherewestand/200400427sm.asp

McConnell, S., & Riggs, J. (1999). The policy challenges of Alzheimer's disease. *Generations,* 23(3), 69–74.

Medicare Payment Advisory Commission. (2003). *Report to the Congress: Medicare payment policy.* Medicare Payment Advisory Commission, Washington, DC.

Medicare Payment Advisory Commission. (2004a). *Report to the Congress: Medicare payment policy.* Medicare Payment Advisory Commission, Washington, DC.

Medicare Payment Advisory Commission. (2004b). *Home health services payment system,* July 13, 2004. Medicare Payment Advisory Commission, Washington, DC.

Medicare Payment Advisory Commission. (2005). *The home health payment system: Presentation to Senate Committee on Finance staff.* March 28, 2003 by Sharon Bee Cheng. Retrieved on December 5, 2005 from http://www.medpac.gov

Medicare Payment Advisory Commission. (2006a). Report to Congress: Increasing the value of Medicare, June. Washington, DC: Medicare Payment Advisory Commission.

Medicare Payment Advisory Commission. (2006b). A data book: Healthcare spending and the Medicare program, June. Washington, DC: Medicare Payment Advisory Commission.

Merton, R. A. (1957). *Social theory and social structure* (Revised ed.). Glencoe, IL: The Free Press.

Metlife Mature Market Institute/National Alliance for Caregiving. (2006). *The MetLife caregiving cost study: Productivity losses to US business.* Westport, CT: The MetLife Mature Market Institute.

Mittelman, M. (2002). Family caregiving for people with Alzheimer's disease: Results of the NYU spouse-caregiver intervention study. *Generations,* 26(1), 104–106.

Mittelman, M. (2004). *The feeling of family caregivers: Dealing with emotional challenges of caring for an individual with Alzheimer's disease.* Retrieved on December 16, 2004 from http://rci.gsw.edu/expalzppt.htm

Mittelman, M., Epstein, C., & Pierzchala, A. (2003). *Counseling the Alzheimer's caregiver: A resource for health care professionals.* Chicago: American Medical Association Press.

Mittelman, M., Ferris, S., Shulman, E., Steinberg, G., Ambinder, A., Mackell, J., & Cohen, J. (1995). A comprehensive support program: Effect on depression in spouse-caregivers of AD patients. *The Gerontologist,* 35(6), 792–802.

Mittelman, M., Ferris, S., Steinberg, G., Shulman, E. M., Ambinder, A., & Cohen, J. (1993). An intervention that delays institutionalization of Alzheimer's disease patients: Treatment of spouse-caregivers. *The Gerontologist,* 33(6), 730–740.

Mittelman, M. S., Roth, D. L., Coon, D. W., Haley, W. E., Zarit, S. H., & Clay, O. J. (2004a). New research: Sustained benefit of supportive intervention for depression symptoms in caregivers of patients with Alzheimer's disease. *American Journal of Psychiatry,* 161(5), 850–857.

Mittelman, M. S., Roth, D. L., Haley, W. E., & Zarit, S. H. (2004b). Effects of a caregiver intervention on negative caregiver approaches to behavior problems in patients with Alzheimer's disease: Results of a randomized trial. *Journals of Gerontology, Series B: Psychological Sciences & Social Sciences,* 59(1), 27.

Mor, V., & Kidder, D. (1985). Cost savings in hospice: Final results of the national hospice study. *Health Services Research,* 20(4), 407–421.

Morrow-Howell, N., Tang, F., Kim, J., Lee, M., & Sherraden, M. (2005). Maximizing the productive engagement of older adults. In: M. L. Wykle, P. J. Whitehouse & D. L. Morris (Eds), *Successful aging through the lifespan: Intergenerational issues in health* (pp. 19–54). New York: Springer Publishing Company.

Mullaly, B. (1997). *Structural social work: Ideology, theory, and practice* (2nd ed.). Don Mills, Ontario: Oxford University Press.

National Alliance for Caregiving. (2004, April 6). *Caregiving in the US*. Retrieved on April 9, 2004 from http://www.caregiving.org/4-6-04release.htm

National Association for Home Care and Hospice. (2006). Basic statistics about home care, updated 2004. Retrieved on December 5, 2006, from: http://www.nahc.org

National Center for Health Statistics. (2006). *Health, United States, 2006*. Hyattsville, MD: US Government Printing Office.

National Hospice and Palliative Care Organization. (2003a). *NHPCO facts and figures (update July 2003)*. Alexandria, VA: National Hospice and Palliative Care Organization.

National Hospice and Palliative Care Organization. (2003b). *2002 NHPCO national data set summary report*. National Hospice and Palliative Care Organization, Alexandria, VA.

National Hospice and Palliative Care Organization. (2004a). *What is hospice and palliative care?* Retrieved on January 2, 2005 from http://www.nhpco.org/i4a/pages/index.cfm?pageid = 3281

National Hospice and Palliative Care Organization. (2004b). *JAMA publishes study examining end-of-life care in US; highest levels of satisfaction provided by hospice care at home (1/06/04)*. Communications alert, January 6, 2004. Retrieved on January 6, 2005 from http://www.nhpco.org/i4a/pages/Index.cfm?pageid = 4178

National Hospice and Palliative Care Organization. (2004c). *Hospice costs Medicare less and patients often live longer new research shows*, September 21, 2004. Retrieved on January 6, 2005 from http://www.nhpco.org/i4a/pages/Index.cfm?pageid = 4343

Newcomer, R., Miller, R., Clay, T., & Fox, P. (1999). Effects of the Medicare Alzheimer's disease demonstration on Medicare expenditures. *Health Care Financing Review, 20*(4), 45–65.

O'Brien, R. L. (2004). Darkness cometh: Personal, social, and economic burdens of Alzheimer's disease. In: R. B. Purtilo & H. A. M. J. ten Have (Eds), *Ethical foundations of palliative care for Alzheimer's disease* (pp. 8–23). Baltimore: Johns Hopkins University Press.

Petersen, A. (2004). Alzheimer's drugs may deserve more time, September 7. Retrieved on September 8, 2004, from http://online.wsj.com/article_print/0,,SB109450918449710610,00.html

Pyenson, B., Connor, S., Fitch, K., & Kinzbrunner, B. (2004). Medicare cost in matched hospice and non-hospice cohorts. *Journal of Pain and Symptom Management, 28*(3), 200–210.

Reisch, M., & Andrews, J. (2002). *The road not taken: A history of radical social work in the United States*. New York: Brunner-Routledge.

Rice, D. P., Fillit, H. M., Max, W., Knopman, W. S., Lloyd, J. R., & Duttagupta, S. (2001). Prevalence, costs, and treatment of Alzheimer's disease and related dementia: A managed care perspective. *American Journal of Managed Care, 7*, 809–818.

Robert Wood Johnson Foundation. (1996). *Chronic care in America: A 21st century challenge*. Retrieved on July 25, 2006 from http://www.rwjf.org/library/chrcare/

Robert Wood Johnson Foundation. (2001). *A portrait of informal caregivers in America 2001*. Princeton, NJ: Robert Wood Johnson Foundation.

Rosack, J. (2006). Geriatric psychiatrists issue Alzheimer's care principles. *Psychiatric News, 41*(15), 6.

Sadick, K., & Wilcock, G. (2003). The increasing burden of Alzheimer disease. *Alzheimer's disease and Associated Disorders, 17*(Suppl. 3), S75–S79.

Santaguida, P. S., Raina, P., Booker, L., Patterson, C., Baldassarre, F., Cowan, D., et al. (2004). Pharmacological treatment of dementia: A summary. Evidence Report/ Technology Assessment No. 97, April. Washington, DC: Agency for Healthcare Research and Quality.

Schulz, R., Belle, S., Czaja, S., McGinnis, K., Stevens, A., & Zhang, S. (2004). Long- term care placement of Dementia patients and caregiver health and well-being. *JAMA, 292*(8), 961–967.

Schulz, R., Burgio, L., Burns, R., Eisdorfer, C., Gallagher-Thompson, D., Gitlin, L., & Mahoney, D. (2003). Resources for enhancing Alzheimer's Caregiver Health (REACH): Overview, site-specific outcomes, and future directions. *The Gerontologist, 43*(4), 514–520.

Sloane, P. D., Zimmerman, S., Suchindran, C., Reed, P., Wang, L., Boustani, M., et al. (2002). The public health impact of Alzheimer's disease, 2000–2050: Potential implication of treatment advances. *Annual Review of Public Health, 23*, 213–231.

Small, G. W., Rabins, P. V., Barry, P. P., Buckholtz, N. S., DeKosky, S. T., Ferris, S. H., et al. (1997). Diagnosis and treatment of Alzheimer's disease and related disorders. Consensus statement of the American Association for Geriatric Psychiatry, the Alzheimer's Association, and the American Geriatrics Society. *JAMA, 278*, 1363–1371.

Society for Human Resource Management. (2003). *HR professionals see more employees struggle with elder care*. Retrieved on December 15, 2003, from http://www.shrm.org/ press/CMS_006639.asp

Stall, S. M., & Firth, K. M. (2001). The National Institute of Aging/National Institutes of Health. In: D. J. Ekerdt (Editor-in-Chief). *Encyclopedia of aging* (Vol. 2, pp. 974–977). New York: Macmillan.

Watt, S., Browne, G., Gafni, A., Roberts, J., & Byrne, C. (1999). Community care for people with chronic conditions: An analysis of nine studies of health and social service utilization in Ontario. *The Milbank Quarterly, 77*(3), 363–392.

Whitehouse, P. J. (2001). The end of Alzheimer's disease. *Alzheimer's Disease and Associated Disorders, 15*(2), 59–62.

World Health Organization. (2004). *Cancer, palliative care*. Retrieved on November 10, 2004 from http://www.who.int/cancer/palliative/en/

World Health Organization. (2008). *Mental health and substance abuse, facts and figures, Alzheimer's disease: The brain killer*. Retrieved on November 18, 2008 from http:// www.searo.who.int/en/Section1174/Section1199/Section1567/Section1823_8066.h

'PROMOTED BY HONG TAO, THE *CHLAMYDIA* HYPOTHESIS HAD BECOME WELL ESTABLISHED ...': UNDERSTANDING THE 2003 SEVERE ACUTE RESPIRATORY SYNDROME (SARS) EPIDEMIC – BUT WHICH ONE?

Frederick Attenborough

ABSTRACT

Purpose – *The aims of this chapter are twofold – first, to develop an understanding of the ways in which primary historical data come to be transformed across generations of popular science histories of emerging epidemics; and second, to develop an understanding of the ways in which those transformations impact on our ability to know what really happened during those epidemics.*

Approach – *The chapter begins with a rhetorical analysis of one particularly influential account of the 2003 severe acute respiratory syndrome (SARS) outbreak. Therein, we learn that the race to discover the outbreak's aetiology was tainted by scientific malpractice; that an*

Understanding Emerging Epidemics: Social and Political Approaches
Advances in Medical Sociology, Volume 11, 183–201
ISSN: 1057-6290/doi:10.1108/S1057-6290(2010)0000011014

esteemed Chinese microbiologist, Dr. Hong, apparently promoted his own, patently false, aetiological discovery, stifled debate on the matter and, in doing so, held the international response to the outbreak back by a number of weeks. But how was this account rhetorically constructed? And how did it engage with Dr. Hong's own research work?

Findings – *Does Hong deserve to be remembered as an inept scientist? Subsequent accounts have been quick to repeat this one, founding text's account, suggesting that 'yes, he does'. This chapter, however, returns to the primary data, examines the ways in which the original account troped those data and moves to suggest that 'no, he does not'.*

Contributions to the field – *Teasing out the more general implications of this particular case study, the chapter concludes with a discussion of the analytical gains that might accrue if other popular scientific histories of emerging epidemics were approached as 'topics' rather than 'resources'.*

INTRODUCTION

How do popular science writers construct their accounts of past emerging epidemics? How do they engage with and interpret their primary data: press conference transcripts, interviews, research articles and so on? Does the imperative of their genre – the telling of an engaging, dramatic story – lead them to foreground certain data and certain *interpretations* of those data at the expense of other data and other interpretations? And what happens after the first such account has been published? How do subsequent accounts relate to that one, founding text? Do they too engage with and interpret the primary data? Or do they simply accept the founding text as a final, definitive account of what *really* happened? These are the questions I want to try and explore in this chapter. In the process, my aims will be twofold: first, to develop an understanding of the ways in which primary historical data come to be transformed across generations of popular science histories of emerging epidemics; and second, to develop an understanding of the ways in which those transformations impact on our ability to know what really happened during those epidemics.

Whilst pursuing those aims, however, I will also be hoping to do something with a little more critical intent. Put simply, I will be looking for *justice*. The object of my care and attention will be a character that appears in many accounts of the 2003 severe acute respiratory syndrome (SARS) outbreak. A character by the name of Dr. Hong Tao. According to those accounts, Dr. Hong was the Chinese microbiologist who sought, but failed (and failed *spectacularly*), to discover the aetiological agent responsible for causing the outbreak. But he did not just fail. For it seems that he also acted to 'promote' his discovery in such a way that other microbiologists in China were subsequently unable to put forward what was, ultimately, the correct aetiological claim. His failure, and his inability to accept his failure, it seems, managed to hold the international response to the outbreak back by a good number of weeks. Reading of his actions during early 2003, it is difficult not to understand Dr. Hong as one of the SARS outbreak's great scientific losers. But does he deserve this reputation? I want to suggest not. In fact, I want to *defend* him. And here, the legal metaphor seems apt. Given the overall aims of this chapter, it seems only fair that it should come to act as something akin to a 'scientific court of appeal'. Whilst seeking to understand how accounts of past epidemics relate to their primary data, we can safely leave our heroes – the Robert Kochs and the Louis Pasteurs of this world – to bask in their own accumulated glory. After all, they would have no interest in such a project. But our scientific losers? Well they would, to a man (and sometimes to a woman), be clamouring for a re-trial. And the very least a sociologist like myself can do is to take up the case of a character like Dr. Hong, asking whether or not he deserves his sentence of a life-long stretch lurking around amongst the discarded refuse in science's back yard.[1]

The case for the defence will be built around a close rhetorical examination of just one particular account of Hong's actions: 'China's missed chance' (CMC). CMC was a 'news focus special report' that appeared in the 18 July 2003 edition of the prestigious journal *Science*. Written by the highly respected science journalist Martin Enserink, it was the first article to tell of the outbreak during the 'post-outbreak' period. The interesting thing about CMC is that in order to understand Hong's SARS laboratory work, in order to incorporate Hong into its overall narrative, it relies on just one piece of material evidence: a research article entitled '*Chlamydia*-like particles and coronavirus-like agents found in dead cases of atypical pneumonia by electron microscopy' (CLA). Written by Dr. Hong and his research colleagues, it was published in the 25 April edition of the *National Medical Journal of China*. That CMC is dependent on CLA in this way generates an interesting analytical opportunity, and one that I seek to take advantage of. It arises because I too have access to CLA.[2] And in the first section of this chapter, CMC's cross-examination commences with a discussion of the ways in which my own understanding of Hong's laboratory work differs from Enserink's. Reading of Hong's actions in CMC it is difficult not to conjure the image of an inept scientist. Yet my own reading leads me to suggest that Hong could, quite plausibly, have been represented in a far more favourable light. In section two, a great deal of attention is given over to understanding how CMC's rhetorical structuring actually enabled Hong's original conviction. Then, in a bid to strengthen the appeal case a little further, the third section explores the ways in which *subsequent accounts* of the SARS outbreak came to relate to, engage with and appropriate CMC. In doing so, two things become clear: first, that CMC was rapidly turned into a 'definitive historical account' of Hong's actions, whilst Hong's *own* account of his *own* actions was completely ignored; and second, that CMC's account was, on a number of occasions, actually *embellished*, with some authors adding their own twists to the tale, accentuating Hong's errors and personal failings to such an extent that CMC begins to appear as if the very model of restraint and fairness. A brief concluding section, the fourth section , looks up from this localised case in order to ask whether these processes might not actually be more general phenomena, inf(l)ecting other (seemingly) factual and (seemingly) unquestionable accounts of past emerging epidemics.

CHINA'S MISSED CHANCE

CMC tells of a race that developed between three scientific research groups during the early weeks of the outbreak. The prize sought by each was the discovery of 'the cause of the new disease' (2003, p. 294). The scientific research groups in question were: a World Health Organisation (WHO) laboratory network led by Dr. Klaus Stöhr, a research team working out of the Academy of Military Sciences (AMMS) in Beijing and led by Dr. Yang Ruifu and, finally, Dr. Hong's research team at the Chinese Centre for Disease Control (CCDC), also in Beijing.

According to Enserink, the group that *really* won this race was the AMMS, led by Dr. Ruifu. 'By the first week of March', he suggests, 'the group had tentative evidence that *a new virus* might indeed be linked to the epidemic' (2003, p. 294). Having 'grow[n] a virus of some sort from the samples in so-called vero cells', 'they [had] observed what looked like coronavirus particles in an electron micrograph'. The team 'also discovered that serum from SARS patients could inhibit the growth of the virus – a key test to show a correlation between an isolated agent and a disease' (2003, p. 295). As Enserink makes clear, having achieved all of this they were 'weeks ahead' of the researchers in the WHO laboratory network (*ibid.*). And yet the AMMS were, nevertheless, to be denied the prize of a 'prominent place in the history of the disease, and perhaps even a publication or two in a prestigious scientific journal' by that very same group (2003, p. 294). For on 16 April, some five weeks after the AMMS had reached the same conclusion, it was the WHO research team that were to receive all the plaudits, announcing at a press conference in front of the world's media that the causal agent was a hitherto unknown coronavirus. 'Looking back' at this episode, Stöhr is quoted as suggesting that 'had the AMMS researchers reported their findings immediately, the larger group [the WHO SARS laboratory network] might have been on the right trail much sooner' (2003, pp. 295–296). How had this situation arisen? Because, according to Enserink, the AMMS 'didn't dare tell the world' about their discovery (2003, p. 294). Their silence, however, was not self-imposed, but forced upon them through the actions of 'an esteemed senior microbiologist and member of the Chinese Academy of Engineering' – Dr. Hong – and the institution for which he worked – the CCDC (*ibid.*). In mid-February, Hong 'proposed that the agent was a new type of *Chlamydia*' (2003, p. 295). And even though 'others suggested that it may have been something different altogether' (*ibid.*), there was apparently no dissuading him: 'promoted by Hong Tao, an esteemed senior microbiologist and member of the Chinese Academy of Engineering, the *Chlamydia* hypothesis had become ... well established' (2003, p. 294). The CCDC, in conjunction with other institutions in China, subsequently forbade any further discussion of the aetiological question, and moved to prevent others from expressing alternate views. In late March, for instance, and 'bolstered by WHO's daily reports and new, more solid data of their own, AMMS scientists reported their findings to the Ministry of Health' (2003, p. 296). The result? 'The department stuck to the *Chlamydia* theory', and set up 'a working group ... to control publicity about SARS pathogen studies' (*ibid.*). Indeed, it was only as late as the last week of April, after the Chinese health minister had been sacked for mishandling the outbreak, that the coronavirus discovery came to receive official acceptance within China (*ibid.*). But by then of course the AMMS team had been pre-empted by the WHO, and it was too late for them to take any credit for the discovery. This, it seems, was 'China's missed chance'.

Everything here centres on the WHO and the AMMS as the champions of the coronavirus aetiological claim. Dr. Hong, on the other hand, concentrates his attentions on a *Chlamydia* bacterium. And, whereas the former groups let their results speak for themselves, Dr. Hong 'promote[s]' his '*Chlamydia* hypothesis'. In a sense, this is a fairly standard popular scientific tale of the 'good' scientists (in this case, microbiologists) who get it right, versus the 'inept' scientist who got it wrong.[3] But what happens when this tale is examined in a little more detail? Presented below is Enserink's interpretation of Hong's article, CLA:

> In a paper in the 25 April *National Medical Journal of China*, Hong reported having found '*Chlamydia*-like particles' in a total of seven patients. (In two, he also noted the presence of a coronavirus which by then had been proven to be the cause of SARS.) But he was not able to actually isolate the microbe or characterise it further, and *Chlamydia* was not found in most SARS patients. Moreover, antibodies to known *Chlamydia* species did not react with the tissue samples. Hong therefore proposed that the agent was a new type of *Chlamydia*, but others suggested that it may have been something different altogether. (2003, p. 295)

Now immediately it seems to me that there is something about this gloss that jars with CMC's overall narrative. For therein, trapped within a parenthesis, is an acknowledgement that Hong had in fact 'noted' the coronavirus too. But before discussing this peculiarity at any great length, I want to present the abstract from the original source document CLA (the most relevant sections have been underlined):

> OBJECTIVE: To explore the causative agents of the atypical pneumonia (also SARS) that occurred recently in some regions of [China]. METHOD: Organ samples of 7 dead cases of SARS were collected from Guangdong, Shanxi, Sichuan Provinces and Beijing for electron microscopic examination. 293 cell lines were inoculated with the materials derived from the lungs in order to isolate the causative agent(s). The agents in the organs and cell cultures were revealed by immunoassay. RESULTS: <u>Both *Chlamydia*-like and coronavirus-like particles were found by electron microscope.</u> Inclusion bodies containing elementary bodies, reticulate antibodies and intermediate bodies of *Chlamydia*-like agent were visualised in multiple organs from the 7 dead cases, including lungs (7 cases), spleens (2 cases), livers (2 cases), kidneys (3 cases) and lymph nodes (1 case), by ultrathin section EM [electron microscope]. In some few sections, coronavirus-like particles were concurrently seen. <u>A coronavirus RNA-polymerase segment (440 bp) was amplified from the lung tissues of two cases.</u> After inoculation with materials from the lung samples, similar *Chlamydia*-like particles were also found in the inoculated 293 cells. Since the *Chlamydia*-like agents visualized in both organs and cell cultures did not react with the genus specific antibodies against *Chlamydia* and monoclonal antibodies against *C. pneumoniae* and *C. psittaci*, the results might well be suggestive of a novel *Chlamydia*-like agent. CONCLUSION: <u>Since the novel *Chlamydia*-like agent was found co-existing with a coronavirus-like agent in the dead cases of SARS, it appears most likely that both agents play some role in the disease. At the present time, however, it is not possible to determine whether these agents interact synergistically, or whether one follows another. This requires further study.</u> (Hong et al., 2003, p. 632)

Not only Enserink's gloss, but also his telling of 'CMC' more generally, starts to appear a little problematic once CLA is examined. Reading through this abstract it seems difficult not to draw the following conclusions: first, that Hong gave his (entirely plausible) coronavirus findings far more attention than Enserink is allowing for; and second, that Hong was far less excited about his (entirely plausible) *Chlamydia* findings than Enserink is allowing for. Hong made it quite clear in CLA that he had not yet ruled out the possibility of the outbreak under investigation having a multifactorial aetiology; that the cases of SARS from which he had received samples might well have been caused by a complex interaction, or 'synergy', between *both* pathogens. But then, if these conclusions can be accepted, it is worth asking the following question: does CLA really support, back up or vindicate *in any way* CMC's tale of the 'good' microbiologists versus the 'inept' microbiologist? I want to suggest not. And the rhetoric through which CMC manages this peculiar 'mismatch' will be the focus of attention in the following section, where, purely for reasons of space, I concentrate on CMC's management of Hong's coronavirus findings.

THE DISCOVERY OF THE CORONAVIRUS

There is one other curiosity about CMC's formulation of CLA that needs some mention here. Every activity detailed within CLA, *including Hong's discovery of the coronavirus*, took place between mid-late February and early March 2003. But if this is the case, then surely Hong's coronavirus findings actually pre-empted *both* the AMMS group (by a few weeks) and the WHO–SARS group (by at least a month). Indeed, if the time period during which Hong's laboratory research took place is taken into account, then Hong can quite easily be cast in the role of microbiological hero! Whether he had adjudged the coronavirus to be the one singular cause or part of a synergistic causal process would, in such a casting, be deemed irrelevant – for he, and he alone, would have been the first microbiologist to see this hitherto unknown coronavirus. The curious thing about CMC's interpretation of CLA, however, is that it possesses a number of rhetorical devices that serve to background just such a version of events.

FINDINGS AND NOTINGS

Consider, for example, the following extract: 'Hong reported having found "*Chlamydia*-like particles" in a total of seven patients. (In two, he also noted the presence of a coronavirus)' (Enserink, 2003, p. 295). Although both sentences seek to capture and represent a process of discovery, they do so in different ways. And this difference, though slight, is highly consequential.

To make this point a little clearer the sentential units can be broken down into their constituent parts: actor, process and goal[4]:

Hong	Reports	Finding	*Chlamydia*
[Actor]	[Process 1]	[Process 2]	[Goal]
Hong	Notes	_____	Coronavirus

In both, the actor quite obviously remains as Hong. The goals, too, remain similar – although differently named entities, they are, nevertheless, entities of a similar, *pathogenic* order. The real difference, the difference that makes a difference, is to be found when the processes are examined. In the first instance, Hong 'reports' on his engagement with *Chlamydia*. 'To report' is to perform not a material, but a mental action process.[5] Considered as an action in and of itself, a report would involve a conscious being sensing a phenomenon before then making that which had been sensed known to others. But in this particular instance the report is a report that a pathogen had been 'found'. And this second process verb, 'to find', immediately implies that some kind of material action process had *also* taken place – a process of doing and not simply of sensing. In order for Hong's 'report' to have become possible, he would have had to have made some kind of material contact with the bacterium through, say, a laboratory instrument. To find, in other words, is to found; to found a relationship, the actor having at least a degree of human interest in the object found. In the second sentence, Hong 'notes the presence of' a coronavirus. To 'note' is to do something very similar to reporting. Both are mental process actions that involve sensing. But unlike in the first sentence, this mental process action is not followed by a material process action. Hong, as a conscious being, simply notes the presence of a phenomenon before making that which he had sensed apparent to others. No material contact with the coronavirus is implied in any of this.

Is this rhetorically significant? I want to suggest that it is. Dr. Hong himself, for instance, suggested in CLA that 'both *Chlamydia*-like and coronavirus-like particles were *found* by electron microscope'. Indeed, not once in CLA does he use the mental process verb 'to note' to describe his coronavirus work. Apart from the electron microscope work in which he 'saw' the coronavirus, everything revolves around material process verbs: to *find*, to *amplify*, to *prepare* and so on. The effect of this 'deletion of materiality' is a definite structuring of the ways in which we, as readers, are able to come to an understanding of Hong's laboratory work. Why? Because as Simpson (2004, p. 23, emphasis added) has noted in relation to process actions:

> Unlike material processes *which have their provenance in the physical world,* mental processes inhabit and reflect the world of consciousness ... the entity 'sensed' in a mental process *is not directly affected by the process, and this makes it of a somewhat different order to the role of Goal in a material process.*

So does the act of 'noting' the presence of something indicate that a scientific discovery has actually been made? Perhaps not. Perhaps it suggests an action that teeters on the edge of not being a discovery at all. To 'note' is merely to acknowledge the presence of an object in passing, remaining at a certain remove from that object before then moving on somewhere else. It is, on Simpson's reading, to leave the entity 'unaffected' by the process. Another way to make the rhetorical significance of Enserink's lexical choices clear is to consider culturally entrenched ways of using language in scientific practice. After all, microbiologists like Dr. Hong do not build their careers around 'notings'. They build them around 'findings'. In microbiology, materiality is everything. So at the very least it seems possible to suggest that a 'noting' does not suggest quite such a clear cut a discovery as a 'finding'. And although previous studies of rhetoric have noted that different process verbs can generate different degrees of 'opacity' when used to portray agency and intention,[6] it seems that here, in CMC, they end up manipulating not human *agency*, but rather, human *interest*. Where CLA indicated that both the coronavirus and the *Chlamydia* findings were of equal ontological standing, leaving their status as discovered objects clear and uncomplicated, CMC erodes this sense of equality via the use of process verbs that evoke differing levels of actorial contact with, and interest in, their end–goal.

HONG'S COGNITIVE BRACKETS

Backgrounding these process actions now, I want to throw something else into relief within that two-sentence extract from CMC – the parenthesis:

> Hong reported having found '*Chlamydia*-like particles' in a total of seven patients. (In two, he also noted the presence of a coronavirus which by then had been proven to be the cause of SARS). (2003, p. 295)

Why is it there? What is its purpose? On the face of it, its stylistic significance seems clear: it serves to surround and completely cut off from the rest of the text the only reference that CMC makes to the fact that Hong found coronavirus as well as *Chlamydia*. That '*Chlamydia*-like particles' – in the plural – were found in all seven of Hong's samples is a point that is left outside the parenthesis. That 'a coronavirus' – in the singular – was noted in just two samples is a point that is placed inside the parenthesis. This, then, is what it does. But it is not at all clear *why* it is made to do what it does *here*. Indeed, the separation is especially curious given that Hong's own research article goes out of its way to avoid making any such separation. The very title of the article – '*Chlamydia*-like and coronavirus-like agents found in dead cases ...' – seeks to draw the two discoveries together. Further, in CLA's conclusions, their entanglement with one another is once again made clear: 'since the novel *Chlamydia*-like agent was found co-existing with a coronavirus-like agent in the dead cases of SARS, it appears most likely that both agents play some role in the disease' (Hong et al., 2003, p. 636). CMC's brackets, however, cut off all links between the two discoveries. And although little has been written about parentheses in rhetorical theory, the concept of enactment, taken from the field of stylistics, helps to make the rhetorical significance of this 'cutting' operation a little clearer.[7] The critical and stylistic assumption underpinning the concept is that literary forms can mime the meanings they seek to express. So, for instance, in Dickens's *Oliver Twist*, a stylistician might note how the following passage seeks to enact movement, noise and confusion *in and as* a description of the actions of movement, noise and confusion:

> Away they ran, pell-mell, helter-skelter, slap-dash, tearing, yelling, screaming, knocking down the passengers as they turn corners, rousing up the dogs, and astonishing the fowls: and streets, squares and courts re-echo with the sound.[8]

My argument is that CMC's brackets work to produce a similar effect in relation to Hong's scientific practice. They enact the 'cognitive brackets' that Hong must have placed around his coronavirus 'noting' in order to come to the final *Chlamydia* conclusion that he ended up 'promoting': Hong dismissed the aetiological significance of the 'noting', and thus the brackets enact the dismissal. Moreover, given what is placed inside – *singular* coronavirus findings – and what is placed outside – *multiple Chlamydia* findings – they start to look less like CMC's own interpretation, and more like a faithful attempt at enactment. The very presence of the parenthesis, the cognitive brackets, is in this way granted an explanation. And although not perhaps entirely convincing to a reader with some first-hand knowledge of CLA, it is at least plausible: Hong's context of discovery, it seems, was a context built around quantitative criteria. Fascinated by the *Chlamydia*-like particles and their abundance in relation to the coronavirus particles, Hong completely overlooked the aetiological significance of the latter. Through the use of the parenthesis, CMC generates a sense that, *even if* we can allow that Hong's coronavirus was a discovery rather than a noting, it was, *nevertheless*, a discovery that Hong himself regarded as secondary and unimportant in relation to *Chlamydia*.

'BY THEN ...'

Things, it seems, could have been very different. And nowhere was this more so than when it came to the question of 'who was first?' CLA could quite easily have been used to index the work of a scientific group that had managed, quite impressively, to pre-empt both the AMMS group (by a few weeks) and the WHO laboratory network (by at least a month). But Enserink manages not to treat CLA in this way. In fact, he manages to treat it in quite the *opposite* way, with the result that Dr. Hong starts to appear as the pre-empted scientist! So how is this reversal achieved? Consider the extract from CMC one final time:

> In a paper in the 25 April *National Medical Journal of China*, Hong reported having found '*Chlamydia*-like particles' in a total of seven patients. (In two, he also noted the presence of a coronavirus which by then had been proven to be the cause of SARS). (Enserink, 2003, p. 295)

In the sentence immediately before the parenthesis the reader watches through Enserink's eyes as a CLA research finding is summarised. According to Enserink, Hong used CLA to 'report' having found *Chlamydia*-like particles. The focalising subject here is Enserink, the focalised object the research article.[9] At no stage during the sentence is there any possibility of observing the actual act of discovery. Because CLA, and not Hong's laboratory work, acts as the focalised object, the reader is placed at a remove from the actual action. The result of this 'distance' is the creation of a temporal lag, a lag between the act of *finding* and the act of *communicating a finding*. At some point in the past, it seems, Hong had found '*Chlamydia*-like particles'. Then, at some point later on, he reported this discovery in a research article. But in actual fact there is no need to be so vague about the timing of all of this. For Enserink had already made clear that the direct act of finding took place 'on 18 February' (2003, p. 295). And, as is clear from the extract presented above, the research article based on those findings was published 'in the 25 April *National Medical Journal of China*'. As a consequence, the article itself had to have been submitted for publication some time between '18 February' and '25 April'.

So much is clear. But when we turn to examine the sentence that appears in the parenthesis, the identity of the focalised object seems a little *un*clear.

The reason for this ambiguity is a lack of any reference to 'reporting', or indeed to any intermediary separating Enserink, our focaliser, from Hong's laboratory work. Is the focalised object Hong's research article? Or his actual laboratory work? Is Enserink watching *a report of* Hong watching the coronavirus, or is he watching Hong watching the coronavirus? To me, the fact that these questions can be asked at all admits the possibility of more than one structural interpretation of the text. In the clause prior to the parenthesis, for instance, such questions would have made no sense: one knew, quite clearly, that the act of *finding* and the act of *communicating the finding* were temporally separate.

For reasons that I hope will become clear, I want to proceed by playing up to my feeling that Enserink is indeed suggesting that he was there, watching Hong in his laboratory. As a result, when he writes that 'in two [samples] he also noted the presence of a coronavirus', we *are* watching through Enserink's eyes as Hong notes, in two patient samples, the presence of coronavirus. The consequence of this immediacy is that any sense of a lag time between the *finding* and the act of *communicating the finding* is lost. In classical rhetorical terms, we no longer watch as Enserink 'tells' of something. Instead, we watch as Enserink 'shows' us an act that appears to be fully present to him. But, if this is so, what we need to ask now is *when* is Enserink's immediacy in this formulation? *When* is he watching Hong doing his noting? A clue here is the deictic marker 'by then' in the second-half of the sentence. It anchors Enserink, the focaliser, as he watches Hong. But if it was 'by then', then when was this 'by then'? Let us run through some of the dates that were mentioned above to try and answer this question. Was 'by then' 18 February, the date when Hong found his *Chlamydia*-like particles? No. It cannot have been. Why? Because 'by then' has to suggest a date after 16 April, that is, the date on which the WHO officially announced that the coronavirus was the causal agent of SARS. By implication, the only way in which Enserink's 'by then' could be referring to 18 February was if it was somehow trying to suggest that Hong, in some bizarrely schizophrenic manoeuvre, had managed to pre-empt himself ('in two he also noted the presence of a coronavirus, which by then he had already discovered …'). Let us reject this possibility.

So what about 25 April, the date on which the article was published? Before answering this question directly, let us imagine for a moment that I was *wrong* in playing up to my suspicion that Enserink had 'told' us of the *Chlamydia* finding, yet 'shown' us, very directly, the coronavirus discovery. Let us imagine, instead, that in both cases he had been focalising Hong's research article. If this were so, then his 'by then' would be a reference to the research article: 'by then [25 April when the article was published] …'. And yet, he surely cannot have been making such a reference. Why? Because in the case of *Chlamydia* he had already admitted that the act of finding took place on '18 February'. He had, in other words, already admitted that the act of finding took place *before* the WHO made their announcement on 16 April. Despite the fact that the article had been published on 25 April, then, the *Chlamydia* findings had been made on 18 February. By implication, if the coronavirus discovery had taken place on or around that same day, or indeed at any point before 16 April, *then irrespective of the date when the article was published,* Enserink would, logically, have had to admit that Hong, in 'noting' the coronavirus, had pre-empted both the AMMS and the WHO laboratory network. What I take from all of this sleuthing around is a proof that Enserink's 'by then' simply *has* to be a reference to the coronavirus discovery, and the coronavirus discovery alone. What I also take from it is a certain confidence that my suspicions were correct: Enserink was indeed playing around with the difference between 'telling' and 'showing' in his reporting of the two discoveries. The coronavirus findings, Enserink would have us believe, were somehow conducted separately and apart from the *Chlamydia* findings.

So, let us ask the question again and, this time, attempt a direct answer: was 'by then' 25 April? No. For the coronavirus findings to have been made and published in a journal on the very same day would, of course, have been impossible. But we are, nevertheless, closer to the correct answer now. For there was in fact a little more time for Enserink to play around with in his reference to 'by then'. As I noted above, and by Enserink's own admission, Hong's article must have been submitted for publication some time between '18 February' and '25 April'. If the coronavirus discovery was already passé by the time the article appeared, then Hong's coronavirus discovery could only have been made in the nine days separating 16 April and 25 April. This, I want to suggest, is the *when* of Enserink's 'by then'. It is, I submit, the only possible way in which his reference to 'by then' could have made any sense at all.

Playing around with a direct focalisation strategy, placing the coronavirus results in a parenthesis and appending those results with the deictic marker 'by then', Enserink brings Hong's coronavirus work forward into a time when it is (was?) already passé. Indeed, this rhetorical strategy is aided by the fact that CMC has already suggested, three paragraphs beforehand, that Hong's *Chlamydia* 'hypothesis' was already 'well established' in China. The coronavirus discovery, we could easily start to suspect, was a 'noting' that came afterwards. And this effect, rather unsurprisingly, does not allow Hong to appear as a very able scientist. Instead of representing 'the first scientist to discover the coronavirus', he now cuts a rather forlorn, buffoon-like figure. 'What', we might conceivably ask based on a reading of CMC, 'was Hong doing dithering over the identity of the causal agent when *by then* everyone knew that the agent was, in fact, a coronavirus?'

If this is indeed what Enserink is suggesting, then it is grossly unfair. *All* the laboratory work reported therein was quite clearly carried out at the same time: February/March 2003. Even a cursory glance at CLA would make this apparent. For whatever else it does, CLA indexes the hard scientific labour that went into its production. As with the AMMS' work, cell lines were inoculated with materials derived from SARS patients, and electron microscope examinations, serological tests and polymerase chain reaction (PCR) tests were conducted. Even by Enserink's account, this kind of work took Ruifu's team a full 12 days – from at least 14 February to at least 26 February. Yet CMC's 'by then' seems to be suggesting that Hong began his coronavirus work after 16 April. If this were so, then in the nine days between 16 April and 25 April, Hong would have had to have done his experimental work, written a five-page scientific report, had it peer-reviewed and then published in China's most prestigious science journal. Put like this, the suggestion starts to appear somewhat implausible.

But if it is so implausible, then why even attempt to suggest that the coronavirus discovery was in some way passé? Because, I submit, it represented the only way in which Enserink could protect CMC's overall story. In order for that story to work, Hong had to be around to make a (patently) false *Chlamydia* claim. Granted, CMC *could* have represented Hong as the microbiologist who saw the coronavirus before anyone else, just as it *could* have represented him as a microbiologist who had taken the coronavirus' presence in patient samples as seriously as that of his other discovery, *Chlamydia*. But if it *had*, then the suggestion that Hong, having made both discoveries, 'promoted' his *Chlamydia* hypothesis whilst ignoring his coronavirus findings would have started to appear a little less believable. At the very least it would have been an idea requiring some further explanation. And that, of course, was precisely the kind of 'further explanation' that Enserink, relying so heavily on the evidence presented in CLA, could not have given.

REPETITION AND EMBELLISHMENT

One final question is the following: *what* happened to CMC after it had been published? For if the fate of Enserink's account was in the hands of later readers, then so too was Hong's reputation. If CMC had been neither read nor cited, then its portrayal of this Chinese microbiologist would have made little impact on our understandings of the SARS outbreak. But the fact is that CMC quickly became a key source for subsequent accounts. As of April 2009, 18 English language scientific research papers containing references to CMC had been published. And whilst it is not *that* unusual for scientific research papers to cite popular scientific texts, the fact that all 18 did so *approvingly*, elevating a work of popular science to the status of 'definitive historical account', is a little unusual. What we find in those accounts is a form of repetition, as in the following research article, written by a research team from the Institute of Medical Virology, Frankfurt, Germany, and published in the *Journal of Clinical Virology*:

> Almost nobody knew at that stage that virologists in Beijing had already discovered a new virus in samples from some of the earliest SARS patients. However, the official line in China at the time was that the novel 'atypical pneumonia' was caused by *Chlamydia* (Enserink, 2003; Berger, Drosten, Doerr, Sturmer, & Preiser, 2004, pp. 13–14)

As might be expected in a scientific research article, actors and their actions are backgrounded, whilst broad processes come to the fore. In this sense, Dr. Hong is 'let off the hook'. And yet, what I find so striking here is the citation strategy. If the metaphor of the 'official line' catches your eye, if it hints at some kind of scientific malpractice, then you have a reputable source to turn to in order to find out more: 'CMC'. But what of Hong's own research article? Despite the fact that the German research team were writing an article of a similar order to Hong's – that is, one that discussed primary scientific knowledge – they eschew any reference to his primary research article in favour of a popular science article that glosses it. This same strategy is at work in each of the 18 research articles: an approving and unquestioning citation of CMC, yet no citation of Hong's research article. There is something else to bear in mind here too. For when the number of citations received by those 18 research articles are added together, a total of 478 citations is generated. At the very least, then, it is possible to suggest that whilst all of those articles would have come into contact with CMC as a definitive historical account, none would necessarily have learnt anything of CLA, that definitive historical account's *primary source.*

But what about popular science accounts? In a sense, they were the accounts that really mattered in mediating an understanding of the outbreak. For most of us today the reality of something like SARS comes to us not through articles in the *Journal of Virology*, but rather, through the filter of journalistic language and imagery. So how did *they* engage with and appropriate CMC? As with the scientific research articles discussed above, a common strategy was *repetition*: each account citing CMC approvingly, and ignoring CLA. The one difference is that there, in the world of popular science, the character of Dr. Hong is suddenly centre-stage. But in those articles another form of appropriation is also apparent: *embellishment*. Consider the following extracts:

> 1. In mid-February, the Institute of Virology also in Beijing, under China's national CDC received two lung tissues … the samples were then divided into three parts: one for Hong Tao, the CDC's chief virologist and CAE member to conduct an electron microscope examination, one for virologist Li Dexin to run the PCR testing and the third for bacterium cultivation purposes. Hong soon claimed, after examining it under the electron microscope, that it was *Chlamydia* – a bacterium notorious for being the pathogen of a common sexually transmitted disease which is not generally fatal – that was the cause of the atypical pneumonia. (Cao, 2004, pp. 262–286)

> 2. The new rumours … came from Guangdong … A senior local scientist maintained that chlamydiae [sic] bacteria had caused the outbreak. The theory was so prevailing that it proved inhibiting in a culture of deference to authority and seniority. When scientists in Beijing identified a new virus in late February, they chose not to say anything about it. (Balasegaram & Schnur, 2006, p. 75)

> 3. The medical community's understanding of the true aetiology of SARS was delayed significantly by a February announcement from a senior scientist at the Chinese Centre for Disease Control that he suspected the infectious agent was *Chlamydia* – a commonly understood bacterial agent that would not have warranted heightened concern of investigation. (Mahmoud & Lemon, 2004, p. 4)

Gone from extract 3, for instance, are any references to Chinese institutions: the CCDC, the Chinese Ministry of Health and so on. It is now Hong, and Hong alone, who stands responsible for the false claim. The all powerful, yet totally inept superman. A line of moral responsibility is drawn, leading straight from this 'senior scientist' to the 'significant delay' in the medical community's attempts to get to grips with the outbreak. Even the identity of Hong's *Chlamydia*-like particles is now characterised in such a way as to make him appear ridiculous. In extract 1, for instance, we are able to laugh at a 'fact' that the cited source, CMC, never mentions: Hong's belief that a sexually transmitted infection could have caused an outbreak of upper respiratory tract disease. And yet the joke, I would suggest, is on the author of extract 1. For there is more than one *Chlamydia* 'bacterium'. Hong, in CLA, merely refers to the viral family Chlamydiaceae, of the class Chlamydiae. Included within this family are two genera: *Chlamydia* and *Chlamydophila*. The species *Chlamydia trachomatis*, which causes 'sexually transmitted disease', is only one of the three *Chlamydia* species, and only one of the nine species included within the overall family Chlamydiaceae. In CLA, Hong never mentions *C. trachomatis*. But he does mention *Chlamydia pneumoniae* and *Chlamydia psittaci*, species which are both known to cause pneumonia-like illness. And finally, consider extract 2. Here, Dr. Hong even has his place of work and his geographical location within China manipulated! Cast in the role of 'local doctor from the rural provinces', Hong-the-simpleton now appears only in order to frustrate the AMMS, the thrusting, big city research group from Beijing.

These repetitions and embellishments perhaps represent the *real* tragedy for Dr. Hong. Whereas CMC at least allowed the reader to catch sight of Hong's double finding – coronavirus *and Chlamydia*-like particles – these accounts do not. Foregrounded in each and every case, and in some cases with an almost *sadistic* pleasure, is the *Chlamydia* discovery and the *Chlamydia* discovery alone. In CMC one could still hear the faint murmurings of a reasonable scientist considering the possibility of the coronavirus. But here, in these texts, that scientist has finally fallen silent.

CONCLUSIONS

In this chapter I have sought to defend Dr. Hong in a hastily assembled scientific court of appeal. I have, in short, been looking for justice. Have I found it? Well, I have made clear the transformations that Hong's account of his own actions underwent at the hands of others. And I have also made clear the extent to which those subsequent accounts can, with a little rhetorical effort, be called into question. That, however, is all I have been able to achieve. Put more accurately, it is all that I *could* have achieved. For the jury in this court is you, dear reader. Have I convinced you? Is Dr. Hong to receive a reprieve? A pardon, perhaps? His fate is in your hands now, not mine.

His fate, but perhaps the fate of others too. For what is perhaps most interesting about this particular episode is the epidemic of *literature* that the epidemic *disease* seems to have generated. Were the rhetorical transformations, appropriations and embellishments at work in this one localised instance unusual? I would suggest not. Indeed, if emerging *disease* epidemics can be said to imply unpredictability and rapid evolutionary mutation, then perhaps historical accounts, in seeking to interpret and to story them, take on some of those very same characteristics: the *disease* epidemic and the *literary* epidemic; the pathogen as tropic and the trope as pathogenic. But then, if this is so, it raises an interesting (rhetorical) question, and one that I want to leave the jury to ponder: who would bet against there being plenty more Dr. Hongs out there, that is, scientists of all kinds, from all eras and all corners of the world, lost in the prison-house of language and in need of sociological representation?

NOTES

1. Here I am paraphrasing Bloor ([1976]1991, p. 30).
2. Hong's research article is available through the U.S. National Library of Medicine's online database, *PubMed*. Having retrieved a copy, I then had the text translated from Chinese to English.
3. That is, 'fairly standard' given the claims of those who study popular science writing: 'many popular science books promote a version of science that is contrasted starkly with the 'other' of science – or at least the 'other' that popular science writers want to identify – namely, foolishness' (Erickson, 2005, p. 148).
4. The distinction between actor, process and goal is drawn from Simpson (2004, pp. 22–23).
5. On the distinction between material and mental action processes, see Simpson (2004, pp. 185–186).
6. In particular, see Potter's (1996) analysis of the construction of factual descriptive accounts, and Marlin's analysis of 'intention-promoting' verbs (1984, pp. 26–29).
7. On the lack of attention to the rhetorical force of the parenthesis in modern literary theory, see Williams (1993).
8. This particular example is taken from Wales (2001, p. 125).
9. The concept of focalisation, drawn from the field of narratology, suggests that all stories are presented in a text through the mediation of a particular 'perspective'. In any study of focalisation, the key question is 'who is the immediate seer here …?' (Toolan, 2001, p. 63).

ACKNOWLEDGMENT

I would like to thank Ananya Mukherjea for her initial, and extremely helpful, debunking of my initial debunking of Enserink's debunking.

REFERENCES

Balasegaram, M., & Schnur, A. (2006). China: From denial to mass mobilization. In: S. Omi (Ed.), *SARS: How a global epidemic was stopped*. Geneva: World Health Organisation Press.
Berger, A., Drosten, C., Doerr, H., Sturmer, M., & Preiser, W. (2004). SARS – paradigm of an emerging viral infection. *Journal of Clinical Virology, 29*, 13–22.
Bloor, D. ([1976] 1991). *Knowledge and social imagery*. London: University of Chicago Press.

Cao, C. (2004). SARS: 'Waterloo' of Chinese science. *China: An International Journal, 2*(2), 262–286.

Enserink, M. (2003). China's missed chance. *Science, 301*, 294–296.

Erickson, M. (2005). *Science, culture and society: Understanding science in the 21st century.* Cambridge: Polity Press.

Hong, T., Wang, J., Sun, Y., Duan, S., Chen, L., Qu, J., et al. (2003). *Chlamydia*-like and coronavirus-like agents found in dead cases of atypical pneumonia by electron microscopy. *Zhonghua Yi Xue Za Zhi, 83*(8), 632–636.

Mahmoud, A., & Lemon, S. (2004). Summary and assessment. In: A. Mahmoud (Ed.), *Learning from SARS*. Washington: National Academies Press.

Marlin, R. (1984). The rhetoric of action description. *Informal Logic, 6*, 26–29.

Potter, J. (1996). *Representing reality*. London: Sage.

Simpson, P. (2004). *Stylistics: A resource book for students*. London: Routledge.

Toolan, M. (2001). *Narrative: A critical linguistic introduction*. London: Routledge.

Wales, K. (2001). *A dictionary of stylistics*. Harlow: Pearson.

Williams, R. (1993). Reading the parenthesis. *SubStance, 22*, 53–66.

THE RHETORIC OF SCIENCE AND STATISTICS IN CLAIMS OF AN AUTISM EPIDEMIC

Victor W. Perez

ABSTRACT

Purpose – *To examine the rhetorical use of scientific medical evidence and diagnoses statistics in claims of an epidemic of childhood autism spectrum disorder.*

Methodology/approach – *Qualitative analysis of the content and dissemination of claims in several venues for social problems construction, including popular media, peer-reviewed scientific literature, and the Internet.*

Findings – *Rhetorical use of etiological evidence, both scientific and experiential, positing a causal link between medical interventions (e.g., vaccines), environmental toxins, and autism is prominent across several arenas for social problems construction. Claims and counterclaims involve statements amiable to or critical of evidence and its relationship to the scientific method. Presentation of diagnoses statistics and covariation with vaccination regimens are integral as a rhetorical device in claims of a true change in prevalence.*

Contribution to the field – *Elucidates how the medicalization of childhood developmental disabilities and increased lay involvement (e.g., parents) in the social problems process were vital for the proliferation of attention and*

Understanding Emerging Epidemics: Social and Political Approaches
Advances in Medical Sociology, Volume 11, 203–221
ISSN: 1057-6290/doi:10.1108/S1057-6290(2010)0000011015

resources directed to autism presently. The fundamental scientific method and the lack of sufficient, valid scientific evidence are not integral to the continuation of the movement that posits vaccines cause autism. The content of these claims is unfettered on the Internet as an arena for claimsmaking, allowing a lay social movement to continue that often stands in opposition to recognized scientific authority and evidence.

INTRODUCTION

Since the late 1990s, much has been written about the increased prevalence of autism spectrum disorder (ASD) diagnoses in children over approximately the past three decades and the potential sources of this increase. To a substantial degree, the controversy over possible links to vaccines and other environmental toxins and the myriad of claims therein propelled "the autism epidemic" to an issue of national and international importance (DeStefano, 2009; Fombonne, 2003; Grinker, 2007; Kirby, 2005; Matson & Minshawi, 2006). Claims of true increases in childhood ASD transcend and interact among several environments for social problems construction (Hilgartner & Bosk, 1988), including familial, political, educational, legal, and medical/scientific arenas, and efforts to promote and dramatize the issue within each of these arenas have been met with efforts to de-dramatize them from within and across their institutional boundaries (Blaxill, 2004; Fombonne, 2008; Hilgartner & Bosk, 1988, p. 62; Kirby, 2005; Moyer & Clignet, 1980).

Some suggest that changes in definition, measurement, and identification of ASD have had important implications for measuring incidence of new diagnoses and the change in overall prevalence in recent decades (Best, 2008a; Fombonne, 2001, 2003, 2005, 2008; Fombonne, Zakarian, Bennett, Meng, & McLean-Heywood, 2006; Grinker, 2007; Johnson, Myers, & The Council on Children with Disabilities, 2007; Normand & Dallery, 2007; Wing, 2005; Yeargin-Allsopp et al., 2003). Among other issues concerning identification of ASD, of particular importance is its expanded diagnostic continuum in widely used clinical manuals such as the *Diagnostic and Statistical Manual of Mental Disorders IV and IV-TR* (APA, 1994, 2000) as a source of an increase in prevalence of childhood ASD, as diagnoses include a broader range of conditions than they did in the past (Fombonne, 2001; Grinker, 2007; Matson & Minshawi, 2006).

Many of the claims of a true increase were facilitated by an increasing cultural preoccupation with medicalizing childhood learning and developmental disabilities (Conrad, 2007; Grinker, 2007; Poulson, 2009). In recent decades, impropriety in various forms of childhood behavior and experience has been redefined and consequently relocated under the jurisdiction of medicine[1] (Conrad, 2007; Conrad & Potter, 2000; Stolzer, 2007) and this has had important implications for understanding and addressing childhood ASD. The diagnostic criteria for a multitude of mental health conditions in the DSM are arguably the most widely accepted and utilized in North America (Matson & Minshawi, 2006, p. 9), and as such ASD has been framed in the realm of medical definition, surveillance, and control (Best, 2008b; Conrad, 2007; Poulson, 2009).

As the social constructionist approach to social problems elucidates, a condition or experience in society does not inherently have qualities or attributes that makes it a social problem. Social problems are putative conditions deemed problematic in a process of social construction through various claimsmaking activities, while in competition with other issues to garner public attention (Best, 1987, 1990, 2008b; Hilgartner & Bosk, 1988; Spector & Kitsuse, 1977). Though there are several avenues for exploring this issue utilizing the social constructionist framework (Best, 2008b; Blumer, 1971; Hilgartner & Bosk, 1988; Spector & Kitsuse, 1977), this research focuses specifically on the rhetorical quality of key claims and counterclaims involving scientific medical evidence and diagnosis statistics (Best, 1987, 1990; Davies, Chapman, & Leask, 2002). Claimsmakers use scientific information not only as objective evidence or grounds for their claims, but also to persuade (Best, 1987, p. 101; Gusfield, 1981). Consequently, the rhetoric of science is deeply embedded in claimsmaking efforts concerning an epidemic of childhood ASD, and as such is a fundamental part of the claimsmaking process in evaluating the validity of the various claims made.

CLAIMS AND COUNTERCLAIMS

There were key claims integral to the initial proliferation of attention given to the increase in prevalence of childhood ASD, and in tandem, were a significant component of the rapid rise of the social movement concerning autism awareness, intervention, and allocation of resources and assistance. These claims have had tremendous impact and involve two primary rhetorical components: the variety of statistics concerning vaccines and ASD prevalence trends and how these numeric estimates convey scientific objectivity and causality, and the generation, dissemination, and interpretation of medical scientific evidence concerning a causal link between vaccines and ASD.

THE RHETORIC OF STATISTICS – "AUTISM IS INCREASING RAPIDLY AND IS NOT RARE"

The importance of the generation, dissemination, and interpretation of childhood ASD diagnosis statistics cannot be overstated. A key claim that the condition of autism is a serious problem that has reached epidemic levels and deserves widespread public attention and resources involves promoting statistics that reveal the rapid increase of those affected and the extent of the condition and its costs to families, schools, and broader society[2] (Best, 1987, 1990, 2001, 2004, 2008a, 2008b). Research estimates current prevalence rates of childhood ASD approximating 60 cases per 10,000 children[3] (Blaxill, 2004; Brock, 2006; Johnson et al., 2007; Newschaffer et al., 2007), rates that may be between three and four times higher than three decades ago (Fombonne, 2003, p. 88), while rates for autism specifically in the United States have shown a 10-fold increase over earlier estimates (Blaxill, 2004, p. 549). A summarization of Centers for Disease Control (CDC) and other research results suggests ASD rates range between 2 and 6 per 1,000 children, or rates between 1 in 500 and 1 in 150 (NIMH, 2008).[4]

Prevalence of ASD diagnosis began to rise in the 1980s, with a more accelerated increase beginning in the early 1990s (Bishop, Whitehouse, Watt, & Line, 2008; Stehr-Green, Tull, Stellfeld, Mortenson, & Simpson, 2003, pp. 101–102), a trend initially gaining widespread attention via a California Department of Developmental Services study suggesting that autism had increased by 273% over that decade in California[5] (Baker, 2008; Gernsbacher, Dawson, & Goldsmith, 2005). Detailed epidemiological record-keeping of diagnoses of childhood ASD began in the early 1990s, often for services in educational settings as related to the Individuals with Disabilities in Education Act and the Americans with Disabilities Act (Boyle, Bertrand, & Yeargin-Allsopp, 1999; Grinker, 2007; Johnson et al., 2007). Consequently, better and more rigorous identification of ASD will lead to an increasing number of diagnoses that, when more accurately and fully recorded, will present itself as a surge of cases (Best, 2001, 2004; Gernsbacher et al., 2005; Grinker, 2007).

These statistics, notably those closer to the 1 in 150 childhood ASD rate, are prominent across advocacy websites and autism-related literature.[6] The rhetorical quality of these claims involving numeric estimates and statistics is important, as it suggests that the data, or quantitative empirical evidence, have scientific objectivity and convey clearly and unequivocally that autism diagnoses have indeed increased rapidly and that the condition is not rare (Best, 1987, 2001, 2004). Furthermore, statistical statements such as "1 in 150" expands the domain of those possibly affected, construing the diagnosis as frequent and appeals to all that any one child is a potential child with autism, thus democratizing the risk. These are important techniques of claims involving numeric estimates to utilize the highest estimates and broaden the base of potential victims of the condition, in turn lending dramatic effect to the issue (Best, 1987, 2008a).

CAUSALITY FROM TREND STATISTICS: *SOMETHING* MUST BE CAUSING THE INCREASE

Several scholars suggest that the rise in diagnoses of childhood ASD is the result of several identification issues: changing diagnostic criteria for childhood ASD as mandated in the DSM; the expanded continuum of diagnoses subsumed under the broader category pervasive developmental disorders (PDD) to include Pervasive Developmental Disorder-Not Otherwise Specified (PDD-NOS) and Asperger's syndrome; diagnostic substitution; and increased awareness and attention and their impact on age at detection, case finding, and educational services (Best, 2008a, pp. 81–82; Fombonne, 2002, 2003, 2008, p. 16; Gillberg, 1999, 2005; Grinker, 2007; Johnson et al., 2007; Matson & Minshawi, 2006; Ouellette-Kuntz et al., 2007; Wazana, Bresnahan, & Kline, 2007; Yeargin-Allsopp et al., 2003).[7]

These factors are interrelated, intersecting in ways that elucidate how the rise in prevalence of diagnoses could be due to changes in how ASD is defined, identified, and measured, and not reflective of a true increase in incidence. In particular, a widening of the possible types of diagnoses now include those who have milder forms of the condition and are more high functioning, including those diagnosed with Asperger's syndrome (Matson & Minshawi, 2006), and those who do not meet all the specific criteria for a diagnosis of autism, but are still considered to have similar developmental difficulties and are consequently diagnosed as PDD-NOS[8] (Best, 2008a; Filipek et al., 1999; Fombonne, 2003, p. 88; NIMH, 2008). Furthermore, social, political, and educational influences on definitions of childhood experience affect how concepts of developmental disability may overlap and replace each other, as social representations of disability categories change over time (Conrad, 2007; Smukler, 2005). Specifically, research demonstrates that prevalence of diagnosis of full-syndrome autism covaried negatively with diagnosis of mental retardation without autism in groups of California children born between 1987 and 1994 (Croen, Grether, Hoogstrate, & Selvin, 2002). Other research suggests the plausibility of diagnostic substitution

(Bishop et al., 2008), with similar phenomena taking place in educational settings, particularly concerning the eligibility of special education resources available for a diagnosis of ASD (Brock, 2006, p. 31).

Thus, increases in prevalence may not reflect true increases in incidence (Grether, 2006), but may reflect broader measurement, better and expanded case identification and record-keeping, and diagnostic substitution. Though some still suggest that changing methodology in ascertainment cannot account for the increase in prevalence rates that have been documented (Blaxill, 2004), what is vital for a social constructionist analysis is the fact that statistics have a strong rhetorical impact on the lay public. Taken at face value, the increased prevalence trends suggest that some new causal agent has made childhood ASD rise exponentially (e.g., increases in vaccinations).[9] As described earlier, the objective, scientific qualities of statistics give us confidence in understanding social issues and the assurance of a well-documented social world from which we can base policy and individual-level decisions. However, all statistics produced and disseminated are based on numerous conceptualization, operationalization, and measurement decisions, in both original and secondary research (Best, 2001, 2004).

MEDICAL INTERVENTIONS IN CHILDHOOD

To a substantial degree, early claims of an autism epidemic involved the hypothesized direct causal links between medical interventions in childhood and the onset or diagnosis of autism thereafter (Bernard, Enayati, Redwood, Roger, & Binstock, 2001; Blaxill, Redwood, & Bernard, 2004; DeStefano, 2009; Fombonne, 2008; Glazer, 2003; Grinker, 2007; Kirby, 2005). These claims involved the notable change in prevalence as evidence of a true increase in childhood ASD and involved assertions of the root causes of autism (and thus the change in prevalence), or at least environmental factors that increase the likelihood of autism developing (Bernard et al., 2001; Blaxill et al., 2004; Kirby, 2005). Those claims carrying the most profound and widespread impact across various institutional arenas involved the toxicity of environmental influences and ill effects of vaccinations such as the measles, mumps, and rubella (MMR) vaccine (Baker, 2008; Fombonne, 2008; Grether, 2006; Poltorak, Leach, Fairhead, & Cassell, 2005) and vaccines containing the preservative thimerosal, which is made up of approximately 50% ethyl mercury (Bernard et al., 2001; Blaxill et al., 2004; Kirby, 2005).[10]

CAUSE OR COINCIDENCE?

In the United States in particular, the focus was on thimerosal in vaccines as the major culprit for advocacy groups and parents in suggesting a causal link between exposure to vaccines and the outcome of autism in their children, when symptoms of autism generally are identified and vaccinations administered at approximately the same time period (Baker, 2008; Doja & Roberts, 2006; Geier, King, Sykes, & Geier, 2008; Katz, 2006; Normand & Dallery, 2007; Offit & Moser, 2009; Shevell & Fombonne, 2006). In confluence with the implementation of more extensive vaccination regimens of young children beginning in the early 1990s (Bernard et al., 2001; Fombonne, 2008; Stehr-Green et al., 2003), medical evidence positing a link between vaccines and ASD (e.g., Wakefield et al., 1998), and a similar time frame for vaccine administration and onset of ASD symptoms, and increased prevalence trends of ASD diagnoses puts forth, on the surface, a dramatic case that vaccines *cause* autism (Baker, 2008). The rhetorical use of co-occurring statistical trends and co-occurring phenomena to suggest causality is an effective way of making a claim to a wider lay public (Best, 2004; Normand & Dallery, 2007).

WHOSE SCIENCE DO WE TRUST?

A number of scientific studies suggest that no strong environmental exposure candidates for autism have been identified as the culprit for increased trends, and the MMR-autism and thimerosal-autism hypotheses are generally unsupported or weak (Baker, 2008; Doja & Roberts, 2006; Fombonne, 2003, p. 88, 2008; Frankish, 2001; Gernsbacher et al., 2005; Grether, 2006; Hviid, Stellfeld, Wohlfahrt, & Melbye, 2003; Institute of Medicine, 2004; Ip, Wong, Ho, Lee, & Wong, 2004; Johnson et al., 2007; Offit, 2008; Schechter & Grether, 2008; Stehr-Green et al., 2003). Though a preponderance of the scientific evidence suggests that there is no causal link between vaccines and the onset of childhood ASD, there is still a large group of parents with the firm belief that vaccines cause autism (Glazer, 2003; Grinker, 2007; Gross, 2009; Johnson et al., 2007).[11]

Major arenas for this debate include academic journals (e.g., *Medical Hypotheses* and *Pediatrics*), advocacy organization websites (e.g., www.safeminds.org and www.neurodiversity.com), and conferences (DAN! conferences and Autism Speaks scientific meetings), as well as Congressional hearings. It is within these realms that some of the most heated rhetorical action takes place concerning scientific *proof* that medical interventions in children can lead to what has been referred to as vaccine-induced autism or vaccine-injury. At this focal point, the actual idea of scientific inquiry and scientific evidence is at the center of the debate, where major principles of the scientific method are being used to challenge one another's findings and alternative sources of evidence are being espoused[12] (Davies et al., 2002; Gross, 2009; Kirby, 2005). From critiquing published articles' research methodology, sample sizes, data sources, and conflicts of interest of scientists/authors, as well as emphasizing the importance of peer-review and the scientific credentials of researchers, most fundamental aspects of the scientific method are being used by more or less two camps to challenge each other: those that posit some causal link between medical interventions and ASD, and those that do not (Fitzpatrick, 2004; Gross, 2009). There are few in the public sphere who are situated in a moderate stance about the state of the knowledge concerning the etiology of ASD, though some prominent advocacy groups do adopt this position.[13]

REQUISITE SOCIAL CONDITIONS

Movements concerning social problems cannot be divorced from the social conditions within which they are embedded and emerge, and their success or failure is heavily determined by their character in the current socio-political atmosphere and their competition with other contemporary social problems (Best, 1987, 1990, 2008b; Hilgartner & Bosk, 1988). It is under particular conditions of contemporary US society that the issue of autism has become characterized as an epidemic, including the medicalization of childhood experiences and consequent changes in claims of causal agents for the onset of ASD (Conrad, 2007; Grinker, 2007; Poulson, 2009), as well as the emphasis on prevention and intervention in medicalized human experience.

MEDICALIZATION OF CHILDHOOD ASD

It is widely suggested that childhood ASD is a neurological disorder, but its diagnosis is based on meeting clinical diagnostic criteria that are phenomenological (Blaxill, 2004; Grether, 2006; Newschaffer et al., 2007; NIMH, 2008; Smukler, 2005). As such, it shares similarities with the diagnosis of other childhood experiences more recently subsumed under the broader jurisdiction of medicine, such as ADHD, whose clinical diagnostic criteria are taken to indicate the presence of some underlying neurological pathology (Conrad, 2007; Molloy & Vasil, 2002; Stolzer, 2007).

Perspectives on the causal origins of autism have been tied to the dominant school of thought in psychiatry and other disciplines studying the condition. With changes in those fields' dominant schools of thought, the explanations for autism also have changed, from one of improper socialization to having a genetic and/or environmental origin (Baker, 2008; Fombonne, 2008; Grinker, 2007; Smukler, 2005). Though not all conditions in the DSM are considered medical, some suggest that "it can be seen as a repository of medicalized categories, especially those having to do with behavior" (Conrad, 2007, p. 48).

These social conditions set the platform for the debate about the increased prevalence of childhood ASD diagnoses by consequently framing the issue in such a way as to direct attention to the more medically oriented possible causes (Baker, 2008; Furedi, 2006), subsequently legitimizing these statements, rather than looking to social influences such as changing measurements and ideas about childhood ASD (though these are often used as counter-arguments to the vaccine-induced hypotheses). Coinciding with the widespread media attention at the time to the Wakefield et al. (1998) study, considered a key catalyst of the vaccine-critical ASD movement (Baker, 2008; Begley, 2009; Kirby, 2005), focus was placed on environmental toxins and medical interventions in childhood that can affect neurological development and functioning (Matson & Minshawi, 2006). As such, the issue was framed from a medicalized perspective, one of disorder (and not simply difference), which also impacted how the issue was rhetorically presented by eager claimsmakers and subsequently dealt with (Baker, 2008; Best, 1987, 2008b; Hilgartner & Bosk, 1988; Molloy & Vasil, 2002; Poulson, 2009).

SCIENTIFIC AGENCY AND PARENT-EXPERTS

As outgrowths of the perspective of medicalization, the contemporary roles of intervention and prevention and their relationship to the agency of parents of children with autism are integral aspects of the current social and cultural zeitgeist concerning childhood developmental difficulties (Baker, 2008; Moldin & Rubenstein, 2006; Ozonoff & Cathcart, 1998; Ryan & Cole, 2009; Stoner & Angell, 2006). Early intervention and treatment for childhood ASD can be effective (Guralnick, 2005; Matson & Minshawi, 2006; Samms-Vaughn & Franklyn-Banton, 2008; Yeargin-Allsopp et al., 2003), but types vary widely and some, such as chelation therapy, are controversial. Nonetheless, the advocacy and activist positions held by many parents has a direct relationship with their involvement and agency in treating their child's ASD (Baker, 2008; Ryan & Cole, 2009; Sabo & Lorenzen, 2008). This is evidenced, for example, on the Autism Research Institute's website:

> the greatest advances in the field of autism occur when professionals collaborate with parents, who are the true experts on what works and what doesn't. As a result, clinicians and researchers affiliated with Defeat Autism Now! do something remarkable: they *listen* to parents and to other health professionals who report success with investigational treatments or who offer ideas about possible interventions. They investigate the scientific basis for these treatments or ideas, often do clinical trials and analytical studies, discuss the results in think tank forums, and extensively evaluate each approach's safety, efficacy, and appropriateness. If a treatment or strategy passes muster, it is formally presented at a think tank and then at a general conference. (Edelson, 2007)

Investigation into the epidemiological breadth of childhood ASD, such as the California-based study described earlier, was prompted largely by the reaction of parents (whose children had ASD) to the Wakefield et al. (1998) study suggesting a link between vaccines and autism (Baker, 2008; Shevell & Fombonne, 2006) and the recommendation of the United States Public Health Service and the American Academy of Pediatrics in July 1999 to remove thimerosal from infant vaccines as a precautionary measure, even though there was no compelling evidence of its harm (DeStefano, 2009). Additionally, though the Wakefield et al. (1998) study was soon after critically challenged and has involved claims of fraud and ethical violations (Begley, 2009; Offit, 2008), the influence of the popular media presenting the alarming prevalence trend statistics and scientific results suggesting the possibility of serious harm being induced to children via vaccines prompted more political, educational, legal, and social movements in a variety of ways involving parents.

Notably, parents of children with ASD utilized this hypothesis to themselves begin generating academic discussions and literature further reinforcing the plausibility of a vaccine–autism causal link, and to offer their own anecdotal experiences as evidence of this link[14] (Baker, 2008; Grinker, 2007; Kirby, 2005). As Baker (2008) noted:

> The hypothesis that thimerosal-containing vaccines could explain the remarkable rise in the prevalence of autism arose not among environmental scientists but among the communities that have emerged over the past 20 years of parents and professionals caring for autistic children. Specifically, parents and clinicians who have framed autism in biomedical terms (such as immune or gastrointestinal dysfunction) have been critical agents in promoting both the concept of the 'autism epidemic' and the primacy of

vaccines as its cause. The passion behind their arguments stems from a long history of advocacy on behalf of their children, often in the face of psychiatric theories perceived as 'parent blaming' and inadequately funded developmental and educational resources in many communities. (p. 248)

Pronouncements of the scientific role of engaged parents are often strong across blogs and advocacy websites, and in the published literature, with proclamations such as "Virtually every step forward of any consequence with respect to the scientific agenda has come from parents. This is a new phenomenon: direct scientific activism by parents using their own professional skills to aggressively take on anyone who makes arguments based on sloppy science to try to make this problem go away" (Mark Blaxill, quoted in Rock, 2004, p. 73). These parties most profoundly impacted were able to strongly vocalize the plausibility of such a causal link and to demand immediate research, social policy changes, and pursue litigation to address the issue (Baker, 2008; Glazer, 2003; Kirby, 2005). Acting as parent-experts on behalf of their children (the patient-victim), they often challenge established medical authorities, provide some level of resistance to dominant medical institutions, and "… assign lay experience a privileged status, and demand institutional, scientific, and cultural affirmation for their representation" of the etiology of their child's ASD (Furedi, 2006, p. 15; Maratea, 2009; Ryan & Cole, 2009).

DISCUSSION

The accumulated evidence suggesting no link of childhood ASD to MMR- or thimerosal-containing vaccines has not slowed the symbolic crusade of many parents and advocacy groups in positing this causal hypothesis, or at least the newer hypotheses of individual genetic susceptibility to vaccines or large quantities of vaccines administered in close time intervals (DeStefano, 2009; Fombonne, 2003; Normand & Dallery, 2007; Gross, 2009). Amidst the often fierce debate and controversy between and among academics, scientists, and parent-advocates/activists regarding diagnosis statistics and the scientific evidence on vaccine-induced autism over the past two decades, there are still notable social movements concerning vaccines, alternative treatments, experiences of celebrities and politicians with children diagnosed with ASD, and litigation involving families of affected children.[15]

Thousands of parents are still involved in litigation with the federal government arguing that thimerosal in vaccines caused their children to develop ASD (DeStefano, 2009; Gross, 2009; Normand & Dallery, 2007).

In 2009, several of the first of these cases were decided and the Office of Special Masters ruled that the scientific empirical evidence demonstrates that thimerosal and MMR vaccines do not have a causal link to autism.[16] As Fombonne (2003) remarked:

> ironically, what has triggered substantial social policy changes in autism appears to have little connection with the state of the science. Whether this will continue to be the case in the future remains to be seen, but further consideration should be given to how and to why the least evidence-based claims have achieved such impressive changes in funding policy. (pp. 88–89)

Having acquired significant social capital in educational realms and widespread public attention, at this point the "true" causes of the apparent increase in diagnosed ASD in childhood are not entirely irrelevant, but certainly not integral to the continuing power of the social movement.

In a relatively short span of time, the movements related to autism (e.g., increasing awareness, allocating educational funds and resources, legal avenues for parents, proclamations for changes to vaccines and other childhood medical interventions and their regimens) have proliferated. This should be the continued focus of sociologists interested in social movements and social problems construction when examining childhood ASD. Sociologists should examine how the issue has been able to sustain dramatic effect across several arenas even though there are strong, scientific counterclaims to the vaccine–autism hypothesis, as well studying how the rhetorical qualities, and the claims themselves, change as the movement progresses.

Autism is still prominently displayed in the venue of the popular media as a pressing issue of epidemic proportions (Gernsbacher et al., 2005). The popular media have, at various times and from a variety of sources, presented several sides of the controversy and debate concerning the increased prevalence of childhood ASD diagnoses and the potential causal factors for that increase, as well as information on new studies, treatments, court cases, etc. (Allen, 2007; DeNoon, 2006; Lilienfeld & Arkowitz, 2007; Martin, 2008; Sachs, 2008; Stobbe, 2007; Wallis, 2007). Within this venue and others, most importantly the Internet, the tension between parent-advocates and scientists, and their respective claims and rhetorical use of scientific information, should continue to be explored in future study (Davies et al., 2002). This chapter suggests that the rhetorical use of science in claims concerning childhood ASD is a major component of the claimsmaking enterprises on all sides of the issue, as evidence is consistently accepted, critiqued, embraced, and rejected in almost cyclical fashion by the various camps (Kirby, 2005). The very ideas of science, evidence, and causality, processes the public may have a limited understanding of (DeStefano, 2009; Offit, 2008), are at question and at the heart of the autism epidemic controversy (Blaxill, 2004). This controversy was grounded in a medicalized view of childhood development and reflects contemporary social and cultural perspectives on disordered human experience.

Furthermore, future research needs to look at how the hyperlinking and networking of the Internet, in addition to the rhetorical component of the claims made there, has a profound influence on the scientific information available and how it is presented and ultimately used by individuals and to facilitate local mobilization and efforts (Davies et al., 2002; Heininger, 2001; Offit, 2008; Schaffer, Kuczynski, & Skinner, 2008). There are numerous websites devoted to the issue of autism, ranging from more moderate informational websites of considerable size and resources (e.g., www.autismspeaks.org), to dynamic blogs where users can discuss and debate the issues of etiology and prevalence (e.g., http://autism.about.com/b/), to those that more strongly pronounce the role of vaccines in causing autism and describe alternative therapies (e.g., www.ageofautism.com, www.generationrescue.org, and www.safeminds.org). Indeed, some regard the Internet as a primary source of information for parents determined to learn more about their child's condition and experiences and mobilize for action (Grinker, 2007; Kirby, 2005; Madge & O'Connor, 2006; Poltorak et al., 2005; Sabo & Lorenzen, 2008; Schaffer et. al, 2008). As such, this is fertile ground for sociologists to analyze the use of the Internet in promoting dramatic effect toward the condition of autism and its function in social movements. The many blogs, advocacy websites, and news sources online (which often permit reactions in the form of blogs after an online article) are arenas with nearly unlimited carrying capacity for individuals and groups with any interest in the issue to promote their point of view through a variety of rhetorical devices and information control (DeStefano, 2009; Maratea, 2008).

NOTES

1. See Conrad and Potter (2000) and Stolzer (2007) for examinations of ADHD.
2. See Ganz (2006) for a comprehensive analysis of costs to families and larger society.
3. ASD include a variety of diagnoses also known as Pervasive Developmental Disorders.

4. During the publication process, the CDC released a newer prevalence estimate of 1 in 110 children diagnosed with an ASD. The rhetorical properties are the same as earlier estimates. See www.cdc.gov/ncbddd/autism/index.html.

5. See Glazer (2003) and Kirby (2005).

6. See www.autismspeaks.org and www.autism.com; also see www.nationalautismassociation.org/autismincreases.php for trend statistics by state. Any number of items in the published scientific and advocacy literature use the rate in introductory statements to describe the scope of the problem. Taken at face value, the 1 in 150 diagnosis rate, or the more current rate of 1 in 110, reflect less than 1% of all children.

7. Blaxill (2004) provides a counter-argument.

8. Some research suggests classifications such as PDD-NOS are the most widely used diagnoses recently (Best, 2008a; Gernsbacher et al., 2005). See Johnson et al. (2007) for a detailed description of the DSM criteria for PDD and ASD.

9. A similar example in recent years involves the apparent substantial increase in young African-American male suicides in the United States. Some argue that accidental and unspecified deaths in the past are now being classified as suicides, making the statistics on completed suicide look like a dramatic, increasing trend, but this trend could be an illusion (Best, 2004).

10. See Grether (2006), Baker (2008), and Fombonne (2008) for critiques of this hypothesis.

11. Some of the most vocal parent advocacy organizations championing this hypothesis include Generation Rescue at www.generationrescue.org, Safe Minds at www.safeminds.org, and The Autism Research Institute at www.autism.com.

12. For example, anecdotal evidence from parents regarding the onset of ASD after vaccination. See McCarthy (2008).

13. See www.autismspeaks.org, the website for the advocacy and awareness group Autism Speaks.

14. For example, see Bernard et al. (2001), Blaxill et al. (2004), and McCarthy (2008).

15. Recent brick and mortar movements concerning vaccines include the Green Our Vaccines march on Washington in June 2008. For information on a variety of alternative treatments, see www.autism.com and www.tacanow.org, and Lemer (2006) for discussion. Celebrities and politicians with children diagnosed with ASD are discussed in Begley (2009), Gross (2009) and Kirby (2005), as well as McCarthy (2007, 2008). Epstein (2005) discusses litigation involving families of affected children and the National Vaccine Injury Compensation Program, as do Normand and Dallery (2007). Furthermore, see www.neurodiversity.com for a wealth of information on recent decisions of the vaccine injury court.

16. See the federal website at www.uscfc.uscourts.gov/node/2718 and www.neurodiversity.com for links to various federal documents.

ACKNOWLEDGMENTS

The author thanks Joel Best and Ray Maratea for helpful suggestions and resources.

REFERENCES

Allen, A. (2007). The autism numbers: Why there's no epidemic. *Slate*, 15 January, viewed 13 November 2008. Available at: www.slate.com/id/2157496/

American Psychiatric Association. (1994). *Diagnostic and statistical manual of mental disorders* (4th ed.). Washington, DC: American Psychiatric Association.

American Psychiatric Association. (2000). *Diagnostic and statistical manual of mental disorders* (4th ed., text revision). Washington, DC: American Psychiatric Association.

Baker, J. P. (2008). Mercury, vaccines, and autism: One controversy, three histories. *American Journal of Public Health*, 98(2), 244–253.

Begley, S. (2009). The vaccine-autism scare. *Newsweek*, 2 March, pp. 43–48.

Bernard, S., Enayati, A., Redwood, L., Roger, H., & Binstock, T. (2001). Autism: A novel form of mercury poisoning. *Medical Hypotheses*, 56(4), 462–471.

Best, J. (1987). Rhetoric in claimsmaking: Constructing the missing children problem. *Social Problems*, 34(2), 101–121.

Best, J. (1990). *Threatened children: Rhetoric and concern about child-victims*. Chicago: University of Chicago Press.

Best, J. (2001). *Damned lies and statistics: Untangling numbers from the media, politicians, and activists*. Berkeley, CA: University of California Press.

Best, J. (2004). *More damned lies and statistics: How numbers confuse public issues*. Berkeley, CA: University of California Press.

Best, J. (2008a). *Stat-spotting: A field guide to identifying dubious data*. Berkeley, CA: University of California Press.

Best, J. (2008b). *Social problems*. New York: W.W. Norton & Company.

Bishop, D. V. M., Whitehouse, A. J. O., Watt, H. J., & Line, E. A. (2008). Autism and diagnostic substitution: Evidence from a study of adults with a history of developmental language disorder. *Developmental Medicine & Child Neurology*, 50(5), 341–345.

Blaxill, M. F. (2004). What's going on: The question of time trends in autism. *Public Health Reports*, 119(6), 536–551.

Blaxill, M. F., Redwood, L., & Bernard, S. (2004). Thimerosal and autism: A plausible hypothesis that should not be dismissed. *Medical Hypotheses*, 62(5), 788–794.

Blumer, H. (1971). Social problems as collective behavior. *Social Problems*, 18(3), 298–306.

Boyle, C. A., Bertrand, J., & Yeargin-Allsopp, M. (1999). Surveillance of autism. *Infants and Young Children*, 12(2), 75–78.

Brock, S. E. (2006). An examination of the changing rates of autism in special education. *The California School Psychologist*, 11, 31–40.

Conrad, P. (2007). *The medicalization of society: On the transformation of human conditions into treatable disorders*. Baltimore, MD: The Johns Hopkins University Press.

Conrad, P., & Potter, D. (2000). From hyperactive children to ADHD adults: Observations on the expansion of medical categories. *Social Problems*, 47(4), 559–582.

Croen, L. A., Grether, J. K., Hoogstrate, J., & Selvin, S. (2002). The changing prevalence of autism in California. *Journal of Autism and Developmental Disorders*, 32(3), 207–215.

Davies, P., Chapman, S., & Leask, J. (2002). Antivaccination activists on the world wide web. *Archives of Disease in Childhood*, 87(1), 22–25.

DeNoon, D. J. (2006). *Researchers question autism 'epidemic'*. Fox News, 3 April, viewed 7 June 2008. Available at: www.foxnews.com/story/0,2933,190393,00.html

DeStefano, F. (2009). Thimerosal containing vaccines: Evidence versus public apprehension. *Expert Opinion on Drug Safety, 8*(1), 1–4.

Doja, A., & Roberts, W. (2006). Immunizations and autism: A review of the literature. *Canadian Journal of Neurological Sciences, 33*(4), 341–346.

Edelson, S. (2007). The Autism Research Institute and Defeat Autism Now!: Who we are, and what we do. *Autism Research Review International, 21*(3), viewed 13 November 2008. Available at: www.autism.com/ari/editorials/ed_aridan.htm.

Epstein, R. A. (2005). It did happen here: Fear and loathing on the vaccine trail. *Health Affairs, 24*(3), 740–743.

Filipek, P. A., Accardo, P. J., Baranek, G. T., Cook, E. H., Jr., Dawson, G., Gordon, B., Gravel, J. S., Johnson, C. P., Kallen, R. J., Levy, S. E., Minshew, N. J., Prizant, B. M., Rapin, I., Rogers, S. J., Stone, W. L., Teplin, S., Tuchman, R. F., & Volkmar, F. R. (1999). The screening and diagnosis of autism spectrum disorders. *Journal of Autism and Developmental Disorders, 29*(6), 439–484.

Fitzpatrick, M. (2004). *MMR and autism.* New York: Routledge.

Fombonne, E. (2001). Is there an epidemic of autism? *Pediatrics, 107*(2), 411–413.

Fombonne, E. (2002). Epidemiological trends in rates of autism. *Molecular Psychiatry, 7*(Suppl. 2), S4–S6.

Fombonne, E. (2003). The prevalence of autism. *JAMA, 289*(1), 87–89.

Fombonne, E. (2005). The changing epidemiology of autism. *Journal of Applied Research in Intellectual Disabilities, 18,* 281–294.

Fombonne, E. (2008). Thimerosal disappears but autism remains. *Archives of General Psychiatry, 65*(1), 15–16.

Fombonne, E., Zakarian, R., Bennett, A., Meng, L., & McLean-Heywood, D. (2006). Pervasive developmental disorders in Montreal, Quebec, Canada: Prevalence and links with immunizations. *Pediatrics, 118*(1), e139–e150.

Frankish, H. (2001). Report finds no link between thimerosal and neurodevelopmental disorders. *The Lancet, 358*(9288), 1163.

Furedi, F. (2006). The end of professional dominance. *Society, 43*(6), 14–18.

Ganz, M. L. (2006). The costs of autism. In: S. O. Moldin & J. L. R. Rubenstein (Eds), *Understanding autism: From basic neuroscience to treatment.* New York: Taylor & Francis.

Geier, D. A., King, P. G., Sykes, L. K., & Geier, M. R. (2008). A comprehensive review of mercury provoked autism. *Indian Journal of Medical Research, 128*(4), 383–411.

Gernsbacher, M. A., Dawson, M., & Goldsmith, H. H. (2005). Three reasons not to believe in an autism epidemic. *Current Directions in Psychological Science, 14*(2), 55–58.

Gillberg, C. (1999). Prevalence of disorders in the autism spectrum. *Infants and Young Children, 12*(2), 64–74.

Glazer, S. (2003). Increase in autism: Is there an epidemic or just better diagnosis? *The CQ Researcher, 13*(23), 545–568.

Grether, J. K. (2006). Epidemiology of autism: Current controversies and research directions. *Clinical Neuroscience Research, 6*(3–4), 119–126.

Grinker, R. R. (2007). *Unstrange minds: Remapping the world of autism.* New York: Basic Books.

Gross, L. (2009). A broken trust: Lessons from the vaccine–autism wars. *PLoS Biology, 7*(5), e1000114, pp. 1–7, viewed 14 July 2009, available at: www.plosbiology.org

Guralnick, M. J. (2005). Early intervention for children with intellectual disabilities: Current knowledge and future prospects. *Journal of Applied Research in Intellectual Disabilities, 18*(4), 313–324.

Gusfield, J. R. (1981). *The culture of public problems: Drinking–driving and the symbolic order.* Chicago: University of Chicago Press.

Heininger, U. (2001). World wide wasting? *Archives of Disease in Childhood, 85*(1), 46.

Hilgartner, S., & Bosk, C. L. (1988). The rise and fall of social problems: A public arenas model. *The American Journal of Sociology, 94*(1), 53–78.

Hviid, A., Stellfeld, M., Wohlfahrt, J., & Melbye, M. (2003). Association between thimerosal-containing vaccine and autism. *JAMA, 290*(13), 1763–1766.

Institute of Medicine. (2004). *Immunization safety review: Vaccines and autism.* Washington, DC: National Academies Press.

Ip, P., Wong, V., Ho, M., Lee, J., & Wong, W. (2004). Mercury exposure in children with autistic spectrum disorder: Case–control study. *Journal of Child Neurology, 19*(6), 431–434.

Johnson, C. P., Myers, S., & The Council on Children with Disabilities. (2007). Identification and evaluation of children with autism spectrum disorders. *Pediatrics, 120*(5), 1183–1215.

Katz, S. L. (2006). Has the measles–mumps–rubella vaccine been fully exonerated? *Pediatrics, 118*, 1744–1745.

Kirby, D. (2005). *Evidence of harm: Mercury in vaccines and the autism epidemic: A medical controversy.* New York: St. Martin's Griffin Press.

Lemer, P. S. (2006). How recent changes have contributed to an epidemic of autism spectrum disorders. *Journal of Behavioral Optometry, 17*(3), 72–77.

Lilienfeld, S. O., & Arkowitz, H. (2007). Is there really an autism epidemic? A closer look at the statistics suggests something more than a simple rise in incidence. *Scientific American, 6* December, viewed 7 June 2008. Available at: www.scientificamerican.com/article.cfm?id=is-there-really-an-autism-epidemic

Madge, C., & O'Connor, H. (2006). Parenting gone wired: Empowerment of new mothers on the internet? *Social & Cultural Geography, 7*(2), 199–220.

Maratea, R. (2008). The e-rise and fall of social problems: The blogosphere as a public arena. *Social Problems, 55*(1), 139–159.

Maratea, R. (2009). Virtual claimsmaking: The role of the Internet in constructing social problems. PhD dissertation, University of Delaware, Newark, DE.

Martin, D. (2008). Vaccine-autism question divides parents, scientists. *CNN*, 24 March, viewed on February 5, 2009. Available at: http://www.cnn.com/2008/HEALTH/conditions/03/24/autismvaccines/index.html

Matson, J. L., & Minshawi, N. F. (2006). *Early intervention for autism spectrum disorders: A critical analysis.* New York: Elsevier.

McCarthy, J. (2007). *Louder than words: A mother's journey in healing autism.* New York: Dutton.

McCarthy, J. (2008). *Mother warriors: A nation of parents healing autism against all odds.* New York: Dutton.

Moldin, S. O., & Rubenstein, J. L. R. (2006). Foreword. In: S. O. Moldin & J. L. R. Rubenstein (Eds), *Understanding autism: From basic neuroscience to treatment.* New York: Taylor & Francis.

Molloy, H., & Vasil, L. (2002). The social construction of Asperger syndrome: The pathologising of difference? *Disability & Society, 17*(6), 659–669.

Moyer, D., & Clignet, R. (1980). Social problems in science and for science. *Science Communication, 2*(1), 93–116.

National Institute of Mental Health. (2008). *Autism spectrum disorders: Pervasive developmental disorders.* U.S. Department of Health and Human Services, viewed 13 November 2008. Available at: www.nimh.nih.gov/health/publications/autism/complete-index.shtml

Newschaffer, C. J., Croen, L. A., Daniels, J., Giarelli, E., Grether, J. K., Levy, S. E., Mandell, D. S., Miller, L. A., Pinto-Martin, J., Reaven, J., Reynolds, A. M., Rice, C. E., Schendel, D., & Windham, G. C. (2007). The epidemiology of autism spectrum disorders. *Annual Review of Public Health*, *28*(1), 235–258.

Normand, M., & Dallery, J. (2007). Mercury rising: Exposing the vaccine–autism myth. *Skeptic*, *13*(3), 32–36.

Offit, P. A. (2008). *Autism's false prophets: Bad science, risky medicine, and the search for a cure.* New York: Columbia University Press.

Offit, P. A., & Moser, C. A. (2009). The problem with Dr. Bob's alternative vaccine schedule. *Pediatrics*, *123*(1), e164–e169.

Ouellette-Kuntz, H., Coo, H., Lloyd, J. E. V., Kasmara, L., Holden, J. J. A., & Lewis, M. E. S. (2007). Trends in special education code assignment for autism: Implications for prevalence estimates. *Journal of Autism and Developmental Disorders*, *37*(10), 1941–1948.

Ozonoff, S., & Cathcart, K. (1998). Effectiveness of a home program intervention for young children with autism. *Journal of Autism and Developmental Disorders*, *28*(1), 25–32.

Poltorak, M., Leach, M., Fairhead, J., & Cassell, J. (2005). 'MMR talk' and vaccination choices: An ethnographic study in Brighton. *Social Science & Medicine*, *61*(3), 709–719.

Poulson, S. (2009). Autism, through a social lens. *Contexts*, *8*(2), 40–45.

Rock, A. (2004). Toxic tipping point. *Mother Jones*, *29*(2), 70–77.

Ryan, S., & Cole, K. R. (2009). From advocate to activist? Mapping the experiences of mothers of children on the autism spectrum. *Journal of Applied Research in Intellectual Disabilities*, *22*(1), 43–53.

Sabo, R. M., & Lorenzen, J. M. (2008). Consumer health websites for parents of children with autism. *Journal of Consumer Health on the Internet*, *12*(1), 37–49.

Sachs, J. S. (2008). *Vaccines: Separating fact from fiction*, CNN, viewed 9 November 2008. Available at: www.cnn.com/2008/HEALTH/family/11/05/par.vaccine.kids

Samms-Vaughan, M., & Franklyn-Banton, L. (2008). The role of early childhood professionals in the early identification of autistic disorder. *International Journal of Early Years Education*, *16*(1), 75–84.

Schaffer, R., Kuczynski, K., & Skinner, D. (2008). Producing genetic knowledge and citizenship through the Internet: Mothers, pediatric genetics, and cybermedicine. *Sociology of Health & Illness*, *30*(1), 145–159.

Schechter, R., & Grether, J. K. (2008). Continuing increases in autism reported to California's developmental services system: Mercury in retrograde. *Archives of General Psychiatry*, *65*(1), 19–24.

Shevell, M., & Fombonne, E. (2006). Autism and MMR vaccination or thimerosal exposure: An urban legend? *Canadian Journal of Neurological Sciences*, *33*(4), 339–340.

Smukler, D. (2005). Unauthorized minds: How 'theory of mind' theory misrepresents autism. *Mental Retardation*, *43*(1), 11–24.

Spector, M., & Kitsuse, J. I. (1977). *Constructing social problems.* Menlo Park, CA: Cummings.

Stehr-Green, P., Tull, P., Stellfeld, M., Mortenson, P., & Simpson, D. (2003). Autism and thimerosal-containing vaccines: Lack of consistent evidence for an association. *American Journal of Preventive Medicine*, *25*(2), 101–106.

Stobbe, M. (2007). *Autism 'epidemic' may all be in the label. MSNBC.* The Associated Press, 4 November, viewed 7 June 2008. Available at: www.msnbc.msn.com/id/21600784

Stolzer, J. M. (2007). The ADHD epidemic in America. *Ethical Human Psychology and Psychiatry*, *9*(2), 109–116.

Stoner, J. B., & Angell, M. E. (2006). Parent perspectives on role engagement: An investigation of parents of children with ASD and their self-reported roles with education professionals. *Focus on Autism and Other Developmental Disabilities, 21*(3), 177–189.

Wakefield, A. J., Murch, S. H., Anthony, A., Linnell, J., Casson, D. M., Malik, M., Berelowitz, M., Dhillon, A. P., Thomson, M. A., Harvey, P., Valentine, A., Davies, S. E., & Walker-Smith, J. A. (1998). Ileal-lymphoid-nodular hyperplasia, non-specific colitis, and pervasive developmental disorder in children. *The Lancet, 351*(9103), 637–641.

Wallis, C. (2007). Is the autism epidemic a myth? *Time,* 12 January, viewed 7 June 2008. Available at: www.time.com/time/magazine/article/0,9171,1576829,00.html

Wazana, A., Bresnahan, M., & Kline, J. (2007). The autism epidemic: Fact or artifact? *Journal of the American Academy of Child and Adolescent Psychiatry, 46*(6), 721–730.

Wing, L. (2005). Reflections on opening Pandora's box. *Journal of Autism and Developmental Disorders, 35*(2), 197–203.

Yeargin-Allsopp, M., Rice, C., Karapurkan, T., Doemberg, N., Boyle, C., & Murphy, C. (2003). The prevalence of autism in a US metropolitan area. *JAMA, 289*(1), 49–55.

PART IV
THE USES AND MISUSES OF
AN EPIDEMIC MODEL FOR
PSYCHIATRIC AND BEHAVIORAL
ISSUES

BIPOLAR DISORDER AND THE MEDICALIZATION OF MOOD: AN EPIDEMICS OF DIAGNOSIS?

Antonio Maturo

ABSTRACT

Purpose – *Over the last years, in the United States there has been significant increase in the consumption of pharmaceuticals for the treatment of mental disorders. More specifically, the number of clinical diagnosis of bipolar disorders in young people has increased by 40 times over the last 10 years. The purpose of this chapter is to analyse the growth of bipolar disorder diagnosis using a sociological frame.*

Methodology/approach – *The methodology is based on the concepts proposed by the 'conflictualist' perspective of medical sociology. Medicalization, that is, the extension of medical categories in everyday life, is the main concept on which the chapter is constructed. The 'syndromization' of the* Diagnostic and Statistical Manual of Mental Disorders *lowers the threshold above which someone may be diagnosed with bipolarism. Moreover, advertisements push people to seek for pharmaceutical treatment for conditions of 'normal' sadness.*

Findings – *This work shows the importance of the analysis of 'medical' phenomena by approaches taken from social sciences. Bipolar disorder*

Understanding Emerging Epidemics: Social and Political Approaches
Advances in Medical Sociology, Volume 11, 225–242
Copyright © 2010 by Emerald Group Publishing Limited
All rights of reproduction in any form reserved
ISSN: 1057-6290/doi:10.1108/S1057-6290(2010)0000011016

can be a terrible and painful disease, but it seems that there is the possibility that it is over-diagnosed.

Contribution to the field – *In this epidemics of diagnosis of bipolar disorder it is central to integrate the medical perspective with other dimensions: the classification of mental disease, the advertisement for drugs and the cultural aspects of a given society.*

1. INTRODUCTION

Over the last years, the United States has had a strong increase in the consumption of pharmaceuticals for the treatment of anxiety, bipolar disorder and depression (Loe, 2008). This 'medicalization of the emotions' is just a part of a larger process of medicalization of everyday life which encompasses many dimensions: sexuality, physical and psychological performance, birth, death, ageing and prevention (Conrad, 2007). The growth of medicalization is fuelled by many forces, not only economic ones (Clarke & Shim, 2009). The American culture, with its emphasis on the pursuit of happiness and on pragmatism, may push the use of psychotropic drugs: a quick and easy answer to sadness (Barker, 2009; Lane, 2007; Satel, 2006; Kleinman, 1988). Yet, the emphasis on the biological aspects of mental disorders removes any link between the socio-economic context and mental and physical health. The main consequence of this trend is the individualization of social problems and the de-politicization of health policy (Illich, 1976). The latest versions of the *Diagnostic and Statistical Manual of Mental Disorders* (*DSM III and IV*), putting symptoms before causes, seem to be part of the same pattern (Horwitz & Wakefield, 2009). Indeed, the 'syndromization' of the *DSM* lowers the threshold above which someone may get a diagnosis of bipolarism (Maturo, 2009). In this scenario, it is not surprising that the incidence of the diagnosis for bipolar disorder increases fast (Moreno et al., 2007). The big number of advertisements of pharmaceuticals contributes to increase the situations in which a person will consider himself/herself as affected by a mood disorder (Murray, 2009).

2. THE 'EPIDEMICS' OF BIPOLAR DISORDER

According to a research published in the *Archives of General Psychiatry* in September 2007, the number of clinical diagnosis of bipolar disorders in young people[1] increased 40 times in 10 years (Moreno et al., 2007). The estimated annual number of youth-office-based visits with a diagnosis of bipolar disorder:

> increased from 25 (1994–1995) to 1003 (2002–2003) visits per 100 000 population, and adult visits with a diagnosis of bipolar disorder increased from 905 to 1679 visits per 100 000 population during this period. (…) most youth (90.6%) and adults (86.4%) received a psychotropic medication during bipolar disorder visits, with comparable rates of mood stabilizers, antipsychotics, and antidepressant prescribed for both age groups. (Moreno et al., 2007, p. 1032)

The prevalence of bipolar disorder in youth would be, according to these figures, 1%. The astonishing increase in paediatric bipolar disorder might be interpreted in two alternative ways: 'either bipolar disorder was historically underdiagnosed in children and adolescents and that problem has now being rectified, or bipolar disorder is currently being overdiagnosed in this age group' (Moreno et al., 2007, p. 1035). Some scholars have no doubts: 'Awareness among general practitioners and psychiatrists that the broad clinical spectrum of bipolar disorders probably affects 5% of the population – rather than the often quoted figure of 1% – is regrettably low' (Smith, Ghaemi, & Craddock, 2008, p. 398). But thankfully: 'childhood bipolar disorder has been regularly featured in the popular press. These developments may have raised clinical and public awareness and promoted appropriate treatment seeking and clinical recognition of the condition at the earlier ages' (Moreno et al., 2007, p. 1036).

An article which pushes for an 'appropriate' treatment seeking is the one of the *New York Times Magazine* of 29 October 2006, six pages dedicated to it. The title of the supplement was: *From Cause to Cure* – taking for granted that BD is the result of one cause. The beginning was like a gothic-novel: 'No matter how much you learn about bipolar disorder, it's still mysterious and frightening …' (p. 24). However, regarding the cause of bipolar disorder, in the main article, *Bipolar Disorder: The Emotional Roller Coaster*, there are not many clues: 'Scientists aren't sure what causes bipolar disorder, but suspect that it may be caused by many different genes acting together, combined with other personal and environmental factors. Brain-imaging studies suggest that the brains of people with bipolar disorder may differ from those of healthy individuals' (p. 24).

But what are the symptoms of bipolar disorder? Referring to the National Institute of Mental Health (NIMH), the (unknown) authors state that in order to have a diagnosis of a manic episode (the basis of BD), elevated mood must occur 'with three or more of the other symptoms most of the day, nearly every day for one week or longer'.

The symptoms include:

> increased energy, activity and restlessness; excessively "high", overly good, euphoric mood; extreme irritability; racing thoughts and talking very fast, jumping from one idea to another; distractibility, can't concentrate well; little sleep needed; unrealistic beliefs in one's abilities and power; poor judgement; spending sprees; a lasting period of behavior that is different from usual; increased sexual drive; abuse of drugs, particularly cocaine, alcohol and sleeping medications; provocative, intrusive or aggressive behavior; denial that anything is wrong. (p. 26)

Without going further into the analysis, it can be noted that the symptoms are very heterogeneous, vague and of different levels. For instance, abuse of sleeping medications is not comparable with distractibility (a quite common condition). Moreover, if one takes cocaine, he/she can expect to experience many of the other symptoms – them being an effect of cocaine taking or of the craving.

But, on the other hand, there are no doubts about the therapy: two pages advertise for a pharmaceutical. In the first page of the advertisements, the ethiological gap, which is the lack of the nexus between causes and effects, is clearly confessed: 'ABILIFY may work by adjusting dopamine activity, instead of completely blocking it and by adjusting serotonin activity. However, the exact way any medicine for bipolar disorder works is unknown' (p. 21). The last four lines of the whole supplement dedicated to bipolar disorder softly suggest that: 'In addition to medications, psychotherapy is useful' (p. 28).

The question at stake here is not the existence of bipolar disorder. Probably, some people really suffer from these symptoms. But, at the same time, I argue that *in the United States there is a strong pressure to enlarge the pathological sphere*. An evidence of that is the increase of the mental conditions considered as pathologies, in the last version of the *DSM* (Horwitz, 2007). Dissatisfaction, anxiety and bad moods may not be ipso facto, that is, automatically, transformed into diseases, but there is a strong spur to consider these conditions as symptoms which could be the sign of something more dangerous (Moynihan & Cassels, 2005). According to Christopher Lane, a research professor at Northwestern University: 'By giving "social phobia" the more patient-friendly name "social anxiety" and by greatly expanding its parameters to cast the problem as one of fear, not avoidance, the *DSM* task forces significantly lowered the bar for the FDA and drug manufacturers' (2007, p. 137).

In the United States, the huge number of commercials for drugs (Murray, 2009) exhorts people to self-observation: 'consumers encouraged by DTC advertising ask their doctor whether they have the disorder they saw in a magazine or on television, and perhaps they request a particular medication' (Conrad, 2007, p. 155). A careful attention on people's body signs is the suggested path for a continuous self-diagnosis process (Murray, 2009). Everyone is a potential patient and therefore an effective consumer.[2]

The bipolar disorder – evoked, advertised and deconstructed into consistent narrative – is an example of the way by which an emotional state can be framed and 'formatted' as a pathology. In other words, the social construction of bipolar disorder lets an undefined sense of illness become a codified and objective entity of disease. A 'label' that can be read and faced and simplified by a pill. Therefore, the 'epidemics' of bipolar disorders could also be the result of the extension of the conditions under which someone can be considered sick, along with a worrisome empirical phenomenon. Indeed, there are few doubts that the last versions of the *DSM* (III and IV) have made difficult to distinguish between depressive disorders and 'normal' sadness (Horwitz & Wakefield, 2009). For this reason, it can be argued that medicine – more or less voluntary – has made possible the medicalization of unhappiness.

3. MEDICALIZATION THEORY

'Once upon a time, plenty of children were unruly, some adults were shy, and bald men wore hats. Now all of these descriptions might be attributed to diseases – entities with names, diagnostic criteria, and an increasing array of therapeutic options'. This is the ironic beginning of the article on medicalization written by McLellan (2007, p. 627).

Medicalization can be described as the process by which medical categories are used to frame and give sense to non-medical aspects of life – non-medical until that moment. Conrad defines medicalization as 'a process by which nonmedical problems become defined and treated as a medical problem' (2007, p. 4). Similarly, Clarke, Mamo, Fishman, Shim, and Fosket (2003, p. 161) see medicalization 'as the processes through which aspects of life outside the jurisdiction of medicine come to be construed as medical problems – one of the most potent social transformations of the last half of the twentieth century in the west'. According to McLellan (2007, p. 627) medicalization refers to 'the process by which certain events or characteristics of everyday life become medical issues, and thus come within the purview of doctors and other health professionals to engage with, study, and treat'.

This concept became popular thanks to the prominent sociologist Ivan Illich. According to Illich (1976), the medical monopoly on health care and on the definition of what can be considered normal and what is pathological has 'expropriated' people from their health. Medicine has colonized aspects of life which once were not considered pathological. Moreover, doctors decide who is sick, who has more chance to become sick and how sick people should be cured.

Illich (1976) is also popular for the concept of iatrogenesis. This concept affirms that the capitalist health-care organization produces pathology, that is, medicine produces illness (*iatros* means *healer* in ancient Greek). Illich distinguishes three kinds of iatrogenesis: clinical iatrogenesis, social iatrogenesis and cultural iatrogenesis. By clinical iatrogenesis, Illich refers to malpractice, clinical errors and collateral effects. The social iatrogenesis derives directly from the organization of care which tends to be pathogenic because medicine creates labels for many conditions which are not pathological in themselves (adolescence, stress and birth). The cultural iatrogenesis has to do mainly with the experience of pain. In Western society, medicine tries to consider pain and sorrow as conditions that should be treated and not as conditions that in some cases are natural answers to difficult situations. Speaking more broadly, according to Illich, illness is a condition 'invented' in order to justify and legitimate the status quo. People would rise up if their pathologies could not be explained as a biological impairment rather than the effect of unhealthy lifestyles caused by an oppressive social system (Bury, 2000).

Even if Illich's proposal depicts a passive subject completely determined by the economic structures, it offers even today an elegant framework to analyse the medicalization process. Indeed, if social iatrogenesis could be considered as the medicalization in its broad sense, because it coincides with the extension of the medical categories into everyday life, cultural iatrogenesis, with its emphasis on internal pain, might be connected with the 'medicalization of unhappiness' simplified by the features of the *Prozac Nation* (Wurtzel, 1995), that is, the growing incapability to accept unpleasant emotions in everyday life (Barker, 2009). Lastly, the clinical medicalization reminds us that drugs also have (many) collateral effects – for instance, the ones on children treated with Ritalin (DeGrandpre, 1999).

We have many examples of medicalization: attention-deficit hyperactivity disorder (ADHD), post-traumatic stress disorder (PTSD), panic attacks, social anxiety, generalized anxiety disorder, erectile dysfunction, breast augmentation, sexuality and andropause. Besides new diagnosis, which *extended* the Foucaultian 'clinical gaze' in new fields (ageing, for instance), we also face the *expansion* of the pathological sphere with regard to bio-physical conditions (Conrad, 2007, p. 24). Examples of expansion are hypertension and cholesterol. A few years ago, a commission modified the definition of high blood pressure (Angell, 2003). We consider hypertension a blood pressure above 140/90 mmHg, but the experts proposed a new disease, or a 'quasi-disease', called pre-hypertension in those whose blood pressure ranged between 120/80 and 140/90 mmHg. For this reason, in one night millions of people became patients and therefore health consumers (Moynihan & Cassels, 2005). This expansion of the definition for a disease opened a new market: the medicalization of prevention.

Paradoxically, the increasing medicalization process is not always promoted by doctors. In some cases, medicalization can also lead to a loss of power and autonomy of the medical profession. According to Metzel (2007) and Hollon (2005), direct-to-consumer advertisements for prescription medication reduce the asymmetry in patient/physician relationship theorized by Parsons (1951) and create a new form of 'empowerment' of the patient.

For this reason medicalization cannot be considered a synonym to the 'professional dominance' proposed by Freidson (1970). According to this scholar, the 'golden age of doctoring' – more or less from the 1950s to the end of the 1970s – was characterized by the physicians' control on the contents of their work. Moreover, they also controlled other health professions (nurses, for instance) and, of course, they had the sovereignty on the scientific territory being the ones who defined what was normal and what was pathological. Not to mention, the power on the patients and the high asymmetry of doctor/patient relationship (Parsons, 1951). In the United States, during the 1980s and 1990s, the rise of managed care weakened the power of the physicians, transferring some power on financial corporations (private insurances and HMOs) (Light, 2000). Together with this shift, also consumerism can be considered as a factor which contributed to a more balanced relationship between the physician and the patient (consumer). The direct-to-consumer advertisements which were deregulated in 1997 in the United States have re-shaped the expectations of the patients in the physician's surgery. In a survey, the FDA found out that 47% of physicians felt pressured by patients to prescribe advertised drugs and 62% of physicians had experienced tension between themselves and their patients due to DTC advertisements (Aikin, 2003). Intra-professionally, it can be noted that the 'Prozac era' was fuelled by family doctors who created the new market of mild disorders and this caused great tension between them and the psychiatrists (Dworkin, 2006). Some scholars indeed propose to substitute medicalization with *pharmacologization* (Conrad, 2000).

4. THE MEDICALIZATION OF UNHAPPINESS

In his famous book *Artificial Happiness*, Ronald W. Dworkin, a science journalist, referring to IMS Health site[3] statistics, describes how from 1988 to 1998 the prescription rate for psychotropic drugs tripled in the United States, with antidepressants accounting for most of the increase. What is surprising, at least at a first glance, is that non-psychiatrists wrote 75% of the new antidepressant prescriptions during that period (Dworkin, 2006, p. 34). This holds true also for more recent times. For example, in 2005 psychiatrists wrote only 29.3% of the total amount of prescriptions (Stagnitti, 2008).

The fact is that, some decades ago, the primary care doctors 'snatched' the battle against unhappiness from the psychiatrists. Primary care doctors, in the 1970s, were able to invent the 'unhappiness disease' (Dworkin, 2006, p. 29):

> Primary care doctors suffered during the twentieth century as their sphere of responsibility shrank and that of specialists grew. Treating unhappiness with drugs reversed this trend, turning the care of unhappiness into a high-tech science that primary care doctors could practice on their own without consulting specialists.

This situation started in the 1960s, when primary care doctors experienced a professional crisis. The big health emergencies had passed, and the rise of a more and more technology-based medicine had decreased their importance (Dworkin, 2006, pp. 29–31). The sign of modernity was represented by huge hospitals and their technological devices (Clarke & Shim, 2009). In this context, the distance between medicine and patients, as noticed by Illich (1976), widened. This period was also characterized by grassroot movements which asked for a de-psychiatrization of mental illness, a less stigmatizing approach to mentally disabled people and a more community-based care (Goffman, 1961, 1963).

The macro-scenario was one of a rapidly changing world with a steady economic growth, but more likely to be anomic. A world which generated anxiety and discontent. Coherently, the patients who entered physician surgery were more sane, but also more unhappy. In some cases, doctors referred the patients to psychiatrists but time after time they realized that they could also do something themselves. Being referred to a psychiatrist was quite stigmatizing at that time (Goffman, 1963) and often patients did not have serious impairment but only bad feelings deriving from everyday troubles; they were *worried wells*.[4] In brief, patients asked to be cured (but not by a psychiatrist) and primary care doctors were looking for new territories. Demands and supply met, no matter from which side you considered them. Yet, there was also a third component in the interaction: pharmaceutical corporations. The prescriptions for tranquilizers like Valium and Librium raised dramatically in the mid-1960s (Dworkin, 2006, pp. 32–34). The advertisements at that time were still directed only to the physicians, and revealed the assumptions pharmaceutical companies wanted to foster: 'While specialist advertisements at the time struck a more sober tone, they nonetheless insisted that tranquilizing anxious patients was the best way of turning them into happy, smiling people' (Lane, 2007, p. 107). The pay-off of the *Serentil* advertisement published in *Medical News* in 1970[5] was quite uncanny: *for the anxiety that comes from not fitting in* and the description of the 'causes' even more:

> The newcomer in town who *can't* make friends. The organization man who *can't* adjust to altered status within his company. The woman who *can't* get along with her new daughter-in-law. The executive who *can't* accept retirement. These common adjustment problems of our society are frequently intolerable for the disordered personality, who often responds with excessive anxiety. Serentil is suggested for *this* type of patient. Not simply because its tranquilizing action can ease anxiety and tension, but because it benefits personality disorders in general. And because it has not been found habituating. (Italics in the original)

However, the advertisement had to be withdrawn by Sandoz because the Subcommittee on Intergovernmental Relations to Study the Safety and Effectiveness of New Drugs considered the advertisement a troubling example of overreach. Indeed, as mesoridazine is a powerful phenothiazine, the Subcommittee decided that it was 'inappropriate for the use for problems of everyday living'.[6]

These examples show that sometimes sadness is a normal reaction to difficult situations. It is natural to experience stress after a loss, for instance, which is a 'good' stress (*eustress*). Trying to cure a normal and maybe 'healthy' sadness by medication means acting on the symptoms pretending that causes do not exist. This attitude is close to the concept of cultural iatrogenesis proposed by Illich (1976), that is, a growing incapability to accept sorrow. Today, as physical suffering due to starvation or wars has declined in rich countries, new needs are emerging. *Cosmetic psychopharmacology* is the label used to indicate pharmaceuticals which act on the level of serotonin circulating in the brain. Increasing the level of serotonin creates

ANTONIO MATURO

positive feelings even if things are going badly in the 'real' world. Prozac might be considered as the hallmark of cosmetic psychopharmacology, even if now there are many drugs which induce artificial happiness. There are also pharmaceuticals which do not affect emotion, but cognition: that is, cognitive enhancers (Miah, 2009; Greely et al., 2008). These drugs increase neuronal activation likely to enhance concentration and memory. According to Rose (2007), the driving force boosting self-enhancement derives from the liberal ideology. Liberalism emphasizes the power of the individual in shaping his/her own destiny. Thanks to our choices we can also shape our future. Not even biology, that is, nature, can be an obstacle to the human will. Maybe the constitutional right to pursue happiness represents a cultural archetype which has justified a heavy use of artificial instruments in order to overcome biological limits. Barker (2009), referring to Kleinman (1988), argues that 'notions of "personal freedom" and "the pursuit of happiness" combine to create a belief among Americans that they have a right to be free of pain. So strong is this belief, in fact, that Americans assume that a lack of suffering is the normative standard to which all Americans are entitled' (Barker, 2009, p. 106).

5. THE EXTENSION OF THE PATHOLOGICAL SPHERE

Up to now we have seen that there are economic forces which lead to pathologizing everyday troubles. We have also noticed that the social representations of health are nowadays, especially in the United States and in rich countries, very close to the ones of happiness. Indeed, the boundaries between the two dimensions are blurred. Since 1997, the legislation on health commercials has less restrictions and this has led to a proliferation of commercials for drugs on television and in newspapers. Finally, we have taken into consideration which roles, economic forces, cultural predispositions and media representations play in the medicalization of everyday life. But what is the role of science in this context? What is the 'position' of the scientific discipline which should shed light on what is normal and what is pathological, that is, psychiatry?

To put it briefly, I am aligned with the words written by Horwitz and Wakefield in describing the onset of the medicalization of mood: 'There is no evidence that pharmaceutical companies had a role in developing *DSM-III* diagnostic criteria. Yet, serendipitously, the new diagnostic model was ideally suited to promoting the pharmaceutical treatment of the conditions it delineated' (2007, p. 182). The *Diagnostic and Statistical Manual of Mental Disorders* is the basis of any mental disorder diagnosis. While the first two editions of the *DSM* were characterized by a strong theoretical view, mainly based on psychoanalysis, the *DSM-III* and, even more, the *DSM-IV* try to be atheoretical and symptom-based. Thus, in the two last versions of the *DSM*, the psychiatric nosography became more and more descriptive and standardized. To define an illness the emphasis is put on symptoms while causes are neglected. The focus of *DSM-III* and *DSM-IV* has therefore shifted from illnesses to disorders and syndromes – the latter being a bunch of symptoms. The key assumption of diagnostic psychiatry is that 'overt symptoms indicate discrete underlying diseases. Whenever enough symptoms are present to meet the criteria for a diagnosis, a particular mental disorder exists' (Horwitz, 2002, p. 106).

There are not any explanatory aims in the *DSM-IV*: symptomatology takes the place of ethiology.

The main consequences of the *DSM-IV* are:

- *Reductionism and proliferation of the disorders*: By shifting from illnesses to syndromes, the complexity of mental illness is reduced, because it coincides with its symptoms. Therefore, in the cure, the symptoms take the place of the causes. Disorders do not imply, as illnesses do, an ethiological model. The emphasis on the symptoms has a pathologizing slippery slope effect; as a matter of fact, disorders grew from 128 in the *DSM-I* to 357 in *DSM-IV* (Blashfield & Fuller, 1996).
- *Likeliness of pharmaceutical treatment*: If disorders become more easily identifiable and recognizable (If 'five (or more) of the following symptoms have been present during the same 2-week period ...'), it becomes easier to associate them to a specific therapy. If the task of psychiatry is to cure the symptoms, then medicines are the best way to do it (the magic bullet). Psychoanalysis treatment is usually long-lasting and tailored on the subject: the opposite of the standardization on which the *DSM-IV* is based (moreover, in a MC regime private insurances are more inclined to pay for rapid drug treatments than for long individual therapies).
- *Having more easily a diagnosis increases the number of patients*: If we are stimulated by TV commercials to make a self-diagnosis just by taking a test in a newspaper or on the net, the chances to pathologize a normal condition increase – therefore, a TV viewer, for instance, easily becomes a patient and a drug consumer.

- *The proliferation of co-morbidity*: If disorders take the place of illnesses, complicated conditions are now represented by a formula, for example – syndrome k + syndrome z + syndrome y – as a result, the therapeutic answer becomes fragmented and de-contextualized.

In the *DSM-IV* it is recognized that a mental disorder should not be confused and identified with subjective unpleasant emotions and feelings resulting from a social stressor (Pearlin, 1989). Nonetheless 'the *DSM* often uses the presence of certain symptoms – exclusive of the context in which they arise and are maintained – to diagnose disorders' (Horwitz, 2007, p. 214).

In the *DSM-IV* the presence of certain symptoms is the basis which allows the physician to make a diagnosis of mental disorder bracketing the causes which have produced the symptoms. Therefore, de facto, *DSM* conflates normality into pathology. It is not only a matter of 'medical dominance' (Freidson, 1970) or 'medical jurisdiction' (Abbott, 1988) into the realm of mental disease; the point is the medical definitional power in deciding what is normal and what is pathological (Brown, 1996). A power which does not have the features of authority, rather than the smoothness of the medical gaze (Foucault, 1963). In other words, the technical tool – the *DSM* – which should be the medium between medical theory and empirical cases is far from being a 'neutral' instrument.

On a different level, Adele Clarke et al. suggest that: 'Computer and information technology and the new social forms co-produced through their design and implementation are the key infrastructural devices of the new genre of meso-institutionalization (…). The techno-organizational innovations of one era become the (often invisible) infrastructure of the next' (2003, p. 165). The *DSM* with its algorithmical narrative and inferential structure – *if* symptoms *then* disease – fits coherently in the biomedical system, playing the role of the neutral infrastructure.

6. SUMMARY: THE SICKSCAPE FRAMEWORK

The last years have been characterized by a progressive extension of the social representations of health and of well-being. The imaginary of health and wellness encompasses aspects which once belonged to everyday life: beauty, ordinary emotions, maleness, intellectual and physical performance (Maturo, 2009). For any deficit in these aspects today we have medical treatment or support.

The reflections carried out up to now might be summarized on the basis of the triad: disease, illness and sickness (Twaddle, 1994; Hoffman, 2002).

Disease can be considered as the bio-medical definition of a pathology; illness coincides with subjective feelings of pain or anxiety; sickness is the way by which society interprets a personal condition. Therefore, if we consider illness as the subjective experience of unease or pain and disease as a physiological disequilibrium, then in the realm of mental health we face an ongoing switch of some 'natural' and ordinary emotions into the sphere of illness and from there into the realm of disease.

Leaving untouched the definition of disease, that is the bio-medical definition of a pathology, a new taxonomy of the triad disease/illness/sickness can be proposed:

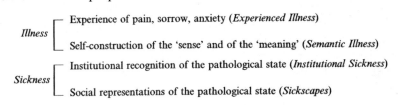

The four terms can be defined in the following ways:

Experienced illness: Any perceptions or feelings of pain, sorrow or anxiety experienced by the subject regardless of the presence of physiological changes detectable by biomedical instruments.

Semantic illness: The sense and meaning a person gives to his/her 'pathological' condition. This interpretation might be linked to an 'objective' view of the condition (disease) but also to the experienced illness. It could also be linked to both dimensions. Semantic illness does not necessarily have any negative connotations (one can wait for death peacefully ...).

Institutional sickness: The sick role, with its connected changes in the everyday life of an individual (exemption from work and normal activities, and legitimacy to stay at home).

Sickscapes: The social representations of illnesses, that is, the social conceptions of the disease (or of the event labelled as 'pathological') held by a population or by a specific social group (subculture). The definition also encompasses also the representations media give of a disease or of an event constructed as pathological.

Applying the above categories on the transformations of the scenario of bipolar disorder, we may summarize our analysis in the following steps:

a. The sickscape fuelled by the media system (direct-to-consumer advertisements for drug with prescription), by scientific discourse (the syndromization of *DSM*), by economic constraints (managed care) and by cultural predispositions (the American right to the 'pursuit of happiness') legitimates the transformation emotion → illness → disease.

b. Therefore, some emotions may be experienced by people as illnesses (experienced illness).

c. People may define their illnesses as something which must be cured (semantic illness).

d. The biomedical and pharmaceutical system creates the framework which facilitates this switch from emotion to illness to disease.

Now, what tentative conclusions may we offer on the basis of this analysis? What kinds of actions could be undertaken in order to resist the increasing medicalization tide?

Durkheim (1897) and Merton (1968) have shown that anomic conditions in which the individuals are unable to attain valued goals produce distress. Other researches, stemming from the work carried out by Engels (1845) until the works by Link and Phelan (2000), have found consistent evidence of the nexus between conditions of economic and social deprivation and individual feelings of discomfort, fatalism and distress. According to evolutionary psychology, stress is a natural answer to grief, loss and difficult situations, that is, stress is an adaptive response and is functional to the survival of the individual in his environment (Pearlin, 1989). On the other hand, as Horwitz (2007) noted, starting from the *DSM-III*, the psychiatric nosography became more and more descriptive and standardized. In order to define an illness the emphasis is now put on symptoms, whereas causes are neglected.

Separating mental disorder and socio-economic context means bracketing the causes and underlining the consequence (Horwitz, 2007). But, in many cases, stress is a normal and 'healthy' answer to a distressful situation – like a divorce, a firing and a bad diagnosis. Indeed, it is likely that situations of high socio-economic deprivation may lead to mental disorders. At the same time, we must be conscious that the pathologization of ordinary emotions and the separation of the disorder from the context (which co-caused the disorder) lead to the treatment of the effects and not of the causes.

The conception of an internal and biological cause for mental disorders neglects any treatment based on the idea that mental disorders are rooted in interpersonal relationships. But, most of all, this trend removes the political aspects of social and health policies. From this point of view, poverty, crime and racism become phenomena that must be fought for reasons related to ethics, law and humanitarism but not in order to improve community health. This may be defined as the medicalization of social service: 'there is a push to medicalize more and more of the needs of social service clients, as a quick and politically viable fix to the complex problems facing various client populations. It is less complicated, for example, to treat juvenile offenders with medications for antisocial personality disorder, than it is to address the underlying social and economic conditions that contribute the juvenile criminal behavioral' (Barker, 2009, p. 101). Moreover, the American health-care system based on private insurances and HMOs encourages this ideology because in many cases drugs are not reimbursed and in most cases they are a less expensive alternative to psychotherapy.

In the mental health sphere a more restrictive policy on advertisement would result in less public spending (Murray, 2009, p. 196). Indeed, a stricter regulation, in this field, could have the effect of reducing simplistic solutions (a pill) for complex situations (sadness for being unemployed, e.g.). It is difficult to find a solution to this situation since the biomedicalization of society has been increasing (Clarke & Shim, 2009). Yet, the growth in health-care costs could be a slowing factor of this trend. Changing the culture of a country is utopistic besides being antidemocratic move. However, I think that setting some limits on the advertisements which have directly to do with people's health may produce some effects, with the passing of time, on the way people relate to their own mind and body.

NOTES

1. Individuals aged 0–19 years.
2. According to a recent document produced by the European Technology Assessment Group (ETAG, 2009), the medicalization of society should be analysed against the background of broad changes in medicine, that is: '(i) the widespread questioning of medical authority by patients and advocacy group, a trend that is arguably reinforced by the rise of the World Wide Web with its countless websites on medical issues, (ii) the new focus on cost control of health care (instead of on access to it), (iii) the commercialisation of medicine (including, for example, the rise of direct-to-consumer marketing, of corporate medicine, and of cosmetic surgery, the shift from the notion of "patient" to that of "consumer", and the emergence of medical markets), and (iv) the rise of modern biotechnology and neurotechnology, which have not only added new approaches to therapy but also changed widespread views of illnesses and disorders and of the human body and mind in general'. (ETAG, p. 58)
3. http://www.imshealth.com/portal/site/imshealth.
4. 'The worried wells are those folks who have medicine cabinets full of every kind of remedy for every imaginable ailment (...) These are the hypochondriacs who are the bane of every doctor's existence. Obsessed with their health, they insist on

providing the physician with every excruciating detail of their imagined symptoms'
(Vasudeva, 2005).
  5. The advertisement is shown in Lane (2007, p. 113).
  6. Quoted in Lane (2007, p. 112).

REFERENCES

Abbott, A. (1988). *The system of professions*. Chicago: University of Chicago Press.
Aikin, K. J. (2003). *Direct-to-consumer advertisement of prescription drugs: Physician survey*.
    Available at: http://www.fda.gov/cder/ddmac/globalsummit2003/sld028.htm. Accessed
    on 15 November 2008.
Angell, M. (2003). *The truth about drug companies. How they deceive us and what to do about it*.
    New York: Random House.
Barker, K. (2009). Medicalization, multiplication of diseases, and human enhancement (round
    table). In: A. Maturo & P. Conrad (Eds), *The medicalization of life, Salute e Società*,
    (Vol. VIII, Is. 2, pp. 99–121).
Blashfield, R. K., & Fuller, K. (1996). Predicting the DSM-V. *The Journal of Nervous and
    Mental Diseases, 184*, 4–7.
Brown, P. (1996). Naming and framing: The social construction of diagnosis and illness.
    In: P. Brown (Ed.), *Perspective in medical sociology* (Chapter 5). Prospect Height, IL:
    Waveland Press.
Bury, M. (2000). On chronic illness and disability. In: C. E. Bird, P. Conrad & A. M. Fremont
    (Eds), *Handbook of medical sociology* (Chapter 12). Upper Saddle River, NJ: Prentice
    Hall.
Clarke, A., Mamo, L., Fishman, J. R., Shim, J. K., & Fosket, J. R. (2003). Biomedicalization:
    Technoscientific transformation of health, illness and U.S. biomedicine. *American
    Sociological Review, 68*, 161–194.
Clarke, A., & Shim, J. R. (2009). Medicalization and biomedicalization revisited: Technoscience
    and transformations of health, illness and biomedicine. In: A. Maturo & P. Conrad
    (Eds), *The medicalization of life, Salute e Società*, (Vol. VIII, Is. 2, pp. 209–242).
Conrad, P. (2000). Medicalization, genetics, and human problems. In: C. E. Bird, P. Conrad &
    A. M. Fremont (Eds), *Handbook of medical sociology* (Chapter 22). Upper Saddle River,
    NJ: Prentice Hall.
Conrad, P. (2007). *The medicalization of society: On the transformation of human conditions into
    treatable disorders*. Baltimore: Johns Hopkins University Press.
DeGrandpre, R. (1999). *Ritalin nation: Rapid-fire culture and the transformation of human
    consciousness*. New York: Norton.
Durkheim, E. (1897). *Le suicide. Étude de sociologie*. Paris: Le Presses Universitarie de France.
Dworkin, R. (2006). *Artificial happiness. The dark side of the new happy class*. New York:
    Carroll & Graf Publisher.
Engels, F. (1845). *Die Lage der arbeitenden Klasse in England*. Berlin: Dietz Verlag.
European Technology Assessment Group (ETAG). (2009). *Human enhancement study, science
    and technology options assessment*. Bruxelles: European Parliament.
Foucault, M. (1963). *Naissance de la clinique. Une archeologie du regard médicale*. Paris: Presses
    Universitaires de France.

Freidson, E. (1970). *Professional dominance: The social structure of medical care.* New York: Atherton Press.

Goffman, E. (1961). *Asylums; essays on the social situation of mental patients and other inmates.* Chicago: Aldine.

Goffman, E. (1963). *Stigma: Notes on the management of spoiled identity.* New Jersey: Prentice-Hall.

Greely, H., Sahakian, B., Harris, J., Kessler, R. C., Gazzaniga, M., Campbell, P., & Farah, M. J. (2008). Towards a responsible use of cognitive-enhancing drugs by the healthy. *Nature, 456,* 702–705.

Hoffman, B. (2002). On the triad disease, illness and sickness. *Journal of Medicine and Philosophy, 6,* 651–673.

Hollon, F. M. (2005). Direct-to-consumer advertising. A haphazard approach to health promotion. *JAMA, 293,* 2030–2033.

Horwitz, A. (2002). *Creating mental illness.* Chicago: Chicago University Press.

Horwitz, A. (2007). Transforming normality into pathology: The *DSM* and the outcomes of stressful social arrangements. *Journal of Health and Social Behavior, 48,* 211–222.

Horwitz, A., & Wakefield, J. (2007). *The loss of sadness. How psychiatry transformed normal sorrow into depressive disorder.* Oxford, NY: Oxford University Press.

Horwitz, A., & Wakefield, J. (2009). The medicalization of sadness: How psychiatry transformed a natural emotion into a mental disorder. In: A. Maturo & P. Conrad (Eds), *The medicalization of life, Salute e Società,* (Vol. VIII, Is. 2, pp. 49–66).

Illich, I. (1976). *Medical nemesis.* New York: Pantheon.

Kleinman, A. (1988). *The illness narratives: Suffering, healing and the human condition.* New York: Basic Books.

Lane, C. (2007). *Shyness. How normal behavior became a sickness.* New Haven: Yale University Press.

Light, D. (2000). The medical profession and organizational change: From professional dominance to countervailing power. In: C. E. Bird, P. Conrad & A. M. Fremont (Eds), *Handbook of medical sociology* (Chapter 14). Upper Saddle River, NJ: Prentice Hall.

Link, B. G., & Phelan, J. C. (2000). Evaluating the fundamental causes explanation for social disparities in health. In: C. E. Bird, P. Conrad & A. M. Fremont (Eds), *Handbook of medical sociology* (Chapter 3). Upper Saddle River, NJ: Prentice Hall.

Loe, M. (2008). The prescription of a new generation. *Context, 7,* 46–49.

Maturo, A. (2009). The shifting borders of medicalization: Perspectives and dilemmas of human enhancement. In: A. Maturo & P. Conrad (Eds), *The medicalization of life, Salute e Società,* (Vol. VIII, Is. 2, pp. 99–121).

McLellan, F. (2007). Medicalisation: A medical nemesis. *The Lancet, 369,* 627–628.

Merton, R. K. (1968). *Social theory and social structure.* New York: Free Press.

Metzel, J. M. (2007). If direct-to-consumer advertisments come to Europe: Lessons from the USA. *The Lancet, 369,* 704–706.

Miah, A. (2009). Medicalization, biomedicalization, or biotechnologization? Biocultural capital and a new social order. In: A. Maturo & P. Conrad (Eds), *The medicalization of life, Salute e Società* (Vol. VIII, Is. 2, pp. 264–268). Milano: FrancoAngeli.

Moreno, C., Laje, G., Blanco, C., Jiang, H., Schmidt, A. B., & Olfson, M. (2007). National trends in the outpatient diagnosis and treatment of bipolar disorder in youth. *Archives of General Psychiatry, 64*(9), 1032–1039.

Moynihan, R., & Cassels, A. (2005). *Selling sickness. How drug companies are turning us into patients.* New York: Nation Books.
Murray, J. (2009). Direct-to-consumer prescription drug advertising in a global context: A comparison between New Zealand and the United States. In: A. Maturo & P. Conrad (Eds), *The medicalization of life, Salute e Società,* (Vol. VIII, Is. 2, pp. 189–207).
Parsons, T. (1951). *The social system.* Glencoe: The Free Press.
Pearlin, L. (1989). The sociological study of stress. *Journal of Health and Social Behavior, 30,* 241–256.
Rose, N. (2007). *The politics of life itself. Biomedicine, power, and subjectivity in the twenty-first century.* Princeton: Princeton University Press.
Satel, S. (2006). *One nation under therapy. How the helping culture is eroding self-reliance.* New York: St. Martin's Griffin.
Smith, D. J., Ghaemi, S. N., & Craddock, N. (2008). The broad clinical spectrum of bipolar disorder: Implications for research and practice. *Journal of Psychopharmacology, 22,* 397–400.
Stagnitti, M. N. (2008). *Antidepressants prescribed by medical doctors in office based and out patient settings by specialty for the US civilian non institutionalized population, 2002 and 2005.* Statistical Brief #206, Agency for Healthcare Research and Quality. Available at http://www.meps.ahrq.gov/mepsweb/data_files/publications/st206/stat206.pdf
Twaddle, A. (1994). Disease, illness and sickness revisited. In: A. Twaddle & L. Nordenfelt (Eds), *Disease, illness and sickness: Three central concepts in the theory of health. Studies on Health and Society* (Vol. 18), Linköping, Sweden.
Vasudeva, P. (2005). Worried sick. *The Telegraph, Calcutta, India* 5 June. Available at http://www.telegraphindia.com/1050705/asp/atleisure/story_4950067.asp. Accessed on 28 July 2009.
Wurtzel, E. (1995). *Prozac nation.* New York: Riverhead.

WHAT EPIDEMIC? THE SOCIAL CONSTRUCTION OF BIPOLAR EPIDEMICS

Kathryn Burrows

ABSTRACT

Purpose – *This chapter explores the changing definition of bipolar disorder, examining how debates within psychiatry actually construct the definition of mental illness, thereby creating the appearance of an emerging epidemic with increasing prevalence.*

Method – *I review the recent psychiatric and epidemiological research to reveal that the intellectual and scientific debates that occur in the psychological laboratory and in survey research are in fact falsely increasing the figures that show that an epidemic of bipolar is emerging.*

Findings – *For centuries, bipolar disorder was equated with severe psychosis and had a prevalence rate between 0.4% and 1.6%. As spectrum and subthreshold conceptions of bipolar disorder become established in official psychiatric diagnostic manuals, however, estimates of the prevalence of bipolar spectrum disorders have risen to almost 25%. I demonstrate that nearly all of this increase is a result of changes in the scientific and intellectual definition of bipolar disorders among psychiatric professionals, and that rates of symptoms are not in fact increasing.*

Understanding Emerging Epidemics: Social and Political Approaches
Advances in Medical Sociology, Volume 11, 243–261
ISSN: 1057-6290/doi:10.1108/S1057-6290(2010)0000011017

Contribution to field – The arbitrariness of diagnostic thresholds naturally leads researchers to argue for lower thresholds. This allows more individuals who were previously considered psychiatrically normal to be reclassified as psychiatrically disordered. Lowering diagnostic thresholds increases the risk of confusing normal elation or sadness with disordered states, increasing the potential of false-positive diagnoses and the false impression of rising rates of disorder.

INTRODUCTION: AN EMERGING EPIDEMIC?

Emil Kraepelin, widely considered the leading psychiatric classifier of the late 19th century (Horwitz, 2002, p. 38), was among the first to write a modern comprehensive nosology of psychiatric disorders.[1] In his classification of mental disease, he focused primarily on two different types of disorders: psychotic disorders, including schizophrenia, and affective disorders, including bipolar disorder (Kraepelin & Diefendorf, 1912).[2] In Kraepelin's time and before, bipolar disorder and its recurrent states of mania, depression, and mixed mood episodes were considered a serious and debilitating mental disease. Vincenzo Chiarugi in Tuscany (1759–1820) wrote: "Mania signifies raving madness. The maniac is like a tiger or a lion, and in this respect mania may be considered as a state opposite to true melancholia" (Angst & Marneros, 2001, p. 7). In modern American psychiatry, bipolar disorder is conceptualized as consisting of two subtypes: bipolar-I and bipolar-II. Both disorders are conceived of as cyclical and pathological mood changes, alternating between depressive lows and euphoric highs, or mania. The cardinal difference between the subtypes is that bipolar-I patients must have experienced at least one episode of mania in addition to depressive episodes, whereas bipolar-II patients need only have a history of hypomanic episodes, which are less severe manifestations of mania. The *Diagnostic and Statistical Manual IV-TR* (*DSM-IV*) estimates the prevalence of bipolar-I disorder to be between 0.4% and 1.6%, and the prevalence of bipolar-II disorder to be approximately 0.5% (American Psychiatric Association, 2000, pp. 382–404).

If we fast forward 100 years from the time Kraepelin first used the term manic-depressive insanity, and only 15 years from the time bipolar-II disorder was introduced into the *DSM-IV* in 1994 (American Psychiatric Association), estimates of the prevalence of disorders on the bipolar spectrum have risen dramatically. Leading bipolar researchers have recently estimated that the population incidence of bipolar-II disorder alone may be as high as 10.9% (Angst et al., 2003, p. 139). The occurrence of subthreshold variants on the bipolar spectrum, less clinically significant than bipolar-II, has been estimated at 9.4% (Angst et al., 2003, p. 139), suggesting that the prevalence of most forms of bipolar illness may be as high as 24.2% (Angst et al., 2003, p. 139). Secondary analyses of the US National Epidemiological Catchment Area Survey of Mental Disorders (ECA) provide evidence that subthreshold cases on the bipolar spectrum are at least four times more prevalent than diagnoses based purely on *DSM-IV* criteria (Judd & Akiskal, 2003, p. 127). Some bipolar researchers who argue for a revision of the diagnostic criteria for bipolar disorders suggest that, under the proposed criteria, up to 30% of patients currently diagnosed with major depressive disorder are actually misdiagnosed bipolar-II patients (Benazzi, 2006, p. 26). Another study found that 61% of outpatients seeking treatment for depression actually met the proposed revised criteria for bipolar-II disorder (Benazzi & Akiskal, 2003, p. 35). Among children and adolescents alone, rates of diagnosis of bipolar disorders have risen 40-fold in the last 10 years (Moreno et al., 2007, p. 1035), and inpatient admissions for bipolar disorder among children doubled in the 5 years between 1995 and 2000 (Harpaz-Rotem, Leslie, Martin, & Rosenheck, 2005, p. 644).

The staggering increase in the diagnosis of, and estimates of the prevalence of, bipolar disorders in the community suggests an alarming epidemic of a family of serious mental disorders. The rapid ascendancy of the estimated prevalence of these disorders foretells a strain on the nations' mental health facilities and services. An epidemic of this scale would result in a marked increase in chronically disabled persons, with an estimated functional recovery rate reported to be as low as 37% over a 2-year period (Tohen et al., 2000, p. 220). The 61% increased risk of death for persons with bipolar disorders (Angst, Angst, & Stassen, 1999, p. 58) would devastate families, the economy, and the social structure. The gravity of this rapidly growing public health crisis inspires understandable apprehension, but there is more to the bipolar epidemic than is immediately apparent.

In this chapter, I argue that there are multiple interpretations of the rise in the estimated prevalence of disorders on the bipolar spectrum. I suggest that these statistics do not in fact represent an increase in the number of people who experience the symptoms described by Kraepelin, and more recently classified as bipolar-I and bipolar-II in the *DSM-IV*. I will explore the social processes and academic debates that have defined and redefined bipolar disorders. Disease classifications are necessarily social products that adhere more or less closely to biological reality. When these classifications, or indeed, the very concept of epidemics, become reified as facts of nature, we lose sight of the origin of these concepts: human beings and the social worlds in which we live (Berger & Luckmann, 1967, p. 89). Human beings who manage competing social, political, economic, and intellectual interests[3] create disease classifications, including those of bipolar disorders. In the rest of this chapter, I will first briefly outline the theoretical concept guiding this work, the social construction of mental illness, as well as the competing paradigm of the biological disease perspective of mental illness. After this quick overview of the intellectual debate that frames the current discussion about bipolar disorders and their ostensible epidemic propor- tions, I will narrow the discussion to focus primarily on two of the social causes, or "culprits," for the apparent epidemic of these disorders.

SOCIAL CONSTRUCTIONS OR BIOLOGICAL ILLNESS?

There is no consensus regarding the "reality" of psychiatric illness categories. Two opposing points of view pit a social constructionist perspective against the disease model of psychiatric illness, which contends that diagnostic categories represent purely biomedical illness (Horwitz, 2002, pp. 5–10). At its most basic level, social construction theories contend that all systems of knowledge and ways of understanding are reflections of culturally specific processes. Our world is inseparable from the social processes that allow us to comprehend and organize that world. Social constructionist scholars do not assume that taken-for-granted categories represent any natural reality, but instead they reflect and respond to shifting social forces (Berger & Luckmann, 1967). The pure social constructionist perspective on mental illness posits that diagnostic categories serve only to classify behavior as deviant or abnormal. Normality, therefore, is culturally created and there exists no universal normality in the same way as there exists no universal morality (Benedict, 1934, p. 73; Hacking, 1986, pp. 12–155). Benedict was one of the first scholars to question psychiatric diagnostic categories as absolute, and asked, "In how far can we regard inability to function socially as diagnostic of abnormality, or in how far is it necessary to regard this as a function of the culture?" (1934, p. 60). Some scholars argue that the entire idea of mental illness is a fallacy, and that attributing problems with living to mental illness is similar to attributing problems to witchcraft, demons, or fate (Szasz, 1960, p. 117). Szasz (1960, p. 118) contends that mental illness is a myth whose function is to disguise and obscure the moral conflicts in human relations. Addressing how the concept of mental illness became accepted and reified as a biological fact, Szasz writes:

> Mental illness, of course, is not literally a thing or physical object, and hence it can exist in only the same way that other theoretical concepts exist. Yet, familiar theories are in the habit of posing, sooner or later, at least to those who come to believe in them, as objective truths or facts. (1960, p. 113)

Opposing the social constructionist perspective[4] is the biological disease paradigm, which is currently in favor within the psychiatric profession. Psychiatric researchers, clinicians, and laypeople alike generally view mental illnesses as biomedical diseases of the brain no different from other illnesses (Horwitz, 2002, p. 5). American psychiatrists do not typically view the disease categories within the *DSM* as simply one, but not the only, way of viewing mental illness (Horwitz, 2002, p. 5). In fact, most mental health professionals regard mental illness categories as defined in the *DSM* as natural entities and not as evolving social constructions (Leshner, 2001, pp. 77–79). This perspective asserts that diseases, both physical and mental, presumably exist in nature as clearly defined entities, regardless of the social meaning attached to them (Horwitz, 2002, p. 5). As diagnostic categories change with the release of new versions of the *DSM*, adherents to the disease model presume that these changes demonstrate that scientific and diagnostic knowledge is getting stronger, not that earlier conceptions or classifications were inaccurate or socially constructed.

The dominance of the biological understanding of mental disorders within American psychiatry is a relatively recent phenomenon. Prior to the publication of the *DSM-III* in 1980, American psychiatric conceptions of mental illness were organized around an environmental and behavioral model of illness, which was informed by psychodynamic and psychoanalytic theories of behavior (Mayes & Horwitz, 2005, p. 249; Wilson, 1993, p. 399). The *DSM-I* and *DSM-II*, unlike their successors, did not provide elaborate classification schemes (Mayes & Horwitz, 2005, p. 249), because within the psychodynamic model of diagnosis, overt symptoms did not reveal disease entities but disguised underlying conflicts between the personality and the environment. In this view of mental illness, mental disorders were not discrete categories with a consistent etiology and treatment, but represented the failure of an individual to adapt to his or her social circumstances. The categorical disease and biological model of mental disorder that gained prominence with the release of the *DSM-III* was prompted in part by a variety of powerful stakeholders who benefited from the disease model, including insurance companies, psychiatric researchers, clinical psychiatrists, and pharmaceutical firms (Horwitz, 2002, pp. 67–77; Mayes & Horwitz, 2005, pp. 253–257).

Whether or not psychiatric disease categories are socially constructed, individuals displaying characteristics understood as being symptomatic of a mental illness, including bipolar disorders, indeed suffer very real distress. The existence of distress should not be confused with the existence of disorder, as one can clearly experience distress without that distress being disordered. Psychiatric diagnostic categories have a profound impact on clinical and community epidemiological studies that attempt to quantify the prevalence of specific mental illnesses. These epidemiological surveys necessarily rely on predetermined categories. However, by reifying and naturalizing these categories, epidemiological studies obscure the social processes that define and redefine what counts as a mental illness. I will now explore two of the social culprits that contribute to the illusion of a bipolar epidemic: the subthreshold and spectrum conception of bipolar disorders, and the expanding definition of mania. As the definition of illnesses expands or contract through social processes, epidemiological studies that quantify disease prevalence will necessarily reflect these social changes. In the case of bipolar disorders, the social redefinition of these disorders has created the impression of an epidemic.

CULPRITS: SUBTHRESHOLDS AND SPECTRUMS

The most recent version of the psychiatric disease classification manual that is used for the diagnosis and treatment of patients, as well as for epidemiological attempts to quantify the prevalence of mental illnesses, is the *DSM-IV-TR*. This manual tends to conceptualize mental illnesses as discrete, non-continuous categories. However, the newer psychiatric literature that is being used to create the anticipated *DSM-V*, scheduled to be released in 2012 (American Psychiatric Association, 2008), relies heavily on conceptions of mental illness as being on a continuum, or spectrum, of illness. This literature examines subthreshold conditions[5] in which a person may meet some, but not all, of the *DSM-IV* diagnostic criteria for a particular disorder. A shift to a broader conception of mental disorders could lead to many more people potentially being placed on a spectrum of mental illness. This has important implications for epidemiological research that suggests that rates of particular illnesses are rising, creating the illusion of an epidemic.

Despite being different concepts, the subthreshold and spectrum movements within psychiatry have a similar impact on epidemiological studies that suggest an impending epidemic of bipolar disorders. Patients are said to have a subthreshold, or subclinical condition, when some, but not all, of the *DSM-IV* criteria for a specific diagnosis are met. A subthreshold presentation might also be identified if a patient meets modified, or reduced, versions of the diagnostic criteria. Including subthreshold symptoms as indicative of mental illness and considering people with these symptoms for inclusion in epidemiological studies that ostensibly count people with the illness may artificially elevate prevalence estimates. For adherents to the medical model of psychiatry, a patient with a subthreshold presentation may represent the beginning of a more serious illness that requires treatment in order to prevent a worsening of the condition. Specifically in the case of bipolar disorders, the identification of subthreshold conditions is considered particularly important because pharmaceutical treatment for those with bipolar disorders, even at the subthreshold level, is typically different than treatment for those with anxiety or depressive disorders (Akiskal & Mallya, 1987, pp. 69–70; Altshuler et al., 1995, p. 1130). However, the expanding definition of illness to include subthreshold conditions merely increases the number of individuals who qualify for a psychiatric diagnosis and treatment. The inclusion of subthreshold conditions in epidemiological studies may provide the appearance that the rates of particular illnesses are rising. However, prevalence rates rise as a direct result of the expansion of the definition of the illness that captures more people in its more inclusive net. For example, in a study that tested expanded definitions of eight psychiatric disorders, looking at subthreshold variants of major depressive disorder, bipolar disorders, eating disorders, generalized anxiety disorder, alcohol abuse, substance abuse, conduct disorder, and ADHD, almost 53% of high-school students in a non-clinical setting met expanded criteria for at least one subthreshold disorder (Lewinsohn et al., 2004, p. 620), far greater than the rates of these disorders when subthreshold conditions are not considered.

The spectrum conception of mental disorders goes one step further than the subthreshold movement, which primarily expands diagnostic categories to include more people with fewer or less severe symptoms. The spectrum model, on the other hand, sees mental illness and health on a continuous scale and not as sets of discrete categories (Lewinsohn et al., 2000, p. 345). Proponents of the spectrum model of mental disorders see both subthreshold and *DSM*-diagnosable conditions as being part of the same bio-psychiatric process. From this perspective, the main difference between points on the spectrum is merely a matter of degree (Cox, Enns, Borger, & Parker, 1999, p. 20).

In addition to bipolar-I and bipolar-II, which are described in the *DSM-IV*, such researchers propose adding a bipolar-1.5 and 2.5 (Akiskal & Pinto, 1999, p. 519), bipolar-III (Akiskal & Mallya, 1987, p. 69), as well as bipolar variants 3.5, IV, and V (Akiskal & Pinto, 1999, pp. 527–532). Still others suggest that certain forms of late-life dementia should be considered as part of the bipolar spectrum, as bipolar-VI (Ng et al., 2008, p. 308). Although scholars disagree about the number of distinct disorders on the spectrum, they all agree that the spectrum includes distinct disorders in addition to subthreshold variants, and that even the distinct disorders seamlessly blend together on the continuum. Angst and Marneros (2001, pp. 13–14) suggest a bipolar spectrum with 10 steps. Their proposed spectrum locates Bipolar-I nearly in the middle of the spectrum, with mixed and schizoaffective type disorders above it, and Bipolar-II and hypomania below it.

The first node on Angst and Marneros' proposed spectrum (2001, p. 14) consists of non-pathological personality types: hyperthymic and cyclothymic temperaments. Akiskal and Mallya (1987, pp. 71–72) suggest characteristics of the hyperthymic personality to be:

- chronic short sleeper (<6 h, including weekends);
- excessive use of denial;
- irritable, cheerful, overoptimistic, or exuberant;
- naïve, overconfident, self-assured, boastful, bombastic, or grandiose;
- vigorous, full of plans, improvident, and rushing off with restless impulse;
- over talkative;
- warm, people seeking, or extraverted;
- overinvolved and meddlesome;
- uninhibited, stimulus seeking, or promiscuous.

In essence, this proposed bipolar spectrum includes a larger variety of human difference than has ever before been considered pathological. What was once normal is now mild disorder. We have certainly all known people with a "hyperthymic temperament" as described above; however, troublesome people have typically been just that – troublesome, but not disordered. Including personality types, even those that are arguably problematic for personal relationships, in the bipolar spectrum, changes the question from "are you bipolar?" to "to what degree are you bipolar?" As definitions of pathological mental illness get more and more broad, it is inevitable that epidemiological estimates of the prevalence of these disorders will rise.

The spectrum conception of mental illness presumes that health and illness are not categorically distinct, but instead lie on a continuum (Horwitz & Wakefield, 2007, p. 126). In this way of thinking, health (or only very mild illness) is on the far left of the continuum, and severe mental illness lies on the far right of the continuum. Most individuals would lie somewhere in between these two extremes. Continuum notions of mental illness conceive virtually the entire population to be ill to some degree (Horwitz & Wakefield, 2007, p. 126). The *DSM-IV* requires a condition to meet three criteria in order to be considered a mental disorder: mental disorders are internal dysfunctions; mental disorders are not an expectable response to particular conditions; and mental disorders are not deviant behavior (American Psychiatric Association, 1994, pp. xxi–xxii; Horwitz, 2002, p. 21). Continuum definitions of bipolar may in fact contradict the *DSM* definition of disorder by not allowing for the concept of healthy and normal variations in mood. For example, disordered mood fluctuations give bipolar sufferers the extreme and dangerous highs of mania, and the profound depth of despair that characterizes depression and suicide. However, normal and healthy variation in mood certainly includes daily joy, even moments of euphoria, and sadness and grief. When normal and healthy fluctuations in mood are pathologized and placed on the bipolar spectrum, the risk for false-positive bipolar diagnoses in clinical practice and epidemiological studies increases. In fact, an alternative way to conceive of the bipolar spectrum is to imagine two continuums: one of healthy mood variation and one of disordered mood variation (Horwitz & Wakefield, 2007, p. 140). Imagining a spectrum of healthy variation as separate from the spectrum of disorder reduces the possibility that people with non-pathological mood states are considered in epidemiological estimates of the rate of bipolar disorders.

Although conceptions of the bipolar spectrum are currently in vogue among bipolar researchers, by no means is there clear agreement within the psychiatric profession that bipolarity should be considered a spectrum disorder. In his *Plea for the Integrity of the Bipolar Disorder Concept*, Baldessarini (2000, p. 5) writes:

> Widespread acceptance of increasingly broad definitions risks weakening or trivializing the core concept of Bipolar disorder, much as what has occurred in the past with schizophrenia, major depression and a growing number of other disorders whose academic and clinical popularity has waxed and waned.

Critics of the spectrum concept of bipolar disorder worry that the inclusion of subthreshold conditions on the bipolar spectrum pathologizes normal behavior as well as trivializes serious illness. In their report about the danger subthreshold variants on the bipolar spectrum pose to research on the causes and treatments of bipolar-I disorder, Soares and Gershon (2000, p. 1) write:

> Increasingly broader definitions of Bipolar disorder are frequently justified under the assumption that these conditions have some resemblance in some of their symptoms and also appear to respond in various degrees to some of their treatments [...] The move towards inclusion of increasingly heterogeneous groups of patients under this diagnostic category threatens to jeopardize clinical research and would be a disservice to the field.

Unfortunately for the integrity of epidemiological estimates of bipolar disorder, the voices of the spectrum critics do not appear to have the same persuasive power as those arguing for an increasingly inclusive spectrum. It is likely that the forthcoming *DSM-V* will even further promote the spectrum conception of bipolar illnesses. This will ensure that epidemiological studies will begin to record an increase in the prevalence of bipolar disorders, as the definitions are expanded and the spectrum becomes reified in the manual.

In their argument for a spectrum conception of psychiatric disorders, Lewinsohn et al. (2004, p. 613) write:

> Under the *DSM-IV*, an individual is determined to have a particular disorder when he or she exceeds a cut-off of a diagnostic algorithm [...] While one hopes that the criteria and cut-off are based on sound empirical and clinical considerations, the fact that these systems are continuously revised and that few are entirely satisfied with them suggests that the determination of the caseness of a disorder is ultimately somewhat arbitrary.

It is this very arbitrariness that makes subthreshold and spectrum movements within psychiatry potential culprits for the appearance of an epidemic. If disease categories are rather arbitrarily constructed and re-constructed, then no epidemiological study that presumes to count the prevalence of a disease in the community can be seen as capturing an immutable, biological fact. Instead, as disease categories themselves are created through social processes, epidemiological estimates reflect only those social processes that have defined the disorder in question. The impact of the definition of disorder on epidemiological studies is striking: estimates of the prevalence of bipolar-I disorder are 1.6% (Kessler et al., 1994, p. 12) but up to 24.2% (Angst et al., 2003, p. 139) for the entire bipolar spectrum.

CULPRIT: EXPANDING MANIA

Threshold and spectrum conceptions of bipolar illness expand the range of symptoms that are considered abnormal, encompassing more people. Subthreshold conditions and the bipolar spectrum work together with the second culprit of bipolar epidemics. The redefinition and weakening of the important symptom of mania also contributes to the illusion of a bipolar epidemic. The key feature that differentiates bipolar-I from bipolar-II and other forms of disorders on the bipolar spectrum is the type of mania experienced by individuals. Individuals with bipolar-I experience mania, which is characterized by non-stop activity, euphoria, racing thoughts, thoughts of grandiosity ("I am Don Juan"), and frequently, psychotic delusions (Akiskal & Pinto, 1999, p. 520). Manic episodes often require hospitalization to prevent dangerous and destructive behavior such as excessive gambling, reckless driving, sexual promiscuity, shopping, impulsive traveling, and drug and alcohol use. Individuals diagnosed with bipolar-II and other bipolar variants experience a less severe form of mania known as hypomania. The *DSM-IV* (American Psychiatric Association, 2000, p. 368) characterizes hypomania as:

(a) periods of elevated or irritable mood (mood changes), which must always be present and must last at least 4 days, different from the usual mood;
(b) three of the following eight symptoms if mood is elevated, four if mood is irritable: inflated self-esteem, decreased need for sleep, more talkativeness, racing thoughts, distractibility, increased goal-directed activity, psycho-motor agitation, and excessive involvement in risky activities;
(c) change in functioning;
(d) observable mood and functioning change;
(e) no marked impairment of functioning and no psychotic symptoms;
(f) symptoms must not be caused by substances, drugs (including antidepressants), or medical disorders.

The identification of hypomania as a psychiatric symptom, rather than a part of normal human experience, was one of the first stages in the broadening of bipolar disorder from a discrete, serious illness to a spectrum disorder ranging from mild to serious distress. Due to its typically relatively benign nature, hypomania is often unrecognized by physicians, and as a result, patients who might meet the criteria for bipolar-II disorder are frequently diagnosed with major depressive disorder instead (Benazzi, 2006, p. 26). For proponents of a spectrum conception of bipolarity, this represents a worrisome and problematic misdiagnosis. The treatment protocols for major depressive disorder, such as the prescription of selective serotonin reuptake inhibitor (SSRI) antidepressants, may actually increase mood cycling in bipolar patients, induce manic episodes, and worsen the course of the disorder (Bhargava Raman et al., 2007, p. 264; Ghaemi, Sachs,

Chiou, Pandurangi, & Goodwin, 1999, p. 136; Goodwin & Jamison, 2007, pp. 25–55). Accordingly, some pro-spectrum researchers argue for a reduction in the number of days that hypomania must be present in order to qualify for a diagnosis of bipolar disorder. Currently, the *DSM-IV* (American Psychiatric Association, 2000, p. 368) requires hypomania symptoms to be present for a minimum of 4 days at least once in a patient's life in order to qualify for a bipolar-II diagnosis. Some psychiatrists suggest that this is too conservative, and that a bipolar disorder may in fact be present if hypomania symptoms are present for 2 days or more (Benazzi, 2006, p. 26; Benazzi & Akiskal, 2003, p. 35; Cassano, Akiskal, Savino, Musetti, & Perugi, 1992, p. 131; Manning, Haykal, Connor, & Akiskal, 1997, p. 105). In arguing for a lower threshold for a patient to meet the criteria for hypomania, Akiskal et al. (2000, p. 5) suggest that most hypomanic episodes last between 1 and 3 days, and they bemoan the "arbitrary" 4-day cutoff currently enshrined in the *DSM-IV*. However, other researchers have found that, at least in children, hypomanic episodes last for a minimum of 4 days, with a mean length of 12 days (Bhargava Raman et al., 2007, p. 264). The key feature that differentiates bipolar disorders from other psychiatric conditions – mania or hypomania – is still contested by leading researchers in the field. The final outcome of this academic debate will significantly affect epidemiological studies that attempt to quantify the number of people with these disorders. As the threshold for hypomania continues to drop, more and more people will potentially be considered as having a variant of bipolar disorder.

In addition to arguing for a reduction in the minimum number of days in which hypomania must be present in order to qualify for a bipolar diagnosis, researchers who are concerned about the under-diagnosis of bipolar disorders propose that revised diagnostic criteria might better capture hypomanic symptoms. They suggest that hypomanic diagnostic criteria that require the presence of an elevated or irritated mood might inappropriately screen out people who may in fact have a bipolar spectrum disorder. In an article about the misdiagnosis of bipolar-II disorder, Benazzi (2006, p. 26) writes, "Because the *DSM-IV* stem question requires remembering periods of elevated or irritable mood, the response to this question by patients with BP II is frequently 'no,' since these periods may be seen as normal mood fluctuations." In other words, patients may under-stand their symptoms to be normal and healthy mood variation, and the current screening criteria may not capture hypomanic symptoms precisely *because* patients do not experience those symptoms as disordered. These patients are then diagnosed with unipolar depression rather than bipolar-II.

In order to reduce the misdiagnosis of pseudo-unipolar depression (Angst et al., 2003, p. 144), some researchers have proposed new diagnostic criteria to screen for hypomania, which would presumably allow many more people to qualify for the diagnosis. In part, the proposed diagnostic criteria (Angst et al., 2003, p. 144) require:

1. Over the last 12 months and, without any special reason, have you, for any length of time:
   - been much more energetic;
   - been more active;
   - been less easily tired;
   - needed less sleep;
   - been more talkative;
   - traveled around more;
   - been busier, etc.?
2. Was this so evident that you had problems with it yourself, it caused you problems with others, or it got you into financial difficulties?
3. Did other people (e.g., family members, partner, etc.) notice these states in you and come to the conclusion that something must be wrong with you?

Proponents of both the expansion of the bipolar spectrum and the redefinition of hypomania argue that the "misdiagnosis" of bipolar disorders, even subthreshold variants, as major depressive disorder can be extremely dangerous to patients. Psychoactive drugs that are prescribed for the treatment of depression may be ineffective, or even dangerous, in treating any bipolar spectrum disorder (Akiskal & Mallya, 1987, p. 70). In this way, the impending bipolar epidemic can be conceived of as a shifting epidemic. By lowering bipolar criteria and expanding the bipolar spectrum, the immediate result will be the reclassification of patients currently diagnosed with depression or anxiety to be diagnosed instead with having bipolar disorders. This in turn will affect epidemiological estimates of the rates of both bipolar disorders and the rates of depression, and in fact this shift is already evident among inpatient admissions for juvenile psychiatric patients (Harpaz-Rotem et al., 2005, p. 644).

The proposed changes in criteria intend to classify behavior that the patient may see as "normal mood fluctuations" (Benazzi, 2006, p. 26) as characteristic of an illness that requires medical treatment, specifically, mood-stabilizing drugs. Patients infrequently seek treatment for hypomanic symptoms because they are frequently seen as a period of improved functioning. Impairment from hypomania, when it occurs, is mild. Persons with hypomanic symptoms seldom complain of, or suffer from, their shifts in energy, activity, and sleep behavior, but tend to experience them as positive. Most such changes, if noticed at all, are likely to be recognized by family and friends (Angst et al., 2003, p. 134). In fact, patients experiencing hypomania function so well they do not recognize it as illness at all (Akiskal & Mallya, 1987, p. 68). The result is that bipolar-II, and other bipolar spectrum disorders, is characterized primarily by a symptom, hypomania, that is generally perceived as non-problematic and a part of normal behavior. This is in contrast to virtually every other disorder in the *DSM-IV*, which requires symptoms to cause either significant distress to the patient or marked dysfunction. As the threshold for what qualifies as hypomania, in both duration and character, continues to drop, bipolar spectrum diagnoses will include even more symptoms that most individuals do not consider marked difficulties. This, in turn, will be reflected in epidemiological estimates of the prevalence of bipolar disorders.

CONCLUSION: WHAT ABOUT
THE DRUG COMPANIES?

Frequently in public discourse about increasing rates of mental illness diagnoses, pharmaceutical companies and their aggressive marketing tactics (Thomson & Trotto, 2002, p. B1), as well as their ties to psychiatrists (Harris, Carey, & Roberts, 2007), are blamed. However, in this chapter I have not directly addressed the pharmaceutical industries' role in rising rates of diagnoses. I want to briefly explore the role of psychoactive drugs in the appearance of a growing bipolar epidemic, but I argue that these drugs have a dialectical relationship with the two main culprits described in this chapter, and are therefore secondary to them.

   Trends in psychiatric diagnoses, or diagnostic fads which could contribute to the illusion of an epidemic, have historically followed the advent of new medication (Akiskal, 1983, p. 271). For example, when Thorazine was invented in the 1950s, it preceded a spike in diagnoses of schizophrenia (Akiskal, 1983, p. 271). Likewise, when lithium was approved for the treatment of bipolar disorder in 1970, rates of bipolar diagnoses rose over those of schizophrenia (Akiskal, 1983, p. 271). In this same vein, when SSRI drugs were made available for the treatment of depression, rates of diagnoses of clinical depression rose dramatically (Horwitz & Wakefield, 2007, p. 183). As the patents for the first-generation SSRI drugs began to expire, which coincided with the advent of atypical antipsychotics and safer anticonvulsant medications with fewer side effects than older medications for the treatment of bipolar-II and subthreshold variants of bipolar disorder, rates of these diagnoses have risen, as have their prescription to patients (Olfson, Blaco, Liu, Moreno, & Laje, 2006, p. 683; Thomas, Conrad, Casler, & Goodman, 2006, p. 65).

Pharmaceutical companies aggressively market drugs directly to consumers (Bell, Kravitz, & Wilkes, 2000, p. 329), which leads to increased prescribing of drugs, even when the prescribing physician does not think the drug is necessary (Hartley, 2002, p. 10). Also contributing to the rates of specific diagnoses, and therefore, drug treatment for these disorders, are ethically and professionally questionable relationships between drug companies and prescribing physicians. For example, it has been widely reported that more than half of the taskforce members who are working on the newest edition of the *DSM*, the *DSM-V*, have ties to the pharmaceutical industry (Parker-Pope, 2008).

However, while the relationship between pharmaceutical companies and rising rates of psychiatric diagnoses is clear, the advent of new drugs alone does not directly increase the rates of diagnoses. Instead, an intervening factor, the redefinition of disorder, and the expansion of conditions that are considered disordered, and therefore eligible for drug treatment, are the direct causes of a spike in diagnoses. Psychiatric drugs have a dialectical relationship with the definition and redefinition of bipolar disorders. For example, of the 64 authors of bipolar papers written after 1990 referenced in this chapter, 20 disclosed ties to drug companies that manufacture psychiatric drugs – a rate of over 31%. Leading bipolar researchers who directly influence and create the definition of bipolar disorders may themselves be influenced by drug companies, but it is this redefinition and expansion of the bipolar spectrum that is the proximal cause of the purported bipolar epidemic. The creation of new drugs may influence the creation of a longer and more inclusive bipolar continuum, and a longer continuum spurs the development of new drugs. This process is particularly poignant in the case of the still-controversial diagnosis of childhood bipolar disorder, in which drug trials for the disorder and the development of effective diagnostic criteria to identity the disorder appear to have occurred nearly simultaneously (Groopman, 2007, p. 30). Certainly a bipolar spectrum that includes more and more people who can be treated with mood-stabilizing drugs is beneficial to the pharmaceutical industry, but the definition of bipolar disorders must first be expanded in order for the industry to accrue these benefits.

The processes described in this chapter of the social construction of bipolar epidemics apply equally to rates of diagnosis of epidemic proportions of other psychiatric conditions such as depression, ADHD, anxiety, autism spectrum disorders, and borderline personality disorder. As human beings enmeshed in complex social environments define and redefine conceptions of the normal and abnormal, epidemiological estimates of the prevalence of these disorders will shift in the direction of these changes. If diagnostic criteria tighten, fewer people will be considered abnormal and epidemiological estimates of the prevalence of those disorders will shrink. However, if diagnostic criteria expand, as in the case of bipolar disorders, more people will be considered disordered, and epidemiological reports will reveal an increase in the rates of affected persons. Epidemiological estimates of disease, especially of psychiatric disorders, do not quantify natural immutable processes. Instead, they reflect the very human social processes that define disorder and that are subject to the social, political, economic, and intellectual whims of human beings.

NOTES

1. One of the earliest known classification systems of mental illness was written in the 10th century by Arabian physician Najab ud-din Unhammad, which included nine major categories of mental disorders (Millon, 2004, p. 38). Mania itself was first described in a non-modern form by Hippocrates in the 4th century B.C. (Healy, 2008, p. 3).

2. Kraepelin's classification used the terms manic-depressive insanity and dementia praecox to refer to those conditions known today as bipolar disorder and schizophrenia. The term schizophrenia appeared in the first edition of the *Diagnostic and Statistical Manual of Mental Disorders* (*DSM-I*) in 1952 (American Psychiatric Association, 1952, pp. 26–28). The term bipolar was first used in 1957 by German psychiatrist Karl Leonhard (Goodwin & Jamison, 2007, p. 9). Throughout this chapter, I will use the modern nomenclature.

3. Not only mental disorders are socially defined; our understanding and classification of many physical diseases and assumedly biological "facts" are strongly influenced by social processes. Two recent papers on this general topic explore the social construction of Lyme disease (Aronowitz, 1991), and the appearance and activity of human sperm and egg cells (Martin, 1991).

4. Not all sociologists use the social constructionist framework to understand the phenomenon of mental illness. Much sociological work in the study of mental illness presumes the biological disease paradigm to guide their work. Examples include work about the relationship between mental health and family status (Umberson & Williams, 1999), class (Muntaner, Borrell, & Chung, 2008), and race (Evans-Campbell, Lincoln, & Takeuchi, 2008).

5. See, for example: Akiskal and Mallya (1987), Angst et al. (2003), Goodwin and Jamison (2007), Judd and Akiskal (2003), Lewinsohn, Shankman, Gau, and Klein (2004), and Lewinsohn, Solomon, Seeley, and Zeiss (2000).

ACKNOWLEDGMENTS

I am grateful to Alan Horwitz, Sarah Rosenfield, and Eunkyung Song for stimulating discussions and thoughtful reviews that greatly enhanced the ideas in this chapter.

REFERENCES

Akiskal, H. S. (1983). The bipolar spectrum: New concepts in classification and diagnosis. *Psychiatry Update: The American Psychiatric Association Annual Review, 2,* 271–291.

Akiskal, H. S., Bourgeois, M. L., Angst, J., Post, R., Moller, H. J., & Hirschfeld, R. (2000). Re-evaluating the prevalence of and diagnostic composition within the broad clinical spectrum of bipolar disorders. *Journal of Affective Disorders, 59,* 5–30.

Akiskal, H. S., & Mallya, G. (1987). Criteria for the soft bipolar spectrum: Treatment implications. *Psychopharmacology Bulletin, 23*(1), 68–73.

Akiskal, H. S., & Pinto, O. (1999). The evolving bipolar spectrum-prototypes I, II, III, and IV. *The Psychiatric Clinics of North America, 22*(3), 517–534.

Altshuler, L. L., Post, R. M., Leverich, G. S., Mikalauskas, K., Rosoff, A., & Ackerman, L. (1995). Anti-depressant-induced mania and cycle acceleration: A controversy revisited. *American Journal of Psychiatry, 152*(8), 1130–1138.

American Psychiatric Association (APA). (1952). *Diagnostic and statistical manual of mental disorders.* Washington, DC: American Psychiatric Association.

American Psychiatric Association (APA). (1994). *Diagnostic and statistical manual of mental disorders* (4th ed.). Washington, DC: American Psychiatric Association.

American Psychiatric Association (APA). (2000). *Diagnostic and statistical manual of mental disorders* (4th ed., text revision). Washington, DC: American Psychiatric Association.

American Psychiatric Association. (APA). (2008). *DSM-V prelude project.* Available at: http:// dsm5.org/index.cfm (accessed November 11, 2008).

Angst, J., Angst, F., & Stassen, H. H. (1999). Suicide risk in patients with major depressive disorder. *Journal of Clinical Psychiatry, 60,* 57–62.

Angst, J., Gamma, A., Benazzi, F., Ajdacic, V., Eich, D., & Rossler, W. (2003). Toward a re-definition of subthreshold bipolarity: Epidemiology and proposed criteria for bipolar-II, minor bipolar disorders and hypomania. *Journal of Affective Disorders, 73*(1–2), 133–146.

Angst, J., & Marneros, A. (2001). Bipolarity from ancient to modern times: Conception, birth, and rebirth. *Journal of Affective Disorders, 67,* 3–19.

Aronowitz, R. (1991). Lyme disease: The social construction of a new disease and its social consequences. *Milbank Quarterly, 69*(1), 79–112.

Baldessarini, R. (2000). A plea for integrity of the bipolar disorder concept. *Bipolar Disorders, 2,* 3–7.

Bell, R. A., Kravitz, R. L., & Wilkes, M. S. (2000). Direct-to-consumer prescription drug advertising, 1989–1998. *The Journal of Family Practice, 49*(4), 329–335.

Benazzi, F. (2006). Bipolar II disorder: Current issues in diagnosis and management. *Psychiatric Times, 23*(9), 26–29.

Benazzi, F., & Akiskal, H. (2003). Refining the evaluation of bipolar-II: Beyond the strict SCID-CV guidelines for hypomania. *Journal of Affective Disorders, 73*(1–2), 33–38.

Benedict, R. (1934). Anthropology and the abnormal. *Journal of General Psychology, 10*, 59–82.

Berger, P. L., & Luckmann, T. (1967). *The social construction of reality.* New York: Anchor.

Bhargava Raman, R. P., Sheshardri, S. P., Janardhan Reddy, Y. C., Girimaji, S. C., Srinath, S., & Raghunandan, V. N. G. P. (2007). Is bipolar II disorder misdiagnosed as major depressive disorder in children? *Journal of Affective Disorders, 98*(3), 263–266.

Cassano, G. B., Akiskal, H. S., Savino, M., Musetti, L., & Perugi, G. (1992). Proposed subtypes of bipolar II and related disorders: With hypomanic episodes (or cyclothymia) and with hyperthymic temperament. *Journal of Affective Disorders, 26*, 127–140.

Cox, B. J., Enns, M. W., Borger, S. C., & Parker, J. D. A. (1999). The nature of the depressive experience in analogue and clinically depressed samples. *Behavior Research and Therapy, 37*, 15–24.

Evans-Campbell, T., Lincoln, K. D., & Takeuchi, D. T. (2008). Race and mental health: Past debates, new opportunities. In: W. R. Avison, J. D. McLeod & B. A. Pescosolido (Eds), *Mental health, social mirror* (pp. 169–189). New York: Springer.

Ghaemi, S., Sachs, G., Chiou, A., Pandurangi, A., & Goodwin, F. (1999). Is bipolar disorder still underdiagnosed? Are antidepressants overutilized? *Journal of Affective Disorders, 52*, 135–144.

Goodwin, F. K., & Jamison, K. R. (2007). *Manic-depressive illness: Bipolar disorders and recurrent depression* (2nd ed.). New York: Oxford University Press.

Groopman, J. (2007). What's normal? The difficulty of diagnosing bipolar disorder in children. *The New Yorker*, April 9.

Hacking, I. (1986). Making up people. In: M. Lock & J. Farquhar (Eds), *Beyond the body proper: Reading the anthropology of material life.* Durham, NC: Duke University Press.

Harpaz-Rotem, I., Leslie, D. L., Martin, A., & Rosenheck, R. A. (2005). Changes in child and adolescent inpatient psychiatric admission diagnoses between 1995 and 2000. *Social Psychiatry and Psychiatric Epidemiology, 40*(8), 642–647.

Harris, G., Carey, B., & Roberts, J. (2007). Psychiatrists, children, and drug industry's role. *New York Times*, May 10. Available at http://www.nytimes.com/2007/05/10/health/10psyche.html (accessed November 22, 2008).

Hartley, J. (2002). Direct-to-patient drug advertising criticized. *General Practitioner, 7*(15), 10–13.

Healy, D. (2008). *Mania: A short history of bipolar disorder.* Baltimore: Johns Hopkins University Press.

Horwitz, A. V. (2002). *Creating mental illness.* Chicago: University of Chicago Press.

Horwitz, A. V., & Wakefield, J. C. (2007). *The loss of sadness.* New York: Oxford University Press.

Judd, L., & Akiskal, H. S. (2003). The prevalence and disability of bipolar spectrum disorders in the US population: Re-analysis of the ECA database taking into account subthreshold cases. *Journal of Affective Disorders, 73*(1–2), 123–131.

Kessler, R., McGonagle, K., Zhao, S., Nelson, C., Hughes, M., Eshieman, S., Wittchen, H., & Kendler, K. (1994). Lifetime and 12-month prevalence of *DSM-IIIR* psychiatric disorders in the United States: Results from the National Comorbidity Survey. *Archives of General. Psychiatry, 5*, 8–19.

Kraepelin, E., & Diefendorf, A. R. (1912). *Clinical psychiatry: A textbook for students and physicians.* London: Macmillan.

Leshner, A. I. (2001). Addiction is a brain disease. *Issues in Science and Technology, 17*(3), 75–80.

Lewinsohn, P., Shankman, S., Gau, J., & Klein, D. (2004). The prevalence and co-morbidity of subthreshold psychiatric conditions. *Psychological Medicine, 34*, 613–621.

Lewinsohn, P., Solomon, A., Seeley, J., & Zeiss, A. (2000). Clinical implications of subthreshold depressive symptoms. *Journal of Abnormal Psychology, 109*(2), 345–351.

Manning, J. S., Haykal, R. F., Connor, P. D., & Akiskal, H. S. (1997). On the nature of depressive and anxious states in a family practice setting: The high prevalence of bipolar II and related disorders in a cohort followed longitudinally. *Comprehensive Psychiatry, 38*(2), 102–108.

Martin, E. (1991). The egg and the sperm: How science has constructed a romance based on stereotypical male–female roles. *Signs, 16*, 485–501.

Mayes, R., & Horwitz, A. (2005). *DSM-III* and the revolution in the classification of mental illness. *Journal of the History of the Behavioral Sciences, 41*(3), 249–267.

Millon, T. (2004). *Masters of the mind: Exploring the story of mental illness from ancient times to the new millennium.* Hoboken, NJ: Wiley.

Moreno, C., Laje, G., Blanco, C., Jiang, H., Schmidt, A. B., & Olfson, M. (2007). National trends in the outpatient diagnosis and treatment in bipolar disorder in youth. *Archives of General Psychiatry, 64*(9), 1032–1039.

Muntaner, C., Borrell, C., & Chung, H. (2008). Class relations, economic inequality and mental health: Why social class matters to the sociology of mental health. In: W. R. Avison, J. D. McLeod & B. A. Pescosolido (Eds), *Mental health, social mirror* (pp. 127–141). New York: Springer.

Ng, B., Camacho, A., Lara, D. R., Brunstein, M. G., Pinto, O. C., & Akiskal, H. S. (2008). A case series on the hypothesized connection between dementia and bipolar spectrum disorders: Bipolar type VI? *Journal of Affective Disorders, 107*, 307–315.

Olfson, M., Blaco, C., Liu, L., Moreno, C., & Laje, G. (2006). National trends in the outpatient treatment of children and adolescents with antipsychotic drugs. *Archives of General Psychiatry, 63*, 679–685.

Parker-Pope, T. (2008). Psychiatry handbook linked to drug industry. *New York Times*, May 6. Available at http://well.blogs.nytimes.com/2008/05/06/psychiatry-handbook-linked-to-drug-industry/ (accessed November 19, 2008).

Soares, J., & Gershon, S. (2000). The diagnostic boundaries of bipolar disorder. *Bipolar Disorders, 2*, 1–2.

Szasz, T. (1960). The myth of mental illness. *American Psychologist, 15*, 113–118.

Thomas, C., Conrad, P., Casler, R., & Goodman, E. (2006). Trends in the use of psychotropic medications among adolescents. *Psychiatric Services, 57*, 63–69.

Thomson, S. C., & Trotto, S. (2002). Washington U hosts program on depression among students. *St Louis Post-Dispatch*, November 13. Available at http://aisweb.wustl.edu/alumni/atwu.nsf/depression (accessed November 18, 2008).

Tohen, M., Hennen, J., Zarate, C. M., Baldessarini, R. J., Strakowski, S. M., Stoll, A. L., Faedda, G. L., Suppes, T., Gebre-Medhin, P., & Cohen, B. M. (2000). Two-year syndromal and functional recovery in 219 cases of first-episode major affective disorder with psychotic features. *American Journal of Psychiatry, 157*(2), 220–228.

Umberson, D., & Williams, K. (1999). Family status and mental health. In: C. S. Aneshensel & J. C. Phelan (Eds), *Handbook of the sociology of mental health* (pp. 225–253). New York: Plenum.

Wilson, M. (1993). *DSM-III* and the transformation of American psychiatry. *American Journal of Psychiatry, 150*(3), 399–410.

THE DEPRESSION EPIDEMIC: HOW SHIFTING DEFINITIONS AND INDUSTRY PRACTICES SHAPE PERCEPTIONS OF DEPRESSION PREVALENCE IN THE UNITED STATES

Sara Kuppin

ABSTRACT

Purpose – *To examine the influence of changing diagnostic tools and the pharmaceutical and health insurance industries' practices on perceptions of depression prevalence in the late 20th and early 21st centuries.*

Approach – *This is a general review of the sociohistorical shifts in depression diagnosis and pharmaceutical and health insurance industry practices during this time period as they impact professional and lay perceptions of changes in depression prevalence.*

Findings – *Shifts in the definition of depression to an increasingly medically oriented, social context-free definition along with the*

Understanding Emerging Epidemics: Social and Political Approaches
Advances in Medical Sociology, Volume 11, 263–279
Copyright © 2010 by Emerald Group Publishing Limited
All rights of reproduction in any form reserved
ISSN: 1057-6290/doi:10.1108/S1057-6290(2010)0000011018

interaction of the pharmaceutical industry, health care, and health insurance industries in the U.S. system of mental health care have become major organizers of professional and lay perceptions of the nature of depression, its treatment, and prevalence. These sociohistorical and economic influences need to be factored into debates on depression prevalence.

Contribution of paper to the field – *This chapter provides an introductory-level synthesis of basic psychiatric epidemiology concepts and social science critiques of professional and lay perceptions of depression prevalence as "epidemic."*

INTRODUCTION

Depression is understood by many as a major public health problem of epidemic proportions (Costello, Erkanali, & Angold, 2006; Horwitz & Wakefield, 2006). In 1999, the U.S. Surgeon General's office published *Mental Health: A Report of the Surgeon General*, stressing the widespread nature of mental illness, with one in five Americans affected by mental illness each year. Mood disorders are depicted as particularly prevalent, ranking among the top 10 causes of disability worldwide, with depression being the most common type (U.S. Health and Human Services, 1999). Many public mental health epidemiologists, treatment advocates, and policy makers express concern over increasing prevalence of depression and the associated suffering and economic cost, particularly with regard to the fact that most who experience "clinically significant" depression do not receive adequate professional treatment (Compton, Conway, Stinson, & Grant, 2006; U.S. Health & Human Services, 1999).

Epidemiologic studies indicate high and rising rates of depressive disorders in the United States and across the world throughout the late 20th and early 21st centuries. After highlighting basic elements of the definitions of depression and epidemic used in epidemiology, this chapter briefly describes these studies. The focus of the chapter, however, is on the historical context of depression diagnosis and its impact on the perception of depression prevalence over this time period. The implications of these shifts for practices in the pharmaceutical and health insurance industries regarding treatment for depression and the significance for examining professional as well as lay perceptions of depression prevalence are discussed.

What is Depression and could there be an Epidemic?

Depression has come to be known by many Americans as a common health condition (Kessler, Chiu, Demler, & Walters, 2005). The term "depression" has entered everyday discourse in the United States (Summerfield, 2006), a fact that is interesting in and of itself, and is explored in depth later in the chapter. But what is "depression?" The term "depression" in epidemiology refers to the medical science term "major depressive episode"[1] as labeled and defined in the following excerpt from the latest edition of the American Psychiatric Association's (2000) *Diagnostic and Statistical Manual (DSM) (version IV-R) of Mental Disorders,*[2] the primary tool used by psychiatrists, other medical doctors, psychologists, other mental health counselors and therapists, and researchers, to define and diagnose mental health disorders:

> Five (or more) of the following symptoms have been present during the same two week period and represent a change from previous functioning; at least one of the symptoms is either (1) depressed mood or (2) loss of interest or pleasure.
>
> (1) Depressed mood most of the day, nearly every day, an indicated by either subjective report (e.g., feels sad or empty) or observation made by others (e.g., appears tearful).
> (2) Markedly diminished interest or pleasure in all, or almost all, activities most of the day, nearly every day (as indicated by subjective account or observation made by others).
> (3) Significant weight loss when not dieting or weight gain (e.g., a change of more than 5% body weight in a month), or decrease or increase in appetite nearly every day.
> (4) Insomnia or hypersomnia nearly every day.
> (5) Psychomotor agitation or retardation nearly every day (observable by others, not merely subjective feelings of restlessness or being slowed down).
> (6) Fatigue or loss of energy nearly every day.
> (7) Feelings of worthlessness or excessive or inappropriate guilt (which may be delusional) nearly every day (not merely self-reproach or guilt about being sick)
> (8) Diminished ability to think or concentrate, or indecisiveness, nearly every day (either by subjective account or as observed by others).
> (9) Recurrent thoughts of death (not just fear of dying), recurrent suicidal ideation without a specific plan, or a suicide attempt or a specific plan for committing suicide.[3]

According to the *DSM-IV-TR* (2000), major depressive episode is a disorder of mood and becomes recurrent "MDD" when a person has had two or more "episodes" of depression.

The U.S. Centers for Disease Control and Prevention (CDC) defines an epidemic as "the occurrence of disease within a specific geographical area or population that is in excess of what is normally expected" (www.cdc.gov/vaccines/about/terms/glossary). This definition of epidemic highlights two key issues that arise in the debate about whether or not there is an epidemic of depression. First, to be an epidemic requires that depression be defined as a disease state. Yet while psychiatry and other branches of medicine tend to frame depression as "MDD" from a medically oriented "disease" perspective, many in the fields of psychology, social psychology, sociology, and others argue depression is best viewed as primarily psychosocial in nature (Conrad, 2005; Gabbard & Kay, 2001; Summerfield, 2006). From this non-medical point of view, while many may report symptoms of depression, symptoms are more likely an indicator of either misidentification of normal emotional experience as disorder (Horwitz & Wakefield, 2007) or indication of a widespread internalization of social ills rather than an individual experience of disease (Blazer, 2005).

The second key question regarding depression's status as an epidemic highlighted in the CDC's definition is, if an epidemic requires occurrence of a condition "in excess of what is normally expected," what is a "normal" amount of depression? Is the number of people found to be depressed in U.S. studies higher than what should be expected? Are those diagnosed in these studies as depressed experiencing abnormal mood disorder or rather the normal ups and downs of life? To label depression an "epidemic" without clarity on how depression exhibits these basic elements of a public health epidemic is problematic and critics of the epidemic perspective of depression warn of broadly defining depressive symptoms as disorder, arguing that to do so is at the expense of acknowledging normal human emotional experience related to stressful life experiences and social circumstances (e.g., poverty and inequality). These perspectives will be discussed in detail after a short review of depression epidemiology and a review of the historical context of depression diagnosis as it relates to efforts to determine changes in prevalence over time.

DEPRESSION EPIDEMIOLOGY

Prevalence is defined as: "The number or proportion of cases or events or conditions in a given population" (www.cdc.gov/reproductivehealth/epiglossary/glossary.htm#P). As is the case in the epidemiologic assessment of any health condition, measuring the prevalence of depression requires that "depression" be accurately and precisely defined. Defining depression is in and of itself subject to controversy as scholars and researchers from a variety of fields subscribe to differing, shifting, though often overlapping definitions.

"Prevalence" and "epidemic" are public health terms designed to specify disease in a population. The mental health treatment community as well as the public health and medical research communities use specific definitions of various "types" of depression as described in the definition of Major Depressive Episode and Disorder featured in the *DSM-IV-TR* (2000). An understanding of how and why depression has come to be defined in medical and public health spheres sheds light on both professional and lay understandings of depression prevalence. However, throughout the rest of the chapter, the use of the term "depression" is often purposefully vague as is necessary to discuss depression from both medical and non-medical perspectives where the definition of the condition and even its nature is contested terrain.

Epidemiologic Studies of Depression Prevalence

Mental health services planning efforts have long depended on community studies in the general population to estimate prevalence of psychiatric disorders such as depression (Patten, 2008; Millman, 2001). After a few early attempts in the first part of the 20th century to measure prevalence of mental disorders which were limited mostly to institutional samples, by mid-century epidemiologic studies were focusing on measuring mental health problems at the population level. These later studies focused on psychiatric classifications and depended on descriptive rather than etiologic foundations (Grob, 1985). However, because of variation in design and classification systems, resulting prevalence estimates vary (Compton et al., 2006).

The Midtown Manhattan and Stirling County studies (Dohrenwend, 1982; Simon et al., 1994) are the most notable of the early community studies. The Stirling County Study of Canadian adults, conducted in three waves (1952, 1970, and 1992), found current prevalence rates of depression at approximately 5% and which remained stable over the study period (Murphy, 2000).[4] The Midtown Manhattan Study began as a cross-sectional study fielded in 1954, adding a follow-up in 1974. Results in 1954 indicated a high (23%) preponderance of "impairment" (defined as clinically significant need for treatment) in adult residents in the study area of Manhattan (Millman, 2001). The later round of data collection in 1974 indicated that for the 695 persons interviewed at both points in time, overall mental health composition remained unchanged (Millman, 2001; Strole & Fischer, 1980).[5]

More recent large epidemiologic studies of mental disorder used a cross-sectional study design to look at prevalence of MDD, including the

Epidemiological Catchment Area (ECA) Study and the National Co-morbidity Survey (NCS). These studies were fielded to yield community-based estimates that could be compared to clinical studies through the use of disorder classifications based on the *DSM-III* (Blazer, 2005). The ECA, conducted in 1980s in five regions across the United States, found 12-month prevalence for MDD to be 2.2% (Robins & Reiger, 1991).[6] The NCS conducted in 1990–1992 and its follow-up National Co-morbidity Replication Survey (NCS-R) conducted in 2001–2002 are currently the gold standard measure of prevalence of mental disorders in psychiatric epidemiology (Kessler et al., 1994; Kessler et al., 2005). Using representative samples of the U.S. population, the NCS estimated 12-month prevalence of MDD to be 8.6% while the later NCS-R indicated a 12-month prevalence of MDD of 6.6% (Kessler et al., 2003).[7,8] A 2006 study analyzing changes in prevalence of major depression between 1991–1992 and 2001–2002 using data from two cross-sectional, representative samples of U.S. population found a more than twofold increase in 12-month prevalence of major depression from 3.33% in 1991–1992 to 7.06% in 2001–2002 (Compton et al., 2006).[9]

In sum, the more recent psychiatric epidemiologic studies indicate a large increase over the second half of the 20th century in the prevalence of mental disorders, including depressive disorders (Compton et al., 2006). This increase in measured prevalence has led to much speculation in scientific and lay circles on what may explain the perceived rise in depression such as whether environmental stressors such as urbanization, changing family structure, economic stresses, and environmental toxins may be responsible for such a trend (Simon et al., 1994; Strole & Fischer, 1980). Although some epidemiologists argue that the perceived increase is likely an artifact of changes in definitions and measurement error rather than a true increase in prevalence (Costello et al., 2006; Simon et al., 1994), others point to the increased recognition and treatment of depressive disorders as partial explanation for this detected increase in prevalence (Kessler et al., 2003). And still others, as discussed in the following section, point to changes in psychiatric diagnostic criteria and their implications for the pharmaceutical and health insurance industries as main drivers in what appears to be a sharp increase in depression prevalence.

History of Psychiatric Diagnosis and Influential Role of the DSM

Contemporary critics of the labeling of depression as an epidemic point to the historical shifts in conceptualization of mental illness from a psychosocial-focused model to the now dominant biomedical model to account for current views of depression as widespread and ever-growing (Blazer, 2005; Horwitz & Wakefield, 2007). While medical sociologists and public health historians trace the concept of depression to Hippocrates (Horwitz & Wakefield, 2007), the term "major depression" did not appear in the medical literature until the mid-20th century (Blazer, 2005). Before then, the relationship of symptomatology to etiology was at the crux of any definition of depression (Grob, 1985; Wilson, 1993).

While a medical perspective on the etiology of mental illness has existed throughout the 20th century, a psychoanalytic school of thought emphasizing a psychosocial etiology of depression dominated by mid-century during which time depression was seen on a continuum of normal to disordered (Luhrmann, 2000). That this was the dominant perspective in psychiatry is evident in the first edition of the *DSM*, published in 1952. This first edition was based heavily in psychoanalytic theory and downplayed biological aspects of mental disorders. It was around this time that the psychiatric treatment community shifted focus from more serious psychotic illness in state-run hospitals to less serious mental health conditions increasingly likely to be treated with psychoanalysis in outpatient settings (Shadish, 1984).

However, with the third edition of the *DSM* (*DSM-III*) (American Psychiatric Association, 1980) comes an important shift in the conceptualization of disorders in psychiatry – this and subsequent editions have taken a symptom-focused approach to diagnosis. With the goal of making the *DSM* accessible for widespread use, the creators of the *DSM-III* attempted to make the manual devoid of reference to etiology to ensure its acceptance and use, since there were and continue to be differences of opinion within and among fields as to the causes of depression (Horwitz, 2002; Horwitz & Wakefield, 2007; Kirk & Kutchins, 1992). A symptom-focused manual also provided standardized definitions that could be operationalized for research purposes to serve the emerging field of psychiatric epidemiology. Because the science on the cause of mental disorders like depression was not definitive and there was disagreement in psychiatry and related fields on etiology, creating a cause- and context-free tool became a central goal in the development of later versions of the manual, and encouraged the symptom-based approach to persist. Subsequently, since making its debut in the 1980 publication of the *DSM-III*, the label MDD has become increasingly common in the psychiatric literature and in diagnostic application (Blazer, 2005).

MEDICALIZING SADNESS

The surge in anti-depressant prescribing is as much a cultural trend as a medical one, reflecting the rise of medicalization and professionalization of everyday life and its problems across Western societies. (Summerfield, 2006, p. 162)

Within and outside of epidemiology there is disagreement as to whether or not depression prevalence is in fact increasing, has reached "epidemic" proportions, or should even be viewed through what is argued to be the often "medicalized" lens of epidemiology. That is to say, whether or not there is an epidemic of depression depends on from which perspective this question is answered. While many critics of an epidemic label for depression acknowledge depression can be a serious, debilitating mental health problem, that there is a "universally valid, pathological entity" in need of medical treatment is perceived as false (Summerfield, 2006). A medically focused, biological definition of depression and the public health frame of epidemic are reflective of the interests of profit-motivated industry rather than health interests of populations.

Supported by findings from the large-scale epidemiologic surveys just discussed, many researchers in the medical and public health arena view depression as a major public health problem with "epidemic" features. Scholars from various fields including sociology, psychology, social work, nursing, and philosophy argue that what appears to be in both professional and lay conceptions as an epidemic of depression is in reality a result of shifts in our social institutions which have influenced our conceptions of what depression is and what to do about it, rather than an accurate assessment of disease rates. What used to be considered part of normal human emotional experience is now, by way of a process termed "medicalization," deemed a medically defined mood disorder. Critics of the *DSM* from a variety of disciplines argue that the manual currently lacks the context necessary to delineate disorder of clinical significance from non-disordered "normal" sadness, resulting in an over-inclusive definition of MDD as the primary contributor to the current overestimates of prevalence of MDD (Conrad, 2005; Horwitz & Wakefield, 2007; Summerfield, 2006).

Defining Medicalization in the Context of Depression

"Medicalization" refers to the process by which the jurisdiction of medicine is increased through the expansion of problems defined by and in terms of the medical establishment (Conrad, 2005). The concept of medicalization, first described in the 1970s, is central to social science critiques of medicine and public health (Aneshensel & Phelan, 1999). Psychiatric illness has long been the subject of medicalization debates, and because of the difficulty in identifying clear-cut biological mechanisms for the diagnosis of various mental disorders, the degree to which the mental is medical remains contested. Yet as depression becomes increasingly framed as a "disease" state, it is represented in professional as well as lay communities as an objectively definable condition regarding the natural function of the body (Bolton, 2008).

In their recent book *The Loss of Sadness: How Psychiatry Transformed Normal Sorrow into Depressive Disorder*, Horwitz and Wakefield (2007) are explicitly concerned with what they view as an over-medicalization of depression encouraged by the current diagnostic tools (e.g., *DSM-IV-R*) used in psychiatry. They write:

> the current 'epidemic' of depression, although a result of many social factors, has been made possible by a changed psychiatric definition of depressive disorder that often allows the classification of sadness as disease, even when it is not. (p. 6)

While acknowledging depressive disorders exist, these authors argue that the "explosion" of diagnosed depression (e.g., MDD) is primarily the result of "conflating the two conceptually distinct categories of normal sadness and depressive disorder" so that those experiencing normal emotional instances of sadness are now classified in epidemiologic studies as depressed. Horwitz and Wakefield argue, as outlined earlier, that the *DSM*'s most recent versions *DSM-IV* (American Psychiatric Association, 1997) and *DSM-IV-TR* (2000) have encouraged this conflation of normal sadness with depressive disorder with their focus on symptomatology without regard to context. From this perspective, the *DSM*'s utility as a research tool aimed at increasing reliability of the depression diagnosis among researchers has come at a cost to the validity of the diagnosis. And, as discussed in the following section, the explosion of diagnosed depression is further driven by the profit interests of industry.

MEDICALIZATION IN PRACTICE: THE ROLE OF INDUSTRY

Pharmaceutical Industry and Depression Prevalence

How is medicalization happening? Is it influencing our perceptions of depression prevalence? The answer to these questions requires an examination of industries' interests and practices – specifically the pharmaceutical and health insurance industries (Conrad, 2005). Each has a potentially useful purpose in society, yet it must be acknowledged that each is also motivated by financial profit and, to further business interests, uses the *DSM* in specific ways which interact to influence professional as well as lay conceptions of depression prevalence.

Early scholars writing about medicalization and mental illness focused on the role of psychiatry as a profession in bringing mental illness back under the umbrella of medical illness for their own professional proprietary purposes. More recently, other forces have become involved in the medicalization of depression, including the proliferation of pharmaceutical companies' research and development of antidepressant medication and subsequent increases in prescription (Olfson et al., 2002; Pincus et al., 1998) along with their ability to market products directly to the public with direct-to-consumer (DTC) advertising (Summerfield, 2006).

In 1997, the U.S. Food and Drug Administration (FDA) approved the use of DTC drug advertisements in popular media. Before this time, pharmaceutical advertising was relegated to publications targeted at medical doctors. By 2000, the pharmaceutical industry was spending over $2 billion annually on DTC advertisements. A lot of this money was and continues to be spent to advertise antidepressants and particularly the selective serotonin reuptake inhibitor (SSRI) antidepressants which have come to be some of the best selling drugs of all time (Lacasse & Leo, 2005).

While pharmaceutical companies began marketing antidepressants to the public at a time when the definition of major depressive episode and disorder in the *DSM-IV-TR* was symptom-focused and void of reference to etiology, DTC advertisements for SSRIs typically feature *DSM*-defined symptoms of MDD in conjunction with explicit reference to (biological) etiology, defining depression as a "chemical imbalance" or lack of normal levels of the neurotransmitter serotonin in the brain.

The structure of these advertisements which typically ask viewers to self-identify "symptoms" and then ask their doctors about the advertised medication, and the subsequent linking in these advertisements of symptoms void of context to a biological etiology (e.g., chemical imbalance), reifies a medicalized definition of depression. Surveys indicate many people get the bulk of their information about mental illness from mass media (Lawrie, 2000; Sieff, 2003), including advertisements. With a medicalized frame of depression dominating public discourse, the lay public becomes ripe for a view of depression as not just a "disease" but one of "epidemic" proportions.

Depression offers a somewhat unique opportunity for the pharmaceutical industry. Medications work on human biology and therefore pharmaceutical companies depend on biological definitions of health problems to sell their products. While the medical and to some degree health insurance industries perpetuate the extreme biological definition purported by the pharmaceutical industry, in reality, science has not borne out the truth of the "chemical imbalance" theory of depression and currently seems to be supporting a complex picture of causality that is biopsychosocial in nature (Lacasse & Leo, 2005). It remains the case that there is no definitive test – no blood test or X-ray – to confirm or deny someone has MDD. This lack of clarity as to etiology, however, provides an opportunity to the pharmaceutical industry of which it has taken full advantage. Because of the uncertainty about cause and the widespread nature of the "symptoms" as defined by the *DSM*, depression diagnosis is more malleable and suggestible – open to interpretation and thus providing opportunity for this industry to expand and morph the definition of what is treatable "illness" to serve their business interests. In this same vein, antidepressants are now approved and advertised for a variety of mental health conditions that, as defined by the current version of the *DSM-IV-TR* (2000), have "symptoms" likely to describe the experience of a large number of viewers.

With the advent of DTC advertising comes the re-framing of patient as consumer, contributing to a new configuration of relationships in which patients are now markets to be tapped or, as just described, markets to be created (Conrad, 2005). Coinciding with advertising of antidepressants directly to the public is an increase in non-advertisement media coverage on the topic. Not only has depression as a topic in scientific literature grown greatly since the term first appeared in the 1970s, but depression and the concern over perceived growth in the prevalence of depression has also become an increasingly common topic for the popular press (Costello et al., 2006; Kuppin, 2006). As depressive disorders began being marketed to the public via DTC advertisements for antidepressant medication, public awareness and concern regarding depression increased. This fact is cited as a benefit of DTC advertising of psychiatric medication by advocates; however, through the lens of antidepressant advertisements, common everyday life experiences or troubles have become framed as disordered, or "sick" and in need of treatment with medication.

Pharmaceutical Companies, Managed Health Care, and Medicine:
How Treatment affects Perceptions of Prevalence

While the pharmaceutical industry's role in the treatment of depression has grown exponentially over the past two decades, the American health insurance industry has also, in tandem with the pharmaceutical industry, greatly influenced depression treatment and perceptions of prevalence by emphasizing a narrow "medicalized" view of depression (Barsky & Borus, 1995; Conrad, 2005). As suggested in the previous section, with advertising of medications and diagnostic criteria directly to the public comes this shift from people seeing themselves and being seen as "patients" to being viewed and viewing themselves as "consumers." Medical sociologist Conrad (2005) writes:

> In our current age, consumers have become increasingly vocal and active in their desire and demand for services. Individuals as consumers rather than patients help shape the scope, and sometimes the demand for, medical treatments for human problems. (p. 9)

This "patient as consumer" frame, supported by DTC advertising, requires a shift in the traditional doctor–patient relationship.

In addition to DTC advertising, depression diagnosis and treatment has become entangled in very practical ways with American health insurance industry practices. Around the time that antidepressants were becoming available in the late 1980s and 1990s is the expansion of managed health care (Kahn, 1990; Kramer, 1993). Managed care prefers faster, least expensive treatment alternatives which, in the case of depression, means medication over psychotherapy. Psychotherapy (e.g., "talk therapy"), a long-time professional treatment option for depressive symptoms, does not fit well with a managed care model – it is not fast, it is not inexpensive, and measuring its effectiveness is more complex than for medication as human variability in therapists can be difficult to account for in outcome studies. To the degree that patients are unable or unwilling to pay for service out of pocket, they must seek the services covered by their health insurance carrier, all of whom, by now, employ at least some managed care practices meaning that health insurance companies have been reluctant to cover psychotherapy costs. With recent mental health parity legislation, insurance companies are being mandated to provide better psychotherapy benefits, but most still have strict limits on coverage unless the mental health problem is deemed by the provider as "biologically-based."

As a result of health insurance structures, physicians are often limited in their practice – what they can diagnose and offer as treatment is somewhat determined by what their patients' health insurance companies define as acceptable. They are also encouraged by insurance companies through fee structures and incentives to select certain diagnoses and treatments over others based on cost. By law, medication must be prescribed by a physician (psychiatric medication cannot be prescribed by a psychologist or other mental health treatment professional). This system structure incentivizes physicians to deem a patient's depression as "biologically-based" as that is what is often required for reimbursement for services rendered.

In addition, managed care has encouraged a reduction in the length of time of physician encounters with patients. In order to profit themselves, doctors must see as many patients as possible to make their practice economically viable. This is very compatible with antidepressant prescription and very incompatible, as discussed, with psychotherapeutic models of mental health care that typically require more time-intensive treatment encounters.

In sum, the health insurance industry, although providing insurance, not medical care, have become important decision-makers regarding what is and is not appropriate treatment for depression. Diagnosis has become entangled in very practical and critical ways with health insurance systems which, in turn, affects the way depression and other mental health treatments are practiced. Therefore, the current and future versions of the *DSM* have and will be more than just a tool for psychiatrists and psychiatric epidemiologists but the basis on which insurance companies decide what services are reimbursable. It is in this way that the interaction of the pharmaceutical industry, health care, and health insurance industries in the U.S. system of mental health care has become a major organizer of our collective perceptions of the nature of depression (as biological), its treatment (with medication), and prevalence (as high and rising).

CONCLUSION: THE DEPRESSION EPIDEMIC AND ITS IMPACT ON THE EXPERIENCE AND TREATMENT OF DEPRESSION

Community studies, rather than uncovering high rates of depressive disorders, simply show that the natural results of acute or chronic stressful experiences could be distressing enough to fit the *DSM* definition of disorder. (Horwitz & Wakefield, 2006, p. 22)

Whether or not they agree with a medical definition of depression, most scholars agree depression is a common and widespread experience. Without doubt quality care, including medication, can range from beneficial to life-saving in the case of depression and other mental health problems. To say depression is not an epidemic is not to argue that it is any less potentially serious a condition, or to argue against the idea that more treatment options need to be made available to those experiencing this debilitating condition. Nor should the idea that depression is "common" be translated to mean that it is not a condition to be taken seriously.

Considering the sociohistorical context of the idea of depression as an epidemic, and the impact of industry on professional and lay perceptions of depression prevalence, questions remain: what is causing this epidemic of depression, whether real or only perceived? What epidemiologic studies are measuring – the number of people experiencing the "symptoms" of the *DSM-IV-TR*-defined MDD – may very well be yielding numbers in the right ballpark, but is this reflective of a level of disorder or disease? Is it an indication of the level of need for treatment? Is it accurate, necessary, or even helpful to view depression as an epidemic? These are the questions being asked by critics of the epidemic perspective of depression, as well as those who question other recent epidemics, such as obesity or autism. Debates about whether or not there is an obesity epidemic, or increasing prevalence of autism, have similar features to the depression debate, including concerns over diagnostic definitions, recognition, and the influence of industry on perceptions of prevalence and treatment need.

To focus on only the biological and genetic individual rather than confronting the overwhelming and difficult-to-affect social problems at the root of much mental suffering is as potentially dangerous as any epidemic in its implications. Critics of an epidemic label for depression warn us of the dangers of over-medicalization of a mental health problem that is in reality most likely a highly complex interaction of human biology, genetics, psychology, and social and physical environments. Answers to the questions highlighted in this chapter regarding the prevalence of depressive symptoms and their implications for the experience and treatment of this mental health problem require continued study and awareness of concerning social structures and forces influencing depression definition, diagnoses, and treatment. A few of the major forces are discussed in this chapter, including the pharmaceutical and health insurance industries. These forces will likely shift and change over time, as will our conceptions of what depression is and what to do about it. Research needs to do the same if public health professionals hope to protect the interests of the ill as well as those of the healthy from untoward influence of industry on the diagnosis and treatment of depressive disorder.

NOTES

1. There are a variety of subtypes of major depressive disorder (MDD) including psychotic depression, melancholic depression, atypical depression, and catatonic depression, as well as other types of depression including postpartum depression, seasonal affect disorder, dysthymia, and bipolar depression.

2. The World Health Organization's International Statistical Classification of Diseases and related Health Problems (ICD-10) uses the label "recurrent depressive disorder".

3. Other important details of the diagnostic criteria include: (1) symptoms cause significant distress or impairment and (2) symptoms are not better accounted for by bereavement.

4. Measured by identified responses to questions on versions 1 and 2 of the structured, lay-administered Depression and Anxiety (DPAX).

5. Measured general mental health using psychiatrists' ratings on global mental health of respondent defined as level of strain in adult role functioning.

6. Measured major depressive disorder as defined in the *DSM-III* with the structured, lay-administered Diagnostic Interview Schedule.

7. Measured major depressive disorder as defined in the *DSM-III-R* with a modified version of the structured, lay-administered Composite International Diagnostic Interview.

8. Measured major depressive disorder as defined in the *DSM-IV* with an expanded version of the Composite International Diagnostic Interview used in the NCS.

9. Both data sets used in the study measured major depressive episode as defined in *DSM-IV* with the Alcohol Use Disorder and Associated Disabilities Interview Schedule *DSM-IV* version.

ACKNOWLEDGMENTS

The preparation of this chapter was supported by National Institutes of Mental Health Research Training Program in Psychiatric Epidemiology Grant #5-T32-MH013043. The author thanks the Psychiatric Epidemiology Training Program Fellows and Faculty at Columbia University in New York City, Vivian Santiago, and Richard Carpiano for their feedback and support.

REFERENCES

American Psychiatric Association. (1980). *Diagnostic and statistical manual of mental disorders* (3rd ed.). Washington, DC: American Psychiatric Association.

American Psychiatric Association. (1997). *Diagnostic statistical manual of mental disorders* (4th ed.). Washington, DC: American Psychiatric Association.

American Psychiatric Association. (2000). *Diagnostic and statistical manual of mental disorders* (4th ed., text revision). Washington, DC: American Psychiatric Association.

Aneshensel, C., & Phelan, J. (1999). The sociology of mental illness: Surveying the field. In: C. Aneshensel & J. Phelan (Eds), *Handbook of sociology of mental health* (pp. 3–17). Dordrecht, Netherlands: Kluwer Academic Publishers.

Barsky, A., & Borus, J. (1995). Somatization and medicalization in the era of managed care. *Journal of the American Medical Association, 274*, 1931–1934.

Blazer, D. (2005). *The age of melancholy*. New York: Routledge.

Bolton, D. (2008). *What is mental disorder?* Oxford: Oxford University Press.

Compton, W., Conway, K., Stinson, F., & Grant, B. (2006). Changes in the prevalence of depression and comorbid substance use disorders in the United States between 1991–1992 and 2001–2002. *American Journal of Psychiatry, 163,* 2141–2147.

Conrad, P. (2005). The shifting engines of medicalization. *Journal of Health and Social Behavior, 46*(1), 3–14.

Costello, E. J., Erkanali, A., & Angold, A. (2006). Is there an epidemic of adolescent depression? *Journal of Child Psychology and Psychiatry, 47*(12), 1263–1271.

Dohrenwend, B., & Dohrenwend, B. S. (1982). Perspectives on the past and future of psychiatric epidemiology. *American Journal of Public Health, 72*(11), 1271–1279.

Gabbard, G., & Kay, J. (2001). The fate of integrated treatment: Whatever happened to the biopsychosocial psychiatrist? *American Journal of Psychiatry, 158*(12), 1956–1963.

Grob, G. (1985). The origins of American psychiatric epidemiology. *American Journal of Public Health, 75*(3), 229–236.

Horwitz, A. (2002). *Creating mental illness.* Chicago: University of Chicago Press.

Horwitz, A., & Wakefield, J. (2006). The epidemic of mental illness: Clinical fact or survey artifact? *Contexts, 5*(1), 19–23.

Horwitz, A., & Wakefield, J. (2007). *The loss of sadness: How psychiatry transformed normal sorrow into depressive disorder.* Oxford: Oxford University Press.

Kahn, D. (1990). The dichotomy of drugs and psychotherapy. *The Psychiatric Clinics of North America, 13*(2), 197–208.

Kessler, R., Berglund, P., Demler, O., Jin, R., Koretz, D., Merikangas, K., Rush, A., Walters, E., & Wang, P. (2003). The epidemiology of major depressive disorder: Results from the Comorbidity Survey Replication (NCS-R). *Journal of the American Medical Association, 289*(23), 3095–3105.

Kessler, R., Chiu, W., Demler, O., & Walters, E. (2005). Prevalence, severity, and comorbidity of 12-month *DSM-IV* disorders in the National Comorbidity Survey Replication. *Archives of General Psychiatry, 62,* 617–627.

Kessler, R., McGonagle, K., Zhao, S., Nelson, C., Hughes, M., & Eshelman, S. (1994). Lifetime and 12-month prevalence of *DSM-III-R* psychiatric disorders in the United States. *Archives of General Psychiatry, 51,* 8–19.

Kirk, S., & Kutchins, H. (1992). *The selling of the DSM*: The rhetoric of science in psychiatry. New York: Aldine.

Kramer, P. (1993). *Listening to Prozac.* New York: Penguin.

Kuppin, S. (2006). *The drug we love to hate: Prozac and representations of medication to treat depression in American newspapers, 1993–2003.* Dissertation Abstracts International, Vol. 67-04, Section: B, p. 1951.

Lacasse, J., & Leo, J. (2005). Serotonin and depression: A disconnect between the advertisements and the scientific literature. *PLoS Medicine, 2*(12), e392.

Lawrie, S. (2000). Newspaper coverage of psychiatric and physical illness. *Psychiatric Bulletin, 24,* 104–106.

Luhrmann, T. (2000). *Of two minds: The growing disorder in American psychiatry.* New York: Alfred A. Knopf.

Millman, E. (2001). The mental health and biosocial context of help-seeking in longitudinal perspective: The Midtown Longitudinal Study, 1954 to 1974. *American Journal of Orthopsychiatry, 71*(4), 450–456.

Murphy, J. (2000). Incidence of depression in the Stirling County Study: Historical and comparative perspectives. *Psychological Medicine, 30,* 505–514.

Olfson, M., Marcus, S., Druss, B., Elinson, L., Tanielian, T., & Pincus, H. (2002). National trends in the outpatient treatment of depression. *Journal of the American Medical Association, 287*(2), 203–209.

Patten, S. (2008). Major depression prevalence is very high, but the syndrome is a poor proxy for community populations' clinical treatment needs. *Canadian Journal of Psychiatry, 53*(7), 411–419.

Pincus, H., Tanielian, T., Marcus, S., Olfson, M., Zarin, D., Thompson, J., & Zito, J. (1998). Prescribing trends in psychotropic medications. *Journal of the American Medical Association, 279*(7), 526–531.

Robins, L., & Reiger, D. (1991). *Psychiatric disorders in America: The Epidemiological Catchment Area Study.* New York: Free Press.

Shadish, W. (1984). Policy research: Lessons from the implementation of deinstitutionalization. *American Psychologist, 39,* 725–738.

Sieff, E. (2003). Media frames and mental illness: The potential impact of negative frames. *Journal of Mental Health, 12*(3), 259–269.

Simon, G., Vonkroff, M., Ustun, B., Gater, R., Gureje, O., & Sartorius, N. (1994). Is the lifetime risk of depression actually increasing? *Journal of Clinical Epidemiology, 48*(9), 1109–1118.

Strole, L., & Fischer, A. (1980). The midtown Manhattan longitudinal study vs. the 'Paradise Lost' doctrine: A controversy joined. *Archives of General Psychiatry, 37,* 209–221.

Summerfield, D. (2006). Depression: Epidemic or pseudo-epidemic? *Journal of the Royal Society of Medicine, 99,* 161–162.

U.S. Department of Health and Human Services. (1999). *Mental health: A report of the surgeon general.* Rockville, MD: U.S. Department of Health and Human Services, Substance Abuse and Mental Health Services Administration, Center for Mental Health Services, National Institutes of Health, National Institute of Mental Health.

Wilson, M. (1993). *DSM III* and the transformation of American psychiatry: A history. *American Journal of Psychiatry, 150*(3), 399–410.

BIOMEDICALIZING MENTAL ILLNESS: THE CASE OF ATTENTION DEFICIT DISORDER

Manuel Vallée

ABSTRACT

Purpose – *The DSM-III reflected American psychiatry's shift from a dynamic approach to a descriptive diagnostic approach. This chapter seeks to elucidate the implications of this shift for the diagnosis and treatment of mental illness.*

Methodology/approach – *To shed light on this issue I analyze the diagnosis and treatment implications of this shift for Attention Deficit Disorder (ADD).*

Findings – *The transition to the diagnostic approach has had three consequences for the handling of ADD, and later Attention Deficit/ Hyperactivity Disorder (ADHD): first, it increased the number of children diagnosed with the disorder; second, it encouraged clinicians to treat the disorder with psychostimulants; and third, it expanded the pool of clinicians who could prescribe stimulants.*

Contribution to the field – *Beyond illuminating the specific cases of ADD and ADHD, this analysis contributes to the medicalization literature by demonstrating that there is more to be studied than merely the expansion*

Understanding Emerging Epidemics: Social and Political Approaches
Advances in Medical Sociology, Volume 11, 281–301
Copyright © 2010 by Emerald Group Publishing Limited
All rights of reproduction in any form reserved
ISSN: 1057-6290/doi:10.1108/S1057-6290(2010)0000011019

or contraction of diagnostic categories. Researchers also have to analyze the implicit assumptions within the diagnostic definitions, which have implications for the prevalence and treatment of illness.

INTRODUCTION

The Diagnostic and Statistical Manual (DSM) is American Psychiatry's main reference manual and provides classifications for all mental disorders recognized by the profession. Prior to 1980, the DSM reflected a dynamic clinical approach, where clinicians were encouraged to identify and address the underlying causes of mental illness. However, the edition released in 1980 (i.e., the DSM-III) differed profoundly from its predecessors as it reflected a symptom-based approach, which bracketed concerns about causes and encouraged clinicians to focus instead on describing and classifying symptoms.

The shift in approach was profound and this chapter examines the implications of the changes for the incidence and treatment of mental illness. To shed light on these issues, I analyze the case of Attention Deficit Disorder (ADD), and argue that the diagnostic approach had three consequences for the handling of ADD: (1) it increased the number of children diagnosed with the disorder, (2) it encouraged clinicians to treat the disorder with psychostimulants, and (3) it expanded the pool of clinicians who could prescribe stimulants.

In the next section I begin the analysis by explaining my conceptual framework. Then, to set the stage for analyzing DSM-III, I provide an overview of DSM-I and DSM-II, followed by an explanation of the changes made for the DSM-III. The third section is devoted to showing how the DSM-III changes impacted the diagnosis and treatment of ADD. The conclusion articulates how this essay helps us understand America's growing mental illness epidemic, as well as it is tendency to address mental illness with psychiatric medications. Additionally, I discuss the implications of this study for the diagnosis and treatment of nonpsychiatric illnesses, and end the chapter by suggesting lines of future research.

CONCEPTUAL FRAMEWORK

Conceptualizing Psychiatric Disease

Historically, sociologists have taken a constructionist approach vis-à-vis mental illness categories, viewing such categories as "culturally specific phenomenon" (Horwitz, 2002, p. 19). Importantly, most constructionists believe that "mental illnesses do not arise in nature but are constituted by social systems of meaning"(Horwitz, 2002, p. 6). In this approach, the mentally ill are not defined by anything they do, but rather by the cultural rules that define what is normal and abnormal behavior, which can vary from country to country and over time. The constructionist approach has much to offer, as it has helped sociologists understand the degree to which psychiatric diagnoses are cultural constructions. At the same time, however, Allan Horwitz argues that a strict constructionist approach is limited, for it fails to consider the biological reality of some disorders, which is particularly salient for the more severe disorders, such as schizophrenia, bipolar disorder, and other psychoses (*ibid.*, p. 9).

To rectify this shortcoming, Horwitz proposes a more nuanced conception of mental illness, one that considers the biological reality as well as the cultural overlay. First, he posits that "mental disorders arise when psychological systems of motivation, memory, cognition, arousal, attachment, and the like are not able to adequately carry out the functions they are designed to perform" (*ibid.*, p. 11). Next, he stresses that the standards of psychological functioning vary from society to society, which leads to differences in what is considered "normal" and "abnormal," as well as differences in the way the societies define their mental disorders.

One advantage of Horwitz's approach is that it enables researchers to analyze the cultural construction of diagnostic concepts without discarding the very real psychological dysfunctions that diagnostic concepts are trying to capture. In turn, this enables researchers to analyze the social forces that shape the diagnostic categories, while remaining sensitive to the patient's lived experience. Another advantage, and one more pertinent to this case, is that Horwitz's model helps us understand how different countries can produce diagnostic concepts (in this case ADD) that target the same symptoms, yet differ profoundly in their definition of those concepts.

In analyzing the United States, Horwitz (2007) argues that American psychiatry overpathologizes daily life, as its diagnostic system attributes all symptoms to biological dysfunctions, which fails to recognize that some symptoms are brought on by social circumstances. In this chapter, I apply Horwitz' insights to the concept of ADD.

The Relationship between Disease Definitions and Medication Usage

Differences in mental illness classifications matter, for how a disease is defined guides clinicians on what to consider as illness, which affects the number of people diagnosed with the disease. Consequently, even the smallest change to disease definitions can have enormous diagnostic implications, as emphasized by two researchers:

> ... by slightly altering the wording of a criterion, the duration for which a symptom must be experienced in order to satisfy a criterion, or the number of criteria used to establish a diagnosis, the prevalence rates in the United States will rise and fall as erratically as the stock market. (Kutchins & Kirk, 1997, p. 244).

Beyond the implications for prevalence, disease definitions are also consequential to medication usage, for the greater the disease prevalence, the greater the potential market for a given pharmaceutical treatment.

An interesting example is Alzheimer's Disease, which went from being an obscure disorder prior to 1980, to being among the top five causes of death in the United States. Fox (1989) attributes the change to a shift in the biomedical conceptualization of Alzheimer's. Specifically, the age criterion was removed from the disease definition, which helped transform what was previously considered senility "into a specific disease with specific pathological characteristics and symptoms." In turn, this shift in conceptualization allowed a greater number of symptomatic people to be diagnosed with the disorder, which greatly expanded the market for treatments (Fox, 1989).

THE DSM HISTORY

While psychoanalysts dominated American psychiatry from the late 1940s through the 1970s, their reign ended in the 1980s, when biological psychiatrists seized the profession's leadership. This transition in power was important because biological psychiatrists held a very different conception of mental illness, which led to significant changes in the DSM and to the treatment of mental illness. In the first half of this section I describe the psychoanalytic conception of mental illness and articulate how it shaped the DSM-I and DSM-II (released in 1952 and 1968, respectively). I then describe the biological psychiatrists' conception of mental illness, and elucidate how it shaped the DSM-III (released in 1980).

DSM-I: Reflecting the Psychodynamic Approach to Mental Illness

From the late 1940s to the late 1970s psychoanalysts dominated American psychiatry as they headed the vast majority of university psychiatry departments, and they held 75% of the committee posts within the American Psychiatric Association (APA; Healy, 2002). Moreover, most American clinicians were psychoanalytically trained and ascribed to dynamic psychiatry, which consisted of three tenets (Healy, 2002; Grob, 1991). First, the approach stipulated that mental illnesses were mainly due to malfunctions of psychological mechanisms, whose role it was to mediate between "instinctual biological drives and the pressures of the external social environment" (Grob 1991, p. 429).

Second, the approach prioritized a dynamic conception of mental illness over a categorical one (Grob, 1991; Wilson, 1993). Categorical understandings are used for nonpsychiatric illnesses (such as chicken pox, measles, mumps, etc.), where disease is either present or it is not. Psychoanalysts believed this conception was ill-suited for mental illness because dysfunctional environments could lead even normal people to migrate from states of wellness to states of illness (Wilson, 1993). Thus, they adhered to a dynamic conception, where mental health was mediated by the surrounding social context.

Third, they believed the psychiatrist's role was to help patients identify and address the social and psychological causes of psychological malfunction (Decker, 2007; Wilson, 1993), as opposed to merely treating the symptoms. Correspondingly, instead of seeing symptoms as something to be classified, they saw symptoms as something to be understood and explained. For example, Karl Menninger[1] argued:

> We must attempt to explain how the observed maladjustment came about and what the meaning of this sudden eccentricity or desperate or aggressive outburst is. What is behind the symptoms? (Menninger 1963, p. 325)

Menninger's perspective is considered to have been the essence of psychodynamic psychiatry: "to understand the meaning of the symptom and undo its psychogenic cause, rather than manipulate the symptom directly (through medication, suggestion, etc.)" (Wilson 1993, p. 400).

The psychodynamic approach was very present in the DSM-I, as suggested by three indicators. First, half the manual was devoted to socially and psychologically caused illnesses. Specifically, the DSM-I mental illness descriptions were arranged into two main categories. The first category listed mental disorders believed to result from or be precipitated by brain dysfunction, which could be brought on by numerous factors, such as infection, brain trauma, drugs, poisons, and alcoholic intoxication (Grob, 1991). The second encompassed disorders considered to result from psychological and/or social causes, and included schizophrenia, antisocial behavior, compulsiveness, stress, drug addiction, and many others (Grob, 1991).

Second, the DSM-I was heavily infused with psychoanalytic concepts, which implicitly attributed mental illness to social and psychological causes. One such concept was the "reaction" term, which was in the name of many mental disorders and implicitly suggested that the illness was a reaction to a dysfunctional environment. An example was the "paranoid reaction" diagnosis, whose name implicitly suggested that symptoms of paranoia were a reaction to a dysfunctional environment. Moreover, in the DSM-I all "functional" psychiatric diagnoses were characterized as "reactions" (Wilson, 1993, p. 401).

And third, the psychodynamic approach manifested itself by the fact mental illness descriptions did not contain symptom checklists. Rather, they consisted of short, general descriptions. These descriptions were intended to heuristically orient the clinician in the diagnostic and treatment process. Specifically, clinicians were encouraged to use the diagnostic concepts to make a general assessment of the patient's condition, which would orient them to the social and/or psychological issues that might be troubling the patient. Importantly, with this approach the initial diagnosis was not set in stone, but rather was subject to change, as the patient maneuvered through the healing process.

DSM-II: Refining the Existing System

In 1968, the APA published the 2nd edition of its Diagnostic Statistical Manual (i.e., DSM-II). For this edition the DSM developers made four changes: (1) they added new mental illness diagnoses, (2) they made minor revisions to preexisting concepts, (3) they attempted to drop references to illness etiology when the etiology was still in doubt, and (4) they encouraged clinicians to use multiple psychiatric diagnoses in a single patient (Kirk & Kutchins, 1992).

While these changes were important, they only amounted to a refinement of psychodynamic approach as the DSM-II continued to use psychoanalytic terms and to provide short, general descriptions of mental disorders (Kirk & Kutchins, 1992). An example was the entry for "Hyperkinetic Reaction to Childhood" (the predecessor to ADD) which read as follows:

> This disorder is characterized by overactivity, restlessness, distractibility, and short attention span, especially in young children; the behavior usually diminishes in adolescence. If this behavior is caused by organic brain damage, it should be diagnosed under the appropriate non-psychotic organic brain syndrome. (American Psychiatric Association, 1968)

Perhaps the most noteworthy item about the DSM-II is that it was intentionally organized to be in direct concordance with the World Health Organization's *International Classification of Disease*.[2] In 1968, the United States government entered into a treaty with the World Health Organization and agreed to use the ICD as its official diagnostic manual for all illnesses (Wilson, 1993). This meant that updates to the ICD would require the APA to update the DSM. Since ICD-8 was slated for release in 1968, the DSM developers worked to ensure that the DSM-II included all diagnostic categories that would be included in the ICD-8, thereby putting the two classification systems in concordance with each other (Kirk & Kutchins, 1992). Further, when it was announced that ICD-9 would be released in 1979, the APA began working on DSM-III, which was released in 1980.

DSM-III: The Shift to a Symptoms-Based Approach

While the DSM-I and DSM-II were developed by psychoanalytically trained clinicians, the DSM-III was developed by research psychiatrists, most of whom were affiliated with Washington University's psychiatry department (Wilson, 1993). That affiliation was significant because the Washington University department had no psychoanalysts (Healy, 2002, p. 295) and held notions that were antithetical to psychodynamic psychiatry.

First, they were at odds with the notion that mental disorders were caused by social and psychological causes, a hypothesis they considered unverifiable. Instead, they preferred to attribute mental illness to biological malfunctions (Klerman, 1978) and "believed that only empirical psychiatric research with a strong focus on biology held any hope for the treatment and improvement of the mentally ill" (Decker, 2007, p. 345). Second, biological psychiatrists had a profoundly different conception of mental illness. Instead of conceptualizing it in dynamic terms, they viewed mental illness in categorical terms – people were either sick or they were not (Klerman, 1978, p. 104). And third, they believed it was asking too much to ask clinicians to identify and treat the underlying causes of disease. Rather, they felt the best clinicians could do was (1) accurately identify symptoms, (2) attribute symptoms to the correct mental disorder categories, and (3) suppress symptoms through symptom-suppressing medications and/or other standardized treatments (Decker, 2007).

This perspective prompted the Washington University group to be very critical of psychoanalysts and their dynamic approach. Moreover, in the 1960s and 1970s the Washington group developed and promoted a descriptive approach to psychiatry, which limited itself to describing the mentally ill and which had an "intentional and explicit concern with diagnosis and classification" (Klerman, 1978, p. 105). Guided by this approach, the developers of DSM-III made two overarching changes to the DSM. First, all mental illness classifications were stripped of any explicit or implicit reference to environmental causes. Essentially, this consisted of removing all psychoanalytic concepts, which implicitly refer to environmental causes. An example is "hyperkinetic reaction to childhood" (found in the DSM-II), which developers changed to "Attention Deficit Disorder." While "hyperkinetic reaction to childhood" implied the syndrome was a result of a dysfunctional environment, such a notion is stripped from "Attention Deficit Disorder," a mental disorder classification that encourages clinicians to focus on the behavioral symptoms and implicitly attributes the cause of symptoms to the child's biology.

Second, the developers introduced standardized criteria for each mental illness. The criteria were lists of the symptoms that clinicians were supposed to observe before giving patients a particular diagnosis. For example, the criteria for "ADD with hyperactivity" stipulated that children had to exhibit three inattention symptoms (drawn from the list shown in Table 1), two symptoms of impulsivity, and two of hyperactivity. Alternatively, the "ADD without hyperactivity" concept required three symptoms of hyperactivity and three symptoms of impulsivity.

DSM-III developers contended that developing such explicit criteria was crucial for standardizing diagnostic practices and increasing the diagnostic consistency between physicians, which, prior to DSM-III, had been mediocre and undermined psychiatry's scientific legitimacy (Kirk & Kutchins, 1992). At the same time, however, providing clinicians with symptom checklists has had important implications for clinical practice, as it encourages clinicians to take a "descriptive" approach, where the focus is on accurately describing the symptoms and classifying them in the appropriate mental illness category (Decker, 2007). Importantly, the descriptive approach encourages clinicians to bracket their concerns about the causes of mental illness, which is a significant departure from the psychoanalysts' focus on the underlying causes of illness. In turn, ignoring the causes of mental illness has important treatment implications as it steers clinicians' away from interventions that could address the underlying causes, and guides them instead toward prescribing psychiatric medications and/or other treatments aimed at suppressing symptoms. In the next section Introduction I elucidate these issues through the case of ADD.

Table 1. Attention Deficit Disorder Criteria for DSM-III.

Inattention	(1) Often fails to finish things he or she starts	(2) Has difficulty sticking to a play activity	(3) Often does not seem to listen	(4) Easily distracted	(5) Has difficulty concentrating on schoolwork or other tasks requiring sustained attention
Hyperactivity	(1) Runs about or climbs on things excessively	(2) Has difficulty sitting still or fidgets excessively	(3) Moves about excessively during sleep	(4) Is always "on the go" or acts as if "driven by motor"	(5) Has difficulty staying seated
Impulsivity	(1) Often acts before thinking	(2) Shifts excessively from one activity to another	(3) Has difficulty organizing work	(4) Needs lots of supervision	(5) Frequently calls out in class

(6) Has difficulty awaiting turn in games or group situations

Source: American Psychiatric Association (1980).

CONSEQUENCES FOR THE TREATMENT OF ADD

While the overarching aim of developing diagnostic criteria was to standardize the diagnosis of ADD, the use of explicit criteria led to two developments, both of which contributed to the rise in psychostimulant usage. First, the criteria has favored a reductionist model of mental illness, which brackets concerns about the underlying cause of symptoms and steers treatment toward the pharmaceutical option. Second, the standardized criteria enables a greater number of practitioners to diagnose ADD, thereby boosting diagnoses and the corresponding psychostimulant prescriptions.

Bracketing Concerns About the Causes

The diagnostic approach brackets three types of causes: (1) psychosocial problems, (2) nutritional factors, and (3) exposures to environmental toxins.

Psychosocial problems include social, emotional, and psychological factors, and were psychiatry's primary focus between 1946 and 1980. An implication of bracketing these causes is that it encourages clinicians to efface the distinction between symptoms caused by an underlying psychological pathology and symptoms that are a normal response to a distressing event or environment (Horwitz, 2002). As Horwitz argues "symptoms of profound grief and immobilization are only signs of depression when they are disproportionate to the situation in which they occur" (*ibid.*, pp. 11–12). Such symptoms are a normal response in the aftermath of a terrorist attack, or other traumatic event. However, this distinction is lost in the diagnostic approach, which is only concerned with the presence or absence of symptoms.

In turn, the focus on symptoms has important consequences for treatment, as it undermines support for treatments that address the underlying cause of the symptoms, while promoting interventions, such as pharmaceuticals, that are geared toward symptom suppression. In the case of ADD, the diagnostic approach undermines support for psychotherapy and behavioral therapies, and clears the way for prescribing Ritalin or other psychostimulants. By comparison, the concern with psychosocial causes is at the center of the French psychiatric approach, as they conceptualize ADHD as a psychosocial disorder and psychosocial therapies are at the core of their ADHD treatment approach.

Besides bracketing the psychosocial causes of mental illness, the diagnostic approach steers clinicians away from considering nutritional causes. Over the last three decades, researchers have linked nutritional deficiencies to a growing number of mental illnesses[3] and this has been particularly true for ADD (as well as Attention Deficit/Hyperactivity Disorder (ADHD), which is ADD's successor), as researchers have repeatedly demonstrated the potential relationship between diet and symptoms of hyperactivity (Boris & Mandel 1994; Conners, 1990; Egger, Carter, Graham, Gumley, & Soothill, 1985; Feingold, 1976). In the 1980s and 1990s, the diet–hyperactivity link was clouded by industry-sponsored research and propaganda (Jacobson & Schardt, 1999). However, in 1999 the Center for Science in the Public Interest (CSPI)[4] reviewed 23 controlled studies, and concluded that 17 supported the diet–hyperactivity link (*ibid.*). Specifically, the studies showed that the behavior of some children is significantly worsened after consuming artificial colors, certain preservatives, and/or allergen-containing foods (such as wheat, eggs, soy, etc.) (Jacobson & Schardt, 1999). Moreover, recent studies have linked ADHD to deficiencies in iron (Konofal et al., 2008) and Omega-3 essential fatty acids (Johnson, Ostlund, Fransson, Kadesjö, & Gillberg, 2008). Despite the mounting evidence, however, nutrition is rarely addressed in clinical practice. Moreover, because the public remains uninformed about the role of nutrition, the situation guarantees that numerous children who could be helped with dietary interventions will instead be treated with medications, thereby artificially inflating demand for psychostimulants.

Exposure to environmental toxins (such as heavy metals, pesticides, solvents, nicotine, and dioxins) is the third potential cause of mental illness that is effectively bracketed by the DSM-III's diagnostic approach. An implication for clinical practice is that the focus on symptoms directs clinicians away from considering or addressing the role toxins might play. Consequently, ignoring the relationship between toxins and mental illness provides two benefits to psychiatric medication manufacturers. First, it means that the affected patients will continue to exhibit symptoms and maintain their dependency on psychiatric medications. Second, it directs attention away from identifying and eliminating the source of those toxins, thereby guaranteeing that more individuals will be exposed, develop the symptoms, and become candidates for psychiatric medications.

Although this is true for many, if not most, psychiatric ailments, it is particularly salient in the case of ADHD as toxicologists have linked numerous neurotoxins to the onset of hyperactivity, impulsivity, and/or attention deficits, the three core symptoms of ADHD. These chemicals include heavy metals (including cadmium, lead, mercury, and manganese), pesticides (including DDT mixtures, organophosphates, and pyrethroids), and solvents (including ethanol, styrene, toluene, trichloroethylene, and xylene), nicotine, dioxins, and PCBs (Schettler, Stein, Reich, Valenti, & Wallinga, 2000). The case for lead is particularly salient as toxicologists have been demonstrating its link to ADHD symptoms and other learning disabilities for over 30 years (Schettler et al., 2000). Relatedly, toxicologists maintain that, when confronted with a child who has ADHD symptoms, the first thing clinicians should do is assess the child for lead exposure and pursue lead chelation if necessary (interview with toxicologist, June 2006).

Despite the mounting evidence, however, mainstream medicine has shown no interest in the relationship between ADHD and environmental toxins. This point is underscored by the fact there is no mention of environmental toxins in practice guidelines dedicated to ADHD, including the 1998 National Institute of Health Conference Statement on the Diagnosis and Treatment of Attention Deficit/Hyperactivity Disorder, and the ADHD clinical practice guidelines produced by the American Academy of Pediatrics (2001) and the American Academy of Child and Adolescent Psychiatry (1997), respectively. This is even true of PCBs, lead, and solvents, the three neurotoxins identified as having a strong causal relationship with ADHD symptoms (Schettler et al., 2000).

The failure to discuss environmental chemicals has steered clinicians away from considering toxins as a potential cause of ADHD symptoms. While DSM-III's diagnostic approach is not the only reason for this situation, its bracketing of causes has played an important role. In defense of the DSM, some might argue that psychiatry never expressed an interest in toxicological research prior to DSM-III. While that is accurate, psychiatrists were previously concerned with the social and psychological causes of mental illness, and thus could have been open to the emerging research on other external causes, such as nutrition and the exposure to environmental toxins.

In summary, the DSM-III's diagnostic approach encourages clinicians to adopt a highly reductionist and brain-blaming conception of ADD. Bracketing the role of social context necessarily attributes the cause to the individual. Likewise, bracketing the patient's psychology (including one's subconscious and psychological biography) encourages clinicians to attribute psychiatric symptoms to faulty biology. Assuming that illness is due to faulty biology, the diagnostic approach steers clinicians away from considering whether nutrition and environmental toxins may be contributing to mental illness, and them clinicians to presume the illness is due to faulty brain chemistry. Consequently, the very framework of this approach effectively channels clinicians to treat patients with brain-targeting drugs, which suppress symptoms by altering the brain's chemistry. Importantly, because the patient's underlying problems are not directly addressed, he/she is left in a state of perpetual dependency vis-à-vis the medications, and the market demand for the products is artificially sustained.

Thus, given the situation, one could argue that the bracketing of psychosocial, environmental toxins, and nutritional causes benefits corporations the most as it inflates market demand for pharmaceutical products, shields producers of environmental toxins, and protects producers of nutritionally suspect items.

Expanding the Pool of Prescribers

Beyond shaping the conception of mental illness, the standardized criteria also expanded the number of clinicians who could diagnose ADHD, and, in turn, prescribe psychostimulants. Specifically, because ADHD is a complicated psychiatric disorder, those who are best prepared to make the diagnosis are clinicians with a specialty in child psychology. However, reducing the diagnostic process to a checklist approach reduced the complexity of making the ADHD diagnosis, thereby encouraging non-specialists to take on suspected ADHD cases. In reflections upon the checklist approach Dr. Diller writes

> When I first began evaluating for ADD I wanted to find out how other doctors dealt with this new group of patients, so I consulted with a fellow ADD specialist nearby. It was no big deal to him: 'Just count the symptoms,' he told me, 'and if they meet criteria, you can treat them' (with medication it was implied). The subtleties and contradictions of behavior and emotions, the interactions of relationships and environment–none of this seemed important to him. It made me wonder why a doctor was needed, if this was all an evaluation required. (Diller 1999, pp. 55–56).

The majority of ADHD cases are now handled by nonpsychiatrists, with pediatricians handling 72%, family physicians handling 13%, and psychiatrists handling 13% (Copeland, Wolraich, Lindgren, Milich, & Woolson, 1987). This development has important implications for treatment because psychiatrists and nonpsychiatrists differ significantly in the way they diagnose and address ADHD. For example, despite the changes brought on by the DSM-III, it is the psychiatrists who are more likely to take a psychodynamic approach to understanding ADHD, which includes understanding how the child's symptoms are related to psychological history and family dynamics. Also, psychiatrists are much more likely to use psychotherapy, behavior modification, and include family members in the therapy process (Rafalovich, 2004). Most nonpsychiatrists, on the other hand, lack training in child psychology and are more likely to ascribe to a biological understanding of ADHD. In addition, they are usually ill-equipped to provide psychotherapy and/or behavior modification, which leads them to treat the child with psychostimulants (Rafalovich, 2004).

DISCUSSION

This analysis has showed that changing to a diagnostic approach has impacted American psychiatry's treatment of ADD and ADHD. Specifically, the diagnostic approach has encouraged clinicians to ignore the cause of ADD and ADHD symptoms. In turn, bracketing the causes has meant clinicians rarely address the underlying cause of illness, and typically treat ADD and ADHD symptoms by prescribing psychostimulants. To be clear, I am not arguing that the switch to the diagnostic approach prompted the original growth in Ritalin consumption, for that trend had started well before the appearance of the DSM-III. Rather, I am arguing that the changes made for the DSM-III concept amplified the preexisting trend by expanding the number of clinicians who could diagnose the disorder and encouraging clinicians address ADD through psychostimulants.

Beyond illuminating the specific cases of ADD and ADHD, this analysis contributes to the medicalization literature by demonstrating that there is more to be studied than merely the expansion or contraction of diagnostic categories. Researchers also have to analyze the clinical approach being used, which has implications for the prevalence and treatment of illness.

The Mental Health Epidemic?

While American psychiatry resisted the diagnostic approach during the 1960s and 1970s, that resistance fell in 1980. Since then, the country has experienced a tremendous growth in the incidence of mental health, with some researchers estimating that each year a quarter of the American population suffers from a mental disorder, and that 50% of the population will come down with a mental disorder at some point in their lives (Kessler et al., 1994). Similarly, the US Surgeon General's report on Mental Health estimates that every year 50 million Americans develop a mental disorder (United States Department of Health and Human Services, 1999). By most accounts, this should qualify as a serious epidemic. However, the numbers are artificially inflated by American psychiatry's refusal to distinguish between symptoms that are a normal reaction to a distressing situation and those that are due to an underlying psychological pathology (Horwitz, 2002).

Outside the United States, the impact of DSM-III has been mixed. Canada, in particular, has warmly received the DSM-III and its diagnostic approach. However, in other countries the reception has been colder. In France, for example, the reception was much cooler as French child psychiatrists maintained that the DSM-III was overly reductionist and inappropriate for the French context (Misès et al., 2002). Moreover, to ward off the possible influence of the DSM-III, the French child psychiatrists developed their own classification system (the French Classification of Child and Adolescent Mental Disorders), which they released in 1983 (Misès et al., 2002). As for the rest of the world, the impact of the DSM-III has been somewhat muted by the existence of the International Classification of Disease (ICD), which is the classification system developed by the World Health Organization. The ICD is the system of choice outside North America, and has, historically, favored a more dynamic approach. However, there are indications that ICD developers are converging toward the DSM model (Healy, 2002, p. 328). If that transpires, the incidence of mental illness in other countries is likely to grow in the same way it has in the United States.

Consequences for Treatment

The clinicians' choice of medical approach also matters profoundly for the treatment of illness, whether in psychiatry or general medicine. If clinicians employ the diagnostic approach, they focus on symptoms, ignore the underlying causes of disease, and are predisposed to treat the condition with symptom-suppressing treatments, such as pharmaceuticals. On the other hand, a more holistic approach tries to understand and address the underlying cause of the symptoms.

While the diagnostic approach is essential in a trauma situation, it is less appropriate for the treatment of chronic illnesses (such as heartburn, high-blood pressure, and arthritis), many of which are caused by diet and other lifestyle choices (exercise, sleep, stress, etc.), and which respond poorly, over the long-term, to symptom-suppressing interventions. Moreover, the weakness of the diagnostic approach has important policy implications, as the inability to identify and address the environmental causes of disease has contributed to America's bloated healthcare system, which currently accounts for nearly 15% of the national budget (OECD, 2008).

Future Lines of Research

Overall, my analysis illuminates the strong synergistic relationship that can exist between diagnostic definitions, the frequency with which a disease is diagnosed and the use of medications to treat it. Moreover, to shed deeper light on the issue, future research could pursue a number of different avenues. First, researchers could compare the American case to countries that use different diagnostic systems. For instance, while American medicine relies on the DSM, the majority of the world uses the ICD. Differences in the way the ICD defines ADHD, as well as other mental illnesses, could well lead to differences in the incidence of diagnosis and psychostimulant consumption.

Second, researchers could analyze more closely the relationship between diagnostic classifications and pharmaceutical company behavior. It might be that a country's use of dynamically oriented disease classifications leads pharmaceutical companies to focus their marketing efforts in America or other countries that employ a diagnostic approach. Or, the existence of the dynamic classification might compel pharmaceutical companies to play a more active role in shaping that country's classification system, by coopting those who are responsible for defining diseases.

A third avenue would be to analyze the extent to which these findings extend to the consumption of other psychiatric medications. In addition to psychostimulants, American children have increased their consumption of many other psychiatric medications (including antidepressants and anti-psychotics[5]) over the last two decades, and it seems this trend was encouraged by American psychiatry's conversion to the diagnostic approach. Further research could compare the ADD case to depression, bipolar disorder and other childhood mental illnesses, and analyze the relationship between changes to definitions of mental disorders and medication usage.

Fourth, researchers should examine the implications of these findings for the pharmaceutical treatment of nonpsychiatric diseases. The onset of most (if not all) nonpsychiatric diseases is influenced by a host of factors (i.e., nutrition, exercise, exposure to pathogens, immune system strength, genetics, environmental toxins, etc.), and it seems that the causal factor(s) to which each disease is attributed will have a significant effect over treatment choice. For instance, if heartburn is understood strictly as a genetic phenomenon, the patient is likely to address it through pharmaceutical treatments. However, if he/she understands that diet and nutrition also contribute to the problem, they are less likely to rely solely, or at all, on pharmaceutical treatments. Thus, future research should carefully analyze the etiological frameworks that are implicitly embedded in diagnostic definitions and elucidate how those frameworks influence disease treatment.

While this article has operated with the underlying assumption that diagnostic definitions influence clinicians, follow-up research should investigate the degree to which they actually do. As well, future research should investigate how clinicians' use of diagnostic definitions is mediated by other institutional structures, such as healthcare systems and culture. With regard to healthcare systems, it could be that managed-care imposes time-constraints on clinical visits, which lead clinicians to rely more on standardized disease definitions than would be the case for physicians in private practice.

Another line of research could analyze the process by which disease classifications are developed, and altered over time. A contribution of this nature is Kirk and Kutchin's *The Selling of DSM: The Rhetoric of Science in Psychiatry* (1992), which masterfully illustrates the political and rhetorical tactics that developers used in constructing and selling the controversial DSM-III. Researchers could build on that work by investigating the process by which specific mental disorder categories (such as ADD, depression, or conduct disorder) are constructed, and focusing their analysis on the developers of those categories. Specifically, researchers could analyze the process by which the developers were selected, the social networks from which developers emerged, and the extent to which those networks shaped the evolution of the mental disorder categories. For example, researchers could map out each developer's institutional affiliations (including ties with universities, governmental agencies, and/or nongovernmental organizations) and analyze the extent to which those relationships influenced the evolution of the mental disorder categories. Similarly, researchers could analyze the developers' relationships with pharmaceutical companies. The pharmaceutical link seems particularly relevant when we consider (1) the strong incentive pharmaceutical manufacturers have over the final version of an illness category and (2) the recent revelation that 56% of DSM-IV developers had financial relationships with one or more pharmaceutical companies (Cosgrove, Krimsky, Vijayaraghavan, & Schneider, 2006).

NOTES

1. Karl Menninger is regarded as having been the most articulate spokesman for the psychosocial perspective during the postwar years of American psychiatry (Wilson, 1993).

2. The ICD is a comprehensive classification of all diseases (psychiatric and nonpsychiatric), injuries, and causes of death. It is used by a wide range of health professionals in countries of varied sizes, cultures, and resources (Kendell, 1991), and was revised periodically, in consultation with health officials from many countries. The intent behind this compendium was to facilitate the standardization of diagnostic practices and the international comparison of morbidity and mortality statistics (Wilson, 1993).

3. For instance, the onset of schizophrenia has been linked to omega-3 deficiencies (Emsley, Myburgh, Oosthuizen, & van Rensburg, 2002; Peet, 2003; Yao et al., 2004), depression has been linked to folate/vitamin B deficiencies (Bell et al., 1991; Young, 2007), with bipolar disorder also linked to omega-3 (Frangou, Lewis, & McCrone, 2006; Stoll et al., 1999) and vitamin B deficiencies (Bell et al., 1990; Hasanah, Khan, Musalmah, & Razali, 1997).

4. CSPI is an award-winning public advocacy nonprofit based in Washington, DC, which specializes in nutrition and health, food safety, alcohol policy, and sound science. http://www.cspinet.org/about/index.html

5. For instance, from 1987 to 1996, the number of American children consuming antidepressants grew from 0.30 to 1.06% of all 6–14 year olds. For 15–18 year olds, the increase was from 0.5 to 2.12% (Olfson, Marcus, Weissman, & Jensen, 2002). As for antipsychotics, the number of children consuming these medications grew from 0.86% in 1996 to 3.96% in 2002 (Cooper et al., 2006).

ACKNOWLEDGMENTS

I thank Catherine Bliss, Ph.D.; Ruha Benjamin, Ph.D.; and Brian Folk, M.A. for their useful comments on an early draft of the chapter. As well, I thank Ananya Mukherjea, Ph.D., for her insightful advice on a later rendition. And finally, I thank my wife, Alise Cappel, for her careful reading of the text throughout the process.

REFERENCES

American Academy of Child and Adolescent Psychiatry. (1997). Practice parameters for the assessment and treatment of children, adolescents, and adults with attention-deficit/ hyperactivity disorder. *Journal of the American Academy of Child and Adolescent Psychiatry, 36*, 85S–121S.

American Academy of Pediatrics. (2001). Clinical practice guideline: Treatment of school-aged child with attention-deficit/hyperactivity disorder. *Pediatrics, 108,* 1033–1044.

American Psychiatric Association. (1968). *Diagnostic and statistical manual of mental disorders* (2nd ed. (DSM-II)). Washington, DC: American Psychiatric Association.

American Psychiatric Association. (1980). *Diagnostic and statistical manual of mental disorders* (3rd ed. (DSM-III)). Washington, DC: American Psychiatric Association.

Bell, I. R., Edman, J. S., Marby, D. W., Satlin, A., Dreier, T., Liptzin, B., & Cole, J. O. (1990). Vitamin B-12 and folate status in acute geropsychiatric inpatients: Affective and cognitive characteristics of a vitamin nondeficient population. *Biological Psychiatry, 27*(2), 125–137.

Bell, I. R., Edman, J. S., Morrow, F. D., Marby, D. W., Mirages, S., Perrone, G., Kayne, H. L., & Cole, J. O. (1991). B complex vitamin patterns in geriatric and young adult inpatients with major depression. *Journal of the American Geriatrics Society, 39*(3), 252–257.

Boris, M., & Mandel, F. S. (1994). Foods and additives are common causes of the attention deficit hyperactivity disorder in children. *Annals of Allergy, 72,* 564–568.

Conners, C. K. (1990). *Feeding the brain: How foods affect children.* New York: Plenum Press.

Cooper, W., Arbogast, P., Ding, H., Hickson, G., Fuchs, C., & Ray, W. (2006). Trends in prescribing of antipsychotic medications for US children. *Ambulatory Pediatrics, 6*(2), 79–83.

Copeland, L., Wolraich, M., Lindgren, S., Milich, R., & Woolson, R. (1987). Pediatricians' reported practices in the assessment and treatment of attention deficit disorders. *Journal of Developmental and Behavioral Pediatrics, 8*(4), 191–197.

Cosgrove, L., Krimsky, S., Vijayaraghavan, M., & Schneider, L. (2006). Financial ties between DSM-IV panel members and the pharmaceutical industry. *Psychotherapy and Psychosomatics, 75,* 154–160.

Decker, H. (2007). How Kraepelinian was Kraepelin? How Kraepelinian are the neo-Kraepelinians? – From Emil Kraepelin to DSM-III. *History of Psychiatry, 18*(3), 337–360.

Diller, L. (1999). *Running on Ritalin: A physician reflects on children, society, and performance in a pill.* New York: Bantam Books.

Egger, J., Carter, C., Graham, P., Gumley, D., & Soothill, J. (1985). Controlled trial of oligoantigenic treatment in the hyperkinetic syndrome. *Lancet, 1,* 540–545.

Emsley, R., Myburgh, C., Oosthuizen, P., & van Rensburg, S. J. (2002). Randomized placebo-controlled study of ethyl-eicosapentaenoic acid as supplemental treatment in schizophrenia. *American Journal of Psychiatry, 159*(9), 1596–1598.

Feingold, B. (1976). Hyperkinesis and learning disabilities linked to the ingestion of artificial food colors and flavors. *Journal of Learning Disabilities, 9,* 19–27.

Fox, P. (1989). From senility to Alzheimer's disease: The rise of the Alzheimer's Disease Movement. *Milbank Quarterly, 67,* 58–101.

Frangou, S., Lewis, M., & McCrone, P. (2006). Efficacy of ethyl-eicosapentaenoic acid in bipolar depression: Randomised double-blind placebo-controlled study. *British Journal of Psychiatry, 188,* 46–50.

Grob, G. (1991). Origins of DSM-I: A study of appearance and reality. *American Journal of Psychiatry, 148*(4), 421–431.

Hasanah, C., Khan, U., Musalmah, M., & Razali, S. (1997). Reduced red-cell folate in mania. *Journal of Affective Disorders, 46,* 95–99.

Healy, D. (2002). *The creation of psychopharmacology.* Cambridge: Harvard University Press.

Horwitz, A. (2002). *Creating mental illness*. Chicago: University of Chicago Press.

Horwitz, A. (2007). Transforming normality into pathology: The DSM and the outcomes of stressful arrangements. *Journal of Health and Social Behavior*, *48*(3), 211–222.

Jacobson, M., & Schardt, D. (1999). *Diet, ADHD, & behavior: A quarter-century review*. Washington, DC: Center for Science in the Public Interest.

Johnson, M., Ostlund, S., Fransson, G., Kadesjö, B., & Gillberg, C. (2008). Omega-3/Omega-6 fatty acids for attention deficit hyperactivity disorder: A randomized placebo-controlled trial in children and adolescents. *Journal of Attention Disorders*, [E-pub ahead of print] Available at: http://online.sagepub.com/cgi/searchresults?src = selected&andorexact fulltext = and&journal_set = spjad&fulltext = johnson+and+omega-3 (Sage Journals Online) [Accessed 20 November 2008].

Kendell, R. (1991). Relationship between the DSM-IV and the ICD-10. *Journal of Abnormal Psychology*, *100*(3), 297–301.

Kessler, R. C., McGonagle, K. A., Zhao, S., Nelson, C. B., Hughes, M., Eshleman, S., Wittchen, H. U., & Kendler, K. S. (1994). Lifetime and 12-month prevalence of DSM-III-R psychiatric disorders in the United States. Results from the National Comorbidity Survey. *Archives of General Psychiatry*, *51*(1), 8–19.

Kirk, S., & Kutchins, H. (1992). *The selling of DSM: The rhetoric of science in psychiatry*. New York: Aldine de Gruyter.

Klerman, G. (1978). The evolution of the scientific nosology. In: J. D. Shershow (Ed.), *Schizophrenia: Science and practice* (pp. 99–121). Cambridge, MA: Harvard University Press.

Konofal, E., Lecendreux, M., Deron, J., Marchand, M., Cortese, S., Zaïm, M., Mouren, M., & Arnulf, I. (2008). Effects of iron supplementation on attention deficit hyperactivity disorder in children. *Pediatric Neurology*, *38*(1), 20–26.

Kutchins, H., & Kirk, S. (1997). *Making us crazy: DSM: The psychiatric bible and the creation of mental disorders*. New York: The Free Press.

Menninger, K. (1963). *The vital balance*. New York: Viking Press.

Misès, R., Quemada, N., Botbol, M., Burzstejn, C., Garrabé, J., Golse, B., Jeammet, P., Plantade, A., Portelli, C., & Thevenot, J. P. (2002). French classification for child and adolescent mental disorders. *Psychopathology*, *35*, 176–180.

OECD (Organisation for Economic Co-operation and Development). (2008). Economic survey of the United States, 2008. (Policy Brief December 2008) [Internet] Washington, DC: OECD (Published December 2008). Available at: www.oecd.org/document/32/0,3343, en_2649_33733_41803296_1_1_1_1,00.html

Olfson, M., Marcus, S., Weissman, M., & Jensen, P. (2002). National trends in the use of psychotropic medications by children. *Journal of the American Academy of Child and Adolescent Psychiatry*, *41*(5), 514–521.

Peet, M. (2003). Eicosapentaenoic acid in the treatment of schizophrenia and depression: Rationale and preliminary double-blind clinical test results. *Prostaglandins, Leukotrienes, and Essential Fatty Acids*, *69*(6), 477–485.

Rafalovich, A. (2004). *Framing ADHD children: A critical examination of the history, discourse, and everyday experience of attention deficit/hyperactivity disorder*. Lanham, MD: Lexington Books.

Schettler, T., Stein, J., Reich, F., Valenti, M., & Wallinga, D. (2000). *Harm's way: Toxic threats to child development*. Cambridge, MA: Greater Boston Physicians for Social Responsibility.

Stoll, A. L., Severus, W. E., Freeman, M. P., Rueter, S., Zboyan, H. A., Diamond, E., Cress, K. K., & Marangell, L. B. (1999). Omega 3 fatty acids in bipolar disorder: A preliminary double-blind, placebo-controlled trial. *Archives of General Psychiatry, 56*(5), 407–412.

United States Department of Health and Human Services. (1999). *Mental health: A report of the surgeon general.* Rockville, MD: United States Department of Health and Human Services.

Wilson, M. (1993). DSM-III and the transformation of American psychiatry: A history. *American Journal of Psychiatry, 150*(3), 399–410.

Yao, J., Magan, S., Sonel, A., Gurklis, J., Sanders, R., & Reddy, R. (2004). Effects of Omega-3 fatty acid on platelet serotonin responsivity in patients with schizophrenia. *Prostaglandins, Leukotrienes, and Essential Fatty Acids, 71*(3), 171–176.

Young, SN. (2007). Folate and depression – A neglected problem. *Journal of Psychiatry Neuroscience, 32*(2), 80–82.

CONTAGIOUS YOUTH: DEVIANCE AND THE MANAGEMENT OF YOUTH SOCIALITY

Mike Jolley

ABSTRACT

Purpose – *The purpose of this chapter is to explore a particular conception of youth deviance and some of its practical implications. This conception is evident in the way that the media and human services construe phenomena like teen violence and "risky" sex in epidemiological terms: as contagious and spreading rapidly through a population.*

Methodology/approach – *This chapter broaches these questions through review and analysis of human services research and literature as well as their practical recommendations.*

Findings – *This chapter argues that the concern over transmission of deviant behaviors or characteristics is linked to anxiety over youth sociality and the spaces it occupies. While historically contingent in their manifestations, causal logics using sociality to explain youth deviance (peer pressure, e.g.) continue to resonate with a medicalized viewpoint of the very category of youth.*

Contribution to the field – *This chapter has contributed to the field through exploring changing conceptions of youth and the sociological question of the medicalization of social problems.*

Understanding Emerging Epidemics: Social and Political Approaches
Advances in Medical Sociology, Volume 11, 303–311
Copyright © 2010 by Emerald Group Publishing Limited
All rights of reproduction in any form reserved
ISSN: 1057-6290/doi:10.1108/S1057-6290(2010)0000011020

INTRODUCTION

Since the mid-19th century, the American discourse of the epidemic has been used to express the extent of youth deviance and to justify intervention into the lives of youth at the collective level. While use of this discourse to describe youth deviance is hardly new, I contend that recent decades have seen an increased emphasis on techniques of intervention that not only target youth collectively but also focus on the very form of youth sociality. Contemporary evidence of this transition can be seen in the language and practice of human services organizations like the Child Welfare League of America (CWLA) as well as in social science research. In this chapter, I will take a critical look at recommendations for more effective youth programming and therapeutic intervention made by the Juvenile Justice Division of the CWLA. These practical recommendations are exemplary of an increased emphasis on the distinct role of sociality in youth deviance, which does not replace the 19th century focus on the collective but rather augments and refines it. I will suggest that this change in American epidemics discourse has been particularly influential to the contemporary constitution of youth as a social and political category as well as for understanding the epidemic as a model or lens through which different objects may be viewed.

CONTEMPORARY DISCOURSE OF THE EPIDEMIC

The American discourse of the epidemic has a long history of application to different kinds of social problems, especially those concerning youth. While concern over contagious disease increased rapidly in the middle to late 19th century so did the legitimacy of the American medical community and their involvement in other areas of reform such as criminal justice and education (King, 1993, Chapter 3). As a result public discussion of social problems and potential solutions took on a more medical tone during this period, making use of concepts like the epidemic and contagion. For example, in *Child Problems* social scientist and reformer George B. Mangold states, "In spite of the theory that the child of the juvenile courts is in need of *formation* instead of *reformation*, it is plainly apparent that a considerable number of children have acquired criminal tendencies. To what extent these are due to natural and inherited traits and instincts and what importance shall be attached to the contagion of an early vicious environment are still unsolved questions" (1913, p. 230). So in addition to infectious diseases like cholera and yellow fever, reformers and social scientists such as Mangold began to describe problems like mental disorders and immorality using the language of the epidemic. Many of these reformers did not conceptually or practically separate the medical from the social; in fact, the two were seen as inextricably linked, an approach that in some ways continues in the present (King, 1993, Chapters 4 and 7). Since the 1980s, the use of epidemics discourse by the media and human services to describe youth social problems has become even more prevalent having been applied to teen pregnancy, violence, substance abuse, and a whole host of other deviant behaviors and attributes (Cook & Laub, 1998, pp. 34–51).

In this context, I take a broadly sociological approach to deviance, one that includes not only legal infractions but is defined in reference to any behavior or attribute deemed outside of the normative concept of American youth. In this broader sense, deviance is dependent on but also constitutive of contemporary conceptions of American youth. This is especially evident in American cultural anxiety over children as the future and as a potentially negative force that must be carefully cultivated and managed.

Two of the most important aspects of this discourse are: (1) the focus on the population or collective and (2) the concern over contagion or transmission. First, the historical and theoretical role of the concept of population is especially important for understanding American epidemics discourse. Briefly, the concept of population entails a move away from focusing solely on the individual and toward a conceptualization of the group or collective as having its own characteristics above and beyond those of its individual members. While this focus on population has a much broader historical and political significance, it is especially important to the modern notion of the epidemic, defined not as much by its effect on individuals as by its distribution throughout a group. Michel Foucault's discussion of this concept and its connection to the formation of the modern nation-state in *The History of Sexuality*, Vol. I (1978) is especially revealing and worth quoting at length.

> One of the great innovations in the techniques of power in the eighteenth century was the emergence of "population" as an economic and political problem: population as wealth, population as manpower or labor capacity, population balanced between its own growth and the resources it commanded. Governments perceived that they were not dealing simply with subjects, or even with a "people", but with a "population," with its specific phenomena and its peculiar variables ...

While Foucault touches on a number of important insights here, the most relevant for my discussion is the idea that populations have their own characteristics and phenomena and that government turns its focus to understanding and managing them. Historically, this is evident in the move away from the clinical treatment of individuals and toward the use of hygiene, sanitation, and urban planning as methods of affecting the environmental causes of various diseases by American public health reformers (Lupton, 1995, pp. 16–20).

It is important to understand that this management of the population is not only repressive and administered by the state but part of a more mobile and productive form of power. So while Foucault saw knowledge of the health of the population as essential, he also pointed to the more localized techniques of power that became linked to the population, techniques that depended on and made use of the "specific phenomena" and "peculiar variables" mentioned above (Foucault, 1978, p. 25). In *The Policing of Families*, Jacques Donzelot captures this productive aspect of power well. Of the changes in the 18th century French family he writes, "What was at issue, then, was *the transition from a government of families to a government through the family* ... [I]t became a relay, an obligatory or voluntary support for social imperatives, conforming to a process that did not consist in abolishing the family register but in *exacerbating its existing tendencies, in exploiting to the maximum its advantages and drawbacks ...*" (Donzelot, 1979, p. 92, emphasis added) In other words, this specific form of power makes use of an existing set of relationships, an approach that is essential to contemporary human services techniques of intervention in their application to youth deviance.

Equally important to epidemics discourse is the concern with contagion or transmission, a concern that again calls into question the divide between the medical and the social. If an epidemic is defined by the specifics of its distribution such as rate and means of transmission, it follows that the study of transmission in human populations must necessarily focus on different forms of contact and mobility. These different forms can be understood: (1) through the model of power mentioned above, as distinctive but immanent characteristics of a population and (2) as inherently social or constituted by human copresence and communicative interaction of one kind or another. So while these different forms of social interaction may be a means of transmission for disease or infection, they may also serve to distribute negative behaviors or attitudes throughout a population. Human services and social science research have come to see social interaction between youth as an important means of transmission for these negative behaviors or attitudes (Gifford-Smith, Dodge, Dishion, & McCord, 2005, pp. 255–265). This problematization of youth sociality is especially obvious in discussions of peer influence as a causal factor and in changes in techniques of intervention such as those discussed by the CWLA.

YOUTH SOCIALITY AND TECHNIQUES OF INTERVENTION

The idea that youth deviance is contagious and transmitted through social interaction has begun to play an important role in the theory and practice of human services. This is evident in the CWLA's concern over the problems that "deviant peer contagion" may cause for youth programming and intervention (Rosch, 2006, p. 1). In a publication by the CWLA's Juvenile Justice Division, Joel Rosch states, "Deviant behavior seems to be contagious, spreading rapidly among adolescents when they associate with other deviant youth, especially in early adolescence" (2006, p.1). This aspect of youth deviance is especially disconcerting for Rosch since, "The typical dominant response to adolescent deviant behavior by public agencies ... is to separate these youth from their families, schools, and communities and place them in programs that increase their contact with youth who show similar problems" (2006, p. 1). He continues on to show the prevalence of grouping deviant youth and some of the techniques for doing so as well as the estimated costs for juvenile justice, mental health, education, and community programs. Some of the ways deviant youth are grouped according to Rosch include: placement in various residential facilities, different forms of group therapy, day treatment programs, social skills training, after school and other community programs, school suspension, alternative schools, and academic tracking. While some of these techniques group youth intentionally and others do so by default, Rosch sees them all as ineffective compared to other forms of intervention like the ones discussed below (Rosch, 2006, pp. 4, 5).

While Rosch laments the overall ineffectiveness of grouping together deviant youth, he also provides some insight into the specific mechanisms through which youth deviance is thought to be transmitted. He sees the process of labeling, the communication and acquisition of norms, the reinforcement of behavior, and "deviancy training" as mechanisms through which youth transmit their deviance. In addition, being grouped with deviant peers may increase opportunities to participate in deviant acts and access to deviant groups, objects, locations, and information according to Rosch. He quotes Dodge, Dishion, and Landsford on this point: "Deviancy training occurs when a peer displays antisocial behavior or talks about it and other peers positively reinforce that behavior by smiling or giving verbal approval and high status to the first peer" (Dodge, Dishion, & Landsford, 2006 in Rosch, 2006, pp. 4, 5). In this formulation, different mechanisms of transmission are understood under the rubric of "peer influence," a concept that structures the alternative forms of intervention recommended by the CWLA (Rosch, 2006, pp. 4, 5).

Having thoroughly problematized the different mechanisms of peer influence as means of transmitting youth deviance, this publication moves on to discuss alternative forms of intervention. I contend that these forms of intervention are reminiscent of the form of power discussed above by Foucault and Donzelot. Rosch states, "[E]vidence suggests that group culture may be engineered to optimize the possibility of establishing prosocial cultural norms ..." (Rosch, 2006, pp. 4, 5). In this case, it is not that the sociality of deviant youth is governed or controlled, but that youth are governed *through* their sociality. In the CWLA schema, this government takes place through two different specific approaches to youth sociality: inclusion or mainstreaming of deviant youth and management of group dynamics.

The first of these approaches is focused on the inclusion or mainstreaming of deviant youth into a more normal or positive, lower risk group of youth. In this approach, human services professionals depend on the normalizing effect of the social group as well as the transmission of more positive cultural norms. So by grouping deviant youth with presumably nondeviant or normal youth, it is assumed that the very fact of their interaction will counteract or prevent future deviance. This may involve a number of different legal/institutional scenarios and take place in different ways. The practice of mainstreaming or including deviant youth in a broader school population is one example of this approach most often associated with youth deviance in educational settings. Some of the other practices discussed by Rosch include "matching deviant youth with well-adjusted peers," "linking at-risk youth with prosocial mentors," and "community programs that combine high- and low-risk youth," all which depend on sociality as a normalizing force (Rosch, 2006, pp. 5, 15, 16)

While this first set of practices tends to focus on characteristics of the group itself and depends on sociality to bring deviant youth into compliance, the second approach is more concerned with the micromanagement of sociality or the minute-to-minute interactions of youth. Here youth are managed through increased adult awareness of the nuances of peer interaction as well as through techniques like "behavior management" and "positive behavior support." Adding structure to group settings and building the "social competence" and interpersonal skills of deviant youth are also seen as effective strategies for modifying the group dynamic. These two approaches are, of course, deeply integrated and it is recommended that practitioners combine different strategies to maximize effectiveness (Rosch, 2006, pp. 5, 15, 16). So while grouping deviant with nondeviant or normal youth is essential, it is also important to Rosch and other advocates of this approach that they be taught and encouraged to interact in certain prescribed ways.

The interlocking character of the different techniques of intervention employed here is actually rather innovative and opposed to what could be considered repressive or exclusionary practices. Of course, some repressive or interventionist practices are still used but they play a supportive rather than primary role. That said, this is a more nuanced, specific, even insidious form of power, one that depends on the "existing tendencies" (Donzelot, 1979, p. 92) of a youth population. It is important to understand that despite their more progressive appearance, these practices are still a means of managing youth deviance or perhaps coercing youth into managing their own deviance. One problematic effect of this approach is the construction of youth as perpetually subject to their sociality and that sociality as transparent and hence open to manipulation. Here the phenomena that emerge from youth social interaction are seen as having their own rules or laws that are accessible to adults and should be used rather than disturbed; however, the possibility that youth themselves might have some awareness or control over these phenomena is not considered. Additionally, this approach takes as given that youth social interaction is uniform and consistent, always taking place in a smooth, uninterrupted fashion rather than being characterized by conflict, negotiation, and struggle. The assumption that deviant youth are not involved in multiple peer groups with a variety of possibly conflicting norms or that they will automatically conform to the norms of a group in which adult human services professionals place them seems almost naïve in this case.

CONCLUSION

In this chapter, I have attempted to show that the approach to youth deviance and practices of intervention advocated by Rosch and the CWLA are exemplary of the influence epidemics discourse has had on the construction of contemporary youth as a category of being. This influence is apparent in the way that the discourse of the epidemic links the category of youth with the concept of risk. In her thorough discussion of the topic, Deborah Lupton discusses the way that youth and other marginalized groups are constituted as a certain kind of subject through this concept. "The 'at risk' label tends either to position members of these social groups as particularly vulnerable, passive, powerless or weak, or as particularly dangerous to themselves or others. In both cases, special attention is directed at these social groups, positioning them in a network of surveillance, monitoring and intervention" (Lupton, 1999, p. 114). Interestingly, risk shares a foundational component with epidemics discourse, the concept of population. Lupton states, "[R]isk is collective, affecting a collective rather than an individual...risk is seen as something that only becomes calculable when it is spread over a population" (Lupton, 1999, p. 95). For centuries risk has been an important category for understanding natural disasters and accidents but since the 19th century has been applied more and more to human beings, "... in their conduct, in their liberty, in the relations between them, *in the fact of their association, in society*" (Ewald, 1991, p. 197, emphasis added). Thus, youth are seen as constantly exposed to risk as well as exposing others through their sociality, a perspective that seems to necessitate the calculability or knowledge of the entire population that Lupton describes.

Rosch's approach to youth deviance depends upon and furthers a set of assumptions about American youth sociality and its vulnerability to calculation and manipulation. These assumptions construct youth as unaware of and subject to the rules or laws of their own sociality. Given that the category of youth is perpetually enmeshed in the problem of risk, and the assessment of risk is by definition based on the potential for a future outcome (Lupton, 1999, p. 92), it follows that there is always some way to justify intervention into the lives of youth. So, while the connection between concern over the population and the specific form of power discussed by Foucault is useful, it does not fully describe the particular convergence of epidemics discourse and youth deviance. Rather than just the regulation of a population that is given, it would seem that what is at issue here is the very constitution of that population through the careful management of sociality. In addition to revealing certain aspects of the way we understand youth deviance, this formulation also informs our understanding of the epidemic as a model or way of viewing certain objects. In this formulation, the epidemic becomes a framework for understanding phenomena at the level of the population and carefully aligning practical techniques of management with those phenomena. This conclusion would also seem to indicate that the recent dismissal of the contemporary importance of the concept of population in the social sciences may be premature (Rose, 2007, pp. 3–4 and pp. 62–63). Instead I suggest that a critical and perhaps more historical exploration of the different contemporary perspectives and techniques of management that rely on the concept of population such as those discussed here would be revealing.

REFERENCES

Cook, P. J., & Laub, J. H. (1998). The unprecedented epidemic in youth violence. In: M. Tonry & M. H. Moore (Eds), *Crime and justice: A review of research*. Chicago: University of Chicago Press.

Dodge, K. A., Dishion, T. J., & Landsford, J. E. (2006). Deviant peer influences in intervention and public policy for youth. *Social Policy Report, 20*(1), 1–19.

Donzelot, J. (1979). *The policing of families*. New York: Pantheon Books.

Ewald, F. (1991). Insurance and risks. In: G. Burchell, C. Gordon & P. Miller (Eds), *The Foucault effect: Studies in governmentality*. London, UK: Harvester Wheatsheaf.

Foucault, M. (1978). *The history of sexuality: An introduction* (Vol. I). New York: Random House.

Gifford-Smith, M., Dodge, K. A., Dishion, T. J., & McCord, J. (2005). Peer influence in children and adolescents: Crossing the bridge from developmental to intervention science. *Journal of Abnormal Child Psychology, 33*(3), 255–265.

King, C. R. (1993). *Children's health in America: A history*. New York: Twayne Publishers.

Lupton, D. (1995). *The imperative of health: Public health and the regulated body*. London, UK: Sage Publications.

Lupton, D. (1999). *Risk*. London, UK: Routledge.

Mangold, G. B. (1913). *Child problems*. New York: The Macmillan Company.

Rosch, J. (2006). Deviant peer contagion: Findings from the Duke executive sessions on Deviant Peer contagion. *The Link: Connecting Juvenile Justice and Child Welfare, 5*(2), 1–17.

Rose, N. (2007). *The politics of life itself: Biomedicine, power, and subjectivity in the twenty-first century*. Princeton, CA: Princeton University Press.

PART V
CASE STUDY OF A NEWLY CONSTRUCTED EPIDEMIC: THREE PERSPECTIVES ON OBESITY

A SOCIAL CHANGE MODEL
OF THE OBESITY EPIDEMIC

Deborah A. Sullivan

ABSTRACT

Purpose – *Obesity has reached epidemic levels in the United States and many other affluent countries and is a growing problem in some developing countries. World Health Organization estimates that the global rate will reach 13 percent by 2015. Because obesity increases the risk of many diseases ranging from type 2 diabetes and asthma to cardiovascular disease and some cancers, it threatens to undermine twentieth-century gains in life expectancy. This chapter offers a theoretical model of obesity that postulates the epidemic is a latent dysfunction of macro-structural changes initiated by industrialization that have decreased the physical activity of everyday life and promoted a nutrition transition to a high-calorie diet.*

Methodology/approach – *Comparative and historical population data are presented that generally support the conceptual model, although some significant cultural differences are found in particular race/ethnic groups.*

Findings – *The finding that structural changes in society created and continue to support the obesity epidemic will make it difficult to control by focusing only on health education campaigns aimed at changing individual behaviors.*

Contribution to the Field – *This chapter offers data and analysis that can support policy making needed to change the structural influences.*

Understanding Emerging Epidemics: Social and Political Approaches
Advances in Medical Sociology, Volume 11, 315–342
ISSN: 1057-6290/doi:10.1108/S1057-6290(2010)0000011021

INTRODUCTION

Although not itself a disease, the level of body fat defined as obesity is a well-documented risk factor for many serious chronic diseases such as type 2 diabetes, cardiovascular disease, and some cancers. This chapter provides an overview of the spreading obesity pandemic. It offers a macro-theoretical model to explain why this epidemic has emerged over the second half of the twentieth century and analyzes historical and comparative population data for the United States to evaluate the usefulness of the model for understanding the causes of the obesity epidemic.

Obesity reached epidemic levels in the United States and some other affluent countries over the past 30 years and is a growing problem in the urban populations of developing countries. The World Health Organization (2008) estimates that approximately 400 million adults aged 15 and over were obese in 2005 and projects the number will reach more than 700 million by 2015. Based on population estimates (U.S. Census Bureau, 2008a), this yields a 2005 global obesity rate of 8 percent that will escalate to 13 percent by 2015. An additional 25 percent of the world's population was overweight in 2005 and that rate is expected to climb to 30 percent over the decade, producing a combined prevalence of 43 percent. There is no sign that this pandemic is abating. World Health Organization estimates that at least 20 million children under age 5 are already overweight. The implications are staggering because of the diseases associated with obesity. The direct medical costs of physician visits, medications, surgeries, and inpatient hospital care for treating the "comorbidities" linked with obesity, such as type 2 diabetes, obstructive sleep apnea, and cardiovascular disease, in the United States was estimated to be $61 billion in 2000 (Centers for Disease Control and Prevention, 2008). Adding indirect costs associated with lost productivity due to sick days, restricted-activity days, and forgone future earnings increased the bill to $117 billion.

Faced with an unfolding epidemic that threatens to undermine the life expectancy gains of the twentieth century and overwhelm health care budgets, researchers have turned their attention to the social epidemiology of obesity. Nationally representative data sets with large samples, such as the National Longitudinal Study of Adolescent Health, a comprehensive 13-year data collection funded by the National Institute of Child Health and Human Development, and the annual National Health and Nutrition Examination Survey of approximately 5,000 persons run by the National Center for Health Statistics, allow multivariate analyses of individual risk factors. The resulting lists of odds ratios and regression coefficients provide a fragmented and inconsistent picture of social, demographic, economic, psychological, and geographic variables associated with obesity, primarily in the United States. Findings so far provide little insight about why obesity is a major problem at this point in time in some places, but not others, or guidance about what to do to control the pandemic. As McDowell (2008) points out, many "risk factors" identified as statistically significant predictors of non-infectious diseases are only "risk markers" of susceptibility to fundamental causes not measured in the multivariate analyses of individual-level data, rather than true causal factors. In other words, by narrowing our focus to individual attributes, we risk seeing only the trees, or the leaves on the trees, and overlooking the forest.

Understanding the social epidemiology of non-infectious conditions such as obesity is especially challenging. Non-infectious diseases lack the single, specific, causal agent that is necessary for an infectious disease to be embodied in a host. The third element of the traditional epidemiological triad, environment, measures a host's exposure to a specific disease agent, as well as external sources of physical, psychological, and social stress that may compromise a host's ability to resist disease. In the absence of a specific causal agent, environmental factors – in all their multilayered complexity – assume greater causal agency. After reviewing theoretical perspectives on social epidemiology and definitions of obesity, I will present a theoretical model and evaluate it using comparative population data to discuss some macro-social changes that have come together to produce the pandemic of obesity at this time in history.

THEORETICAL PERSPECTIVES

Geoffrey Rose's seminal 1985 article, "Sick Individuals and Sick Populations," provides valuable guidance for thinking about the social epidemiology of obesity. Rose distinguishes two dimensions within the etiology of disease. The first, the "causes of cases," refers to explanations of why some individuals in a society are susceptible to a particular disease, while others are not. Most epidemiological research seeks to identify and measure these individual risk factors. The second, the causes of incidence (new cases) and prevalence (total cases), involves explanations of why one population has a higher rate of a disease than another. Both dimensions reflect Durkheim's conception of the "social facts" in a society that exist outside the individual and constrain some types of behavior, at the same time they facilitate other types of behavior. These social facts include cultural norms, values, beliefs, technologies, and the social structure created by economic, political, and other institutions, as well social groups and the statuses and roles of individuals in these groups. If we only look for the social facts that cause individual cases, we overlook the equally, if not more, important public health question of the social facts that determine prevalence. Rose cautions that the causes of population incidence can be different than the causes of cases. Understanding the causes of prevalence of obesity is particularly important because the rates of obesity vary widely across populations, indicating that this epidemic cannot be fully understood by focusing on the causes of cases.

Rose warns that analyses of individual-level data assume that what is common in a population is "normal." When everyone is exposed to the same disease-causing agents, analyses of individual-level "risk factors" only identify markers of susceptibility to these agents, not the causal agents. To identify the causal agents in such circumstances Rose urges us to go beyond the limits of individual analyses and consider the determinants of a population's incidence or prevalence rates. He illustrates the value of population analyses by comparing data for Finland where coronary heart disease is very common and Japan where it is not. Although separate individual-level analyses in these and other countries show no statistically significant relationship between diet, serum cholesterol level, and coronary heart disease, population-level data tell a different story about the causal importance of diet that would be missed, if only individual-level data are examined.

Critics charge that Rose ignores the cumulative effects of the life course and multiple risk exposure (Frohlich & Potvin, 2008). Multilevel theoretical models have been proposed that include the contextual influence of the social and physical environment (Kaplan, 2004). Glass and McAtee (2006) build on epidemiology's metaphorical causal stream from distal social factors to proximate individual factors in three dimensions that include the interactions between social context and biology over the flow of time across the life course. The necessary longitudinal individual- and contextual-level data to test such complex models do not yet exist. More importantly, the central focus of these models ultimately is the causes of cases, not the causes of population prevalence.

Fig. 1 offers a social change model of population obesity. The model postulates that the increasing prevalence of obesity is a latent dysfunction of macro-social changes launched slowly 250 years ago with the beginning of industrialization in Western Europe and North America. These changes – urbanization, increased agricultural productivity, expanded division of

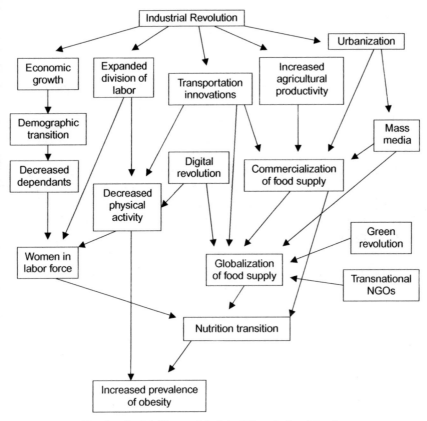

Fig. 1. Social Change Model of Population Obesity.

labor, economic growth, and transportation innovations – gradually gained momentum in the nineteenth and early twentieth centuries. The emergence of mass media, the green revolution, the digital revolution, and transnational nongovernmental organizations helped to accelerate the macro-changes in the second half of the twentieth century and spread them to new regions where obesity is now emerging as a problem alongside under-nutrition. The initial macro-changes created by industrialization precipitated other social changes including the demographic transition, women's increased labor force participation, and the commercialization and globalization of the food supply. Together these macro-changes decreased the physical activity of everyday life and promoted a transition to a diet high in fat, sugar, volume, and calories. The result is an increased prevalence of obesity. This conceptual, structural-functional model guides the analysis of population data presented in this chapter.

OVERWEIGHT, OBESITY, AND COMORBIDITIES

Adults are defined as overweight if their body mass index (BMI) is between 25 and 29.9 and obese if it is 30 or more. BMI is calculated by dividing weight in kilograms by the square of height in meters. An adult with a BMI of 30 who is 5 feet 6 inches weighs about 186 pounds, while an adult with the same BMI who is 5 feet 9 inches weighs about 203 pounds. Both overweight and obese adults are at higher risk than normal-weight adults for the comorbidities in Table 1. Health risks increase steeply at higher BMI scores. As a result, adults with BMIs of 40 or more are classified as "morbidly

Table 1.   A Partial List of Health Risks Associated with Excessive Body Fat.

Physical Health	Emotional Health	Social Health
Osteoarthritis	Depression	Stigma
Hypertension	Low self-esteem	Negative stereotyping (lack self-control, lazy, etc.)
Dyslipidemia	Negative body image	Lower education attainment
Gallbladder disease	Anxiety	Workplace discrimination in hiring, wages, promotion
Diabetes	Eating disorders	Lower marriage rates
Hyperinsulinemia	Higher risk of suicide	Teasing and bullying
Nonalcoholic fatty liver disease	Less satisfied with partners and work	Social marginalization
Urinary stress incontinence	Lower levels of self-reported happiness	
Gastroesophageal reflux	Shame	
Sleep apnea	Substance abuse	
Asthma		
Coronary heart disease		
Stroke		
Anemia		
Neoplasia		
Endometrial, breast, and colon cancer		
Infertility		
Pregnancy complications		

obese" or class III "extreme obesity." Unless they are very short, adults with a BMI of 40 weigh about 100 pounds above the top of the normal weight category.

The BMI classification provides only a crude estimate of the health risks of excessive weight because it neither distinguishes muscle and bone weight from fat weight, nor takes into account other associated health risk variables such as cholesterol and blood glucose levels that independently influence health risks at the individual level. For example, the BMI tends to overestimate body fat in muscular, fit individuals and underestimate body fat in older individuals and others who have lost muscle mass and bone density due to diminished physical activity. The BMI also does not takes into account the additional health risks of fat that is disproportionately concentrated in the abdominal area (Pischon, Boeing, & Hoffmann, 2008). Despite these shortcomings, the BMI is a strong predictor of the prevalence of many chronic diseases in a population (Table 1). Obesity is associated with more chronic morbidity than smoking or poverty (Sturm & Wells, 2001). It is also associated with increased mortality (Flegal, Graubard, Williamson, & Gail, 2005). The mortality relationship is stronger among adults under age 70 than above it, underscoring the substantial contribution of obesity to premature mortality.

THE GLOBAL OBESITY EPIDEMIC

Obesity increased at an exponential rate in the United States and some other developed countries over the past 30 years. It is now increasing rapidly in subpopulations of many developing countries. While obesity is more prevalent in affluent countries than in most developing countries, there is wide variation (Fig. 2). Japan and South Korea have the lowest rates, while the United States has the highest rate, 34 percent in 2006.

The United States has been at the forefront of the global epidemic for more than 30 years. No other Western country has an obesity rate nearly as high as the United States, although virtually all are experiencing an increase in prevalence. In recent years some, such as the United Kingdom, have had more rapid rates of increase than the United States. Prevalence remains lower in these countries at this time only because their rates of obesity in the 1980s were at most half that of the United States.

Rates of obesity are also high in the Eastern Mediterranean region, except in the very poorest countries (World Health Organization, 2004, p. 27). The most affluent of these countries have rates as high as the United States.

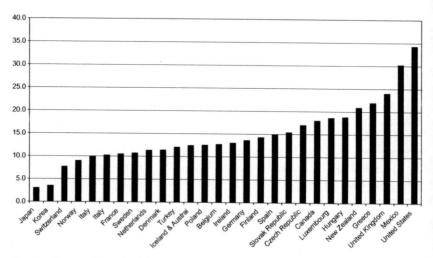

Fig. 2. Percent Obese in Selected OECD Countries, 2002–2006. *Source:* Organisation for Economic Co-Operation and Development (OECD) (2009).

An article in the *Saudi Medical Journal* reports a prevalence rate of 44 percent among adult females and 26 percent among adult males (Al-Nozha, Al-Mazrou, Al-Maatouq, & Arafah, 2005). A similar substantial sex difference is present in most of the other countries in the region as well.

Data on developing countries' obesity rates should be interpreted with caution. Most sample surveys in these countries over-represent urban populations where a greater range of food choice is available, often at lower cost than in rural areas because of government subsidies. Moreover, many jobs in urban areas require less physical activity than farming. Weight classifications and the age groups used in these studies vary as well. These limitations notwithstanding, there is an obvious association between the prevalence of obesity and level of economic productivity, as hypothesized in the social change model. Economies in transition such as Mexico, Brazil, Argentina, and Venezuela have prevalence rates in the range of European societies (Fig. 3). Less affluent developing countries increasingly face the health problems of obesity in urban subpopulations at the same time that chronic under-nutrition continues to be their major problem. Rates of obesity are rising among urban women in the least affluent countries of Africa, where most of the world's undernourished population resides (World Health Organization, 2004, p. 21).

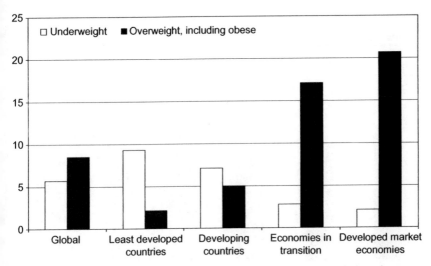

Fig. 3. Percent Underweight and Overweight by Level of Economic Development.
Source: www.fao.org/FOCUS/E/obesity/obes2.htm.

It is equally evident that obesity is not solely a function of economic growth. Not only do some affluent developed countries have relatively low levels of overweight and obesity, there also are significant differences among developing societies. Rates tend to be substantially lower in Asian societies than in Latin American societies at the same level of economic productivity, suggesting the importance of cultural and structural differences in these societies besides their level of economic productivity. Examining the distribution of obesity across subpopulations within one society can help identify other social facts that influence the prevalence of obesity in a population.

OBESITY IN THE UNITED STATES

The proportion of adults who are overweight, but not obese, according to the standard BMI classification discussed previously, has been stable since 1960 in United States (Fig. 4). The age-adjusted rate has remained between 32 and 34 percent. In stark contrast, the proportion of American adults who are obese almost tripled as it increased from 13 to 34 percent over the same time period. Moreover, the rate of increase has been steeper for higher levels

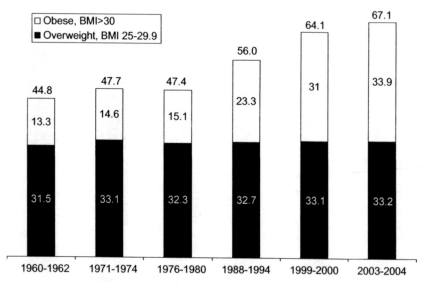

Fig. 4. Age-Adjusted Percent of Overweight and Obesity Among Adults 20–74 Years of Age: United States, 1960–2004. *Source:* National Center for Health Statistics (2007a, p. 40).

of obesity than lower levels (Fig. 5). As a result, 1 in 20 American adults are now classified as morbidly obese because they have a BMI of 40 or more (Ogden et al., 2006) and the subgroup of them with the most extreme level of morbid obesity, measured by a BMI of 50 or more, comprises an increasing share of this population. To put this in perspective, a 5 foot 6 inch tall adult would have to weigh 309 pounds to reach a BMI of 50, while a 5 foot 9 inch tall adult would have to weigh 338 pounds.

The rapid increase in the prevalence of morbid levels of obesity is a major public health challenge. Approximately three of every four adults with a BMI of 40 or more have one of the physical comorbidities listed in Table 1 and a substantial portion of them has two or more (Must, Spadano, Coakley, & Field, 1999). The likelihood of having physical comorbidities increases steeply as the degree of obesity increases (McTigue, Larson, Valoski, & Burke, 2006). Similarly, the likelihood of premature mortality, much of which is mediated through diabetes, hypertension, and hyperlipidemia, increases as the degree of obesity increases. Fontaine and associates (2003) estimate that the life expectancy of 20-year-old white men with BMIs of 45 or more is reduced 13 years compared to those with a BMI of 24,

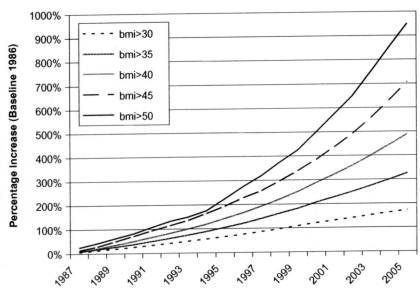

Fig. 5. Rate of Increase in Obesity by BMI Categories Since 1986. *Source:* Sturm (2007).

which is near the top of the normal range; the life expectancy of white women of the same age and weight status is reduced 8 years.

The report that the 2005–2006 obesity rate is not significantly different than the 2003–2004 rate (Ogden, Carroll, McDowell, & Flegal, 2007) could be interpreted as evidence that the obesity epidemic is beginning to wane in the United States. However, the dramatic increase in the prevalence of obese children and adolescents since the mid-1960s in Fig. 6 argues that a decline in adult obesity in the near future is highly unlikely without effective early intervention. Weight status in adolescence is a strong predictor of weight status in adulthood (Crossman, Sullivan, & Benin, 2006). Being overweight in adolescence increases the odds of being overweight or obese six years later as young adults by 832 percent, while being obese in adolescence increases the odds 2,492 percent. Weight in adolescence remains the strongest predictor of young adult weight even when numerous other variables such as parental weight, physical activity, and eating patterns are included in the analysis. In general, the prevalence of obesity increases with age until the early sixties when it begins to decline (National Center for Health Statistics, 2007a).

These findings indicate that the overall distribution of weight in the American adult population is moving into a higher range as the proportion

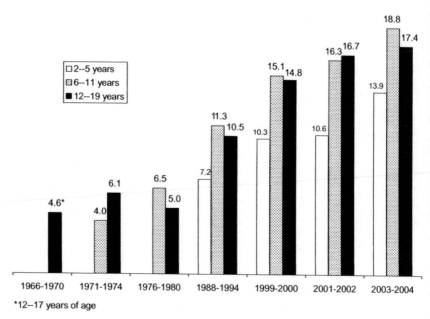

*12--17 years of age

Fig. 6.   Percent of Obese Children by Age Group: United States, 1966–2004. *Source*:
National Center for Health Statistics (2007a).

of adults in the normal BMI range shrinks and the proportion in the
morbidly obese range increases. Not only is a much higher percent of adults
obese today than 45 years ago, the obese population today also is heavier on
average than it was in the 1960s and 1970s. Given the increased health risks
associated with higher levels of excessive weight, the shifting distribution of
body weight in the population underscores the importance of considering
the causes of prevalence, rather than only the causes of cases.

Gender

Obesity is more prevalent among women than men in the United States
(Fig. 7). The gap is narrowing because the prevalence among men tripled
between 1960 and 2004, while the prevalence among women only doubled.
With a few exceptions such as France, Denmark, and Argentina, other
countries have gender differences in the same direction, although the size of
the gap varies widely (World Health Organization, 2004). It is very small in

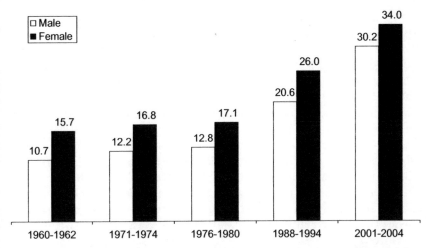

Fig. 7. Age-Adjusted Percent of Obesity Among Adults 20–74 Years of Age by Sex: United States, 1960–2004. *Source:* National Center for Health Statistics (2007a).

some countries such as Finland, Germany, and Canada and large in most of Latin America, African countries with estimated data such as Egypt, and some of the more affluent Middle Eastern countries. Multivariate analyses of longitudinal individual data for the United States indicate that the relationships between adolescent weight status and various individual risk factors differ in significant ways by gender (Crossman et al., 2006). Only a small part of this difference is attributable to the later onset of puberty in boys compared to girls. The rest points to social facts such as gender roles and norms as important determinants of body weight at the population level.

The narrowing of the obesity gender gap in the United States and many other post-industrial, affluent societies, while it remains high in the least industrialized, developing countries, supports several hypotheses about the impact of industrialization and globalization embedded in the social change model of obesity in Fig. 1. Industrialization increased the division of labor by creating low-skill, factory jobs that offered employment opportunities for farm girls and lower-class domestic workers and immigrants beginning in the nineteenth century. The resulting increase in economic productivity, along with public policy that mandated universal education of women as well as men, fueled an expansion of retail, office, and other urban, service sector jobs such as nursing and teaching from the late 1800s through the mid-1900s. These jobs offered an attractive safety net for unmarried middle class women at a time when middle and upper class women were not expected to work if they were married. Over the same time period, the rising standard of living, along with public health reforms, greatly reduced infant and child mortality and supported a transition to lower fertility. The reduction in time spent raising young children by the mid-twentieth century lowered the major structural obstacle to middle class women's employment outside the home. And, as more middle class women acquired not only high school diplomas, but also college and post-baccalaureate degrees, they faced high "opportunity costs" from forgone earnings, if they did not enter the paid labor force. The stagnation of men's earnings and growing income inequality between the top 5 percent of households and the rest of the population in the United States since the 1970s (U.S. Census Bureau, 2000), together with the rising cost of sending children to college, provided additional incentive for more middle class women to enter the workforce.

These macro-changes led to significant changes in women's roles and social institutions. The demographic transition to low fertility was virtually complete in European and North American societies by the 1970s when middle class women, followed by an increasing number of highly educated, upper class women, flooded into the paid labor force, mostly into service sector positions that ranged from pink collar secretary and hairdresser jobs to managerial and professional jobs. The increased participation of more affluent women in the paid labor force in turn increased the employment opportunities of lower-class women in jobs that offer substitute services for women's traditional domestic roles of childcare, housecleaning, and meal preparation.

The transition from an industrial to post-industrial society also transformed the lives of American men. The integration of the global economy in the second half of the twentieth century, combined with the digital revolution and innovations in transportation, manufacturing, and agricultural technology, encouraged the transfer of low-skill, labor-intensive jobs to developing countries. The impact on the occupational distribution of American men was substantial. Employment in the most physically strenuous, traditionally male occupations of farming, forestry, fishing, and heavy equipment operation declined dramatically over the last 25 years (U.S. Bureau of Labor Statistics, 2009a). Men today are much less likely to work in physically demanding jobs. Similar to women, they increasingly work in such sedentary occupations as managerial and professional jobs, sales, and service sector jobs. This relatively recent structural change in men's occupational distribution has increased their vulnerability to obesity.

Women's rapid movement into the paid labor force in the United States since the 1960s also contributed directly to the nutrition transition. About 76 percent of all American women 25–54 years of age are now in the labor force (U.S. Bureau of Labor Statistics, 2009b). With less time available for meal preparation, working men and women and their dependent children consume more processed "convenience" foods that are heavily advertised and more profitable for the international commercial food industries that grew out of the industrialization of agriculture. They also eat more food away from home. The amount of money spent on food consumed away from home as a percent of all food expenditures doubled from 1960 to 1998 from 20 to 40 percent and continued to increase to 42 percent by 2007 (U.S. Department of Agriculture, 2008). These changes in food consumption result in a diet that is much higher in saturated fat, sugar, volume, and calories. Both the decline of physically demanding jobs and the nutrition transition that have resulted from industrialization are proximate structural predictors of the obesity epidemic in Fig. 1.

Race/Ethnicity and Immigration Status

The prevalence of obesity is increasing among all race/ethnic groups in the United States. It is increasing faster among non-Hispanic white men than among African American and Hispanic men (Fig. 8). A higher proportion of the latter two groups continue to work in physically demanding jobs such as construction and farming, while non-Hispanic white men have been moving more rapidly into service sector jobs (U.S. Bureau of Labor Statistics, 2007). Unemployment is also significantly higher for African American and Hispanic men (U.S. Bureau of Labor Statistics, 2009c). All other things being equal, higher rates of unemployment should reduce food consumption. African American men are also much more likely to serve in the military where physical fitness is stressed (Segal & Segal, 2004, p. 20) and 5 percent of adult African American men, compared to less than 1 percent of White men, are incarcerated (Farley & Haaga, 2005). Incarceration not only restricts dietary options, it also gives inmates opportunity and motivation to strengthen their bodies. Extreme body-building practices have become sufficiently common that some prison systems have removed weight lifting equipment because of concerns about the physical threat that these "bulked-up" inmates pose to other inmates and guards.

While there are no longer significant differences in the prevalence of obesity between men in the largest racial/ethnic groups in the United States,

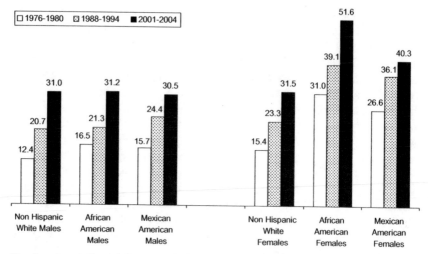

Fig. 8. Age-Adjusted Percent of Obesity Among Adults 20–74 Years of Age by Race/Ethnicity: United States, 1976–2004. *Source:* National Center for Health Statistics (2007a).

the disparities between women have increased. More than half of African American women are now obese. Almost 14 percent were morbidly obese in 1999–2002, up from 7.9 in 1988–1994 (Wang & Beydoun, 2007). African American women's rate of morbid obesity is more than double Non-Hispanic white women and Mexican American women and more than four times men's rates. Neither the structural social change model in Fig. 1, nor the socioeconomic effects discussed in the next section explains the higher rates of excessive weight among African American women. Different cultural standards about female body weight likely play a role. One can also speculate that the high rates of unemployment and incarceration among African American men reduce African American women's perception of their chances of finding an acceptable spouse and encourage some to turn to food for comfort.

Fig. 9 compares the 2006 rates of obesity and overweight in the adult population by race/ethnicity. American Indians and Native Hawaiian/Pacific Islanders have an obesity prevalence that is almost as high as African Americans. In contrast to African Americans, Hispanics, and non-Hispanic whites, the prevalence is higher for Native American men (38 percent) than women (29 percent) (Office of Minority Health, 2008). The reversed gender gap in this population points to a different set of structural influences on

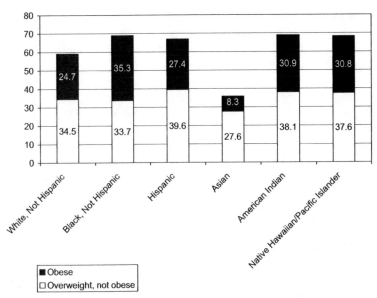

Fig. 9. Age-Adjusted Rates of Overweight/Not Obese and Obesity Among Adults Age 18 and Over by Race/Ethnicity: United States, 2006. *Note:* Data are for single race categories. *Source:* National Center for Health Statistics (2007b). Table 31. Available at http://www.cdc.gov/nchs/data/series/sr_10/sr10_235.pdf.

body weight than those included in Fig. 1. Following the influx of Europeans, government policies broke down the traditional social structure of indigenous tribes and left many Native Americans isolated on reservations and mired in poverty. Most have been marginalized from the industrial revolution and the ongoing digital revolution. Unemployment, estimated to be 48 percent on the Navajo Nation (Choudhary, 2006), is extremely high and reduces the physical activity associated with employment. Alcoholism is a widespread social problem and contributes to excessive weight gain. Food choices are limited and unlikely to include expensive fresh fruit and vegetables. Similar structural problems and cultural differences may contribute to the high obesity of Native Hawaiians and Pacific Islanders. Obesity is also high in the indigenous populations of other lands seized by Europeans, including Aboriginal Canadians (Katzmarzyk, 2008), Aboriginal Australians (Australian Bureau of Statistics, 2008), and Maoris (New Zealand Ministry of Health, 2008). Like alcoholism, obesity has become a major health problem in indigenous populations that transcends national borders. Although it may not be created by the structural variables in Fig. 1, obesity in indigenous populations is influenced by structural variables as well as cultural variables that are particular to these populations' histories.

In stark contrast to other minority groups, Asian Americans, approximately 64 percent of whom are foreign born (U.S. Census Bureau, 2008b), have significantly lower rates of excessive weight, mirroring the lower rates in their countries of origin. Unlike Hispanic immigrants, Asian immigrants and their children have high levels of education, although there are variations by country of origin and refugee status. Nearly half of all Asian Americans who are 25 years of age and older have a bachelor's degree and one in five have a post-baccalaureate degree (U.S. Census Bureau, 2006). Not only does their educational attainment exceed that of non-Hispanic whites and other minorities, Asian Americans' median income is also higher.

Undoubtedly the greater resources that come with higher socioeconomic status, discussed in the next section, contribute to the lower level of excessive weight among Asian Americans, but there is evidence of cultural effects as well. Research on Asian American adolescents finds that greater accultura-tion, measured by years in the United States or being born in this country, increases the likelihood of obesity (Popkin & Udry, 1998). The positive association between duration of residence and prevalence of obesity is also found among adult immigrants and persists when sociodemographic factors are controlled (Mita, McCarthy, Phillips, & Wee, 2004). The most substantial increase in the prevalence of obesity occurs after 10 years of residence. These findings suggest that the cumulative process of accultura-tion, which involves adopting the dietary norms of American culture and the more sedentary lifestyle created by a post-industrial social structure, reaches an important threshold around 10 years of residence when most immigrants are fairly well assimilated into American society.

Socioeconomic Status

The low rate of obesity among Asian Americans, the population with the highest levels of education and income in the United States, points to socioeconomic status as a determinant of body weight. Unlike international comparisons that show a positive association between gross national income and obesity, socioeconomic status is inversely related to obesity within the United States population. The prevalence is higher for subpopulations with

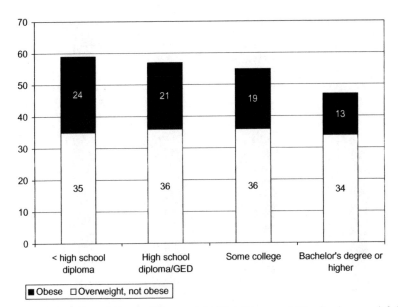

Fig. 10. Age-Adjusted Rates of Overweight/Not Obese and Obesity Among Adults Age 18 and Over by Education: United States, 2006. *Source:* National Center for Health Statistics (2007b). Table 31. Available at http://www.cdc.gov/nchs/data/ series/sr_10/sr10_235.pdf.

lower educational attainment (Fig. 10). The same is true for low-income populations (Fig. 11). However, consistent with the social change model in Fig. 1, the difference in the rate of obesity by income has narrowed considerably over the last 35 years as an increasing proportion of low-income workers is employed in less physically demanding service sector jobs such as fast food, retail, and health care that are expanding in number, while employment in physically demanding jobs such as farming, forestry, mining, and fishing declines.

Socioeconomic measures account for much, but not all, of the variance in obesity among race/ethnic groups. When socioeconomic status and race/ethnicity are both included in individual-level analyses, the association between socioeconomic status and obesity differs in some complex ways by race/ethnicity and gender. For example, more education is generally associated with lower odds of obesity, but Wang and Beydoun (2007) report that African American women with less than a high school education have a lower rate of obesity than those with more education. Similarly, despite the strong inverse association between socioeconomic status and

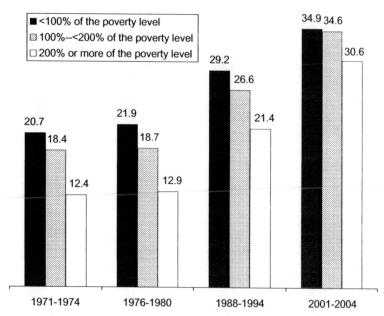

Fig. 11. Age-Adjusted Percent of Obesity Among Adults 20–74 Years of Age by Poverty Status: United States, 1971–2004. *Source:* National Center for Health Statistics (2007a).

obesity among non-Hispanic white adolescent females, African American adolescent females from families with the highest socioeconomic status are more likely to be obese than those from families with the lowest socioeconomic status. These findings again point to social facts not included in the structural model in Fig. 1, including differences in cultural beliefs, values, norms, and social and physical environmental context that remain between race/ethnic groups after socioeconomic differences are taken into account.

The inverse relationship between education and obesity in individual-level analyses is usually interpreted as evidence of the protective impact of greater knowledge about health and nutrition. However, the relatively higher level of educational attainment in the United States population compared to many other affluent countries and all other developing countries has not proven to be protective at the population level where it is overshadowed by structural and cultural factors that promote obesity.

Other Structural Determinants of Obesity

Industrialization's demand for labor fueled urbanization, but urbanization would not have been possible without the increased agricultural productivity from mechanization that freed an increasing proportion of population from the need to grow food. Expanding urban populations increased the demand for commercially available food. Innovations in transportation supported the commercialization and commodificaton of food as well as urbanization by reducing the physical activity needed to move food and other goods to market, workers to jobs, and people to schools, retail businesses, and other destinations. Transportation innovations, along with digital technology, increased agricultural productivity from the Green revolution, and commercial supply chains, also facilitated the globalization of the food supply that paved the way for the nutrition transition. Even in the absence of industrialization, transnational institutions that emerged after World War II, such as the World Bank, the International Monetary Fund, and the Food and Agricultural Organization, pushed developing countries to adopt more efficient agricultural technologies. These powerful nongovernmental organizations advocate the production of export commodity crops such as sugar, coffee, and palm oil as a development strategy. As a result, global food production increased faster than global population, driving down the cost of food, particularly in more affluent countries with relatively open import policies.

The impact of these macro-changes on the cost of food in the United States is evident in Fig. 12. Since 1950, the percent of disposable income spent on food declined from over 20 percent to under 10 percent. An increasing share of that money is spent on food consumed away from home that is higher in calories to appeal to consumer preference for the taste of sweet, the texture of fat, and "value-sizing." The lower cost of food and the increased consumption of heavily processed convenience foods and restaurant meals contributed to the nutrition transition and imbalance between calories of energy consumed and calories of energy expended.

Surveys reveal that men's average calorie consumption increased from 2,450 to 2,618 between 1971 and 2000, while women's average consumption increased from 1,542 to 1,877 (Centers for Disease Control and Prevention, 2004). Given that one pound of body weight approximately equals 3,500 calories, a woman already eating enough calories to sustain body weight would gain almost three pounds per month from the additional energy intake and a man would gain almost a pound and a half, unless their energy expenditure increased by a corresponding amount. This has not been the

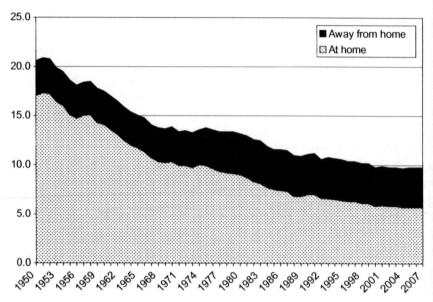

Fig. 12. Food Expenditures as a Percent of Disposable Personal Income in the United States, 1950–2007. *Source:* U.S. Department of Agriculture (2008).

case for most Americans as the economy transitioned to service sector jobs, transportation reduced physical activity, and the digital revolution created more sedentary work and leisure activities. Nearly one-third of adolescents and 55 percent of the adults do not meet the minimum recommended 30 minutes of moderately intense activity at least five days a week (Institute of Medicine, 2005a).

Institutional Responses

The Surgeon General issued a warning about the obesity epidemic in 2001. The Institute of Medicine (2005b, 2007) followed with reports on childhood obesity that urge government, businesses, schools, and families to recognize the problem of obesity and promote increased physical activity and healthy food consumption. With the exception of recommendations to improve the nutritional quality of school lunches and develop guidelines for both the built environment and marketing food to children, the recommendations individualize the social problem of obesity. They assume that if people are educated about obesity, they will make healthy choices.

Industry has also announced corporate policies to join the campaign against obesity (Ludwig & Nestle, 2008). McDonald's wants to "empower individuals to make informed choices ..." PepsiCo helps "kids lead healthier lives by offering product choices ..." Kraft "gives back to communities" by "helping children and their families make healthy food choices ..." These statements also individualize obesity as a problem of poor personal choices, rather than a social problem created by an environment saturated with inexpensive, high-calorie commercial food products that are aggressively marketed.

Most physicians similarly view obesity as an individual problem that does not respond well to lifestyle interventions or existing drugs. Many are reluctant to spend time counseling patients to lose weight (Loureiro & Naygo, 2006) and available prescription drugs reduce baseline weight only by an average of 2.9–4.6 percent per year (Simons-Morton, Obarzanek, & Cutler, 2006). The lack of more effective medical therapies drove an estimated 205,000 people to undergo bariatric surgery in the United States in 2007 (American Society for Metabolic & Bariatric Surgery, 2008). These procedures limit the amount of food a stomach can hold. Some also limit calorie absorption. Because of risks, patients must be morbidly obese or have a BMI of 35 or more with a comorbidity. This is still a large pool of potential patients and the number of procedures is increasing exponentially. In the short term, bariatric surgery dramatically reduces weight and some comorbidities such as type 2 diabetes and coronary heart disease in the majority of patients who change their eating and exercise habits after surgery. The long-term effectiveness, benefits, and risks are still unknown.

CONCLUSION

Bariatric surgery is too far "downstream" to stop the flood of obesity. It has the potential, however, to reduce the physical and economic toll of some comorbidities. No drug yet available promises as much. The irony is that bariatric surgery only reduces the impact of these secondary diseases if patients commit to radical behavioral changes in their diet and physical activity. Whether the post-surgical population will be able to sustain such changes, while living in a society with a social structure and culture that continues to promote obesity, remains to be seen.

Public education campaigns aimed at reducing obesity by promoting behavioral changes in eating and exercise are likely to have little sustained impact. Rose warns that efforts to change individual risk behaviors that are normative in the cultural and social context rarely succeed. Unlike antismoking campaigns that urge people to quit or never start smoking by stigmatizing the unhealthy behavior, anti-obesity campaigns urge people to change dietary and activity preferences that were adopted in a social context where obesity is already highly stigmatized. Many Americans want to lose weight; they spent $55 billion on weight-loss products and services in 2006 (Marketdata Enterprises, 2007). When their efforts fail, as is most often the case, they blame themselves for their lack of self-discipline and overlook the upstream social facts of their everyday lives.

Changing eating and activity behavior is a daunting task. People have to make constant decisions about eating and physical activity in a structural context that promotes obesity. The products offered by the commercial food industry reflect dominant population choices that likely draw on innate food preferences evolved in times of periodic famines. Expecting that the commercial food industry will voluntarily eliminate profitable, but unhealthy, products that appeal to customers and give them an edge in a highly competitive market is unreasonable and a violation of their fiduciary responsibility to shareholders. The industry produces what consumers demand within the context of government regulations. As a major payer for the cumulative health problems caused by obesity, the government has a public fiduciary responsibility and a moral obligation to regulate unhealthy products, despite the great reluctance of elected leaders who are more responsive to industry lobbyists than the public good. We need to reframe obesity as a social problem, not merely an individual problem, and look for ways to make "upstream" changes in the structural determinants of obesity, including adopting government regulations of unhealthy food products.

Policies to create built-environments that encourage a higher level of physical activity are an obvious upstream strategy, but not one likely to have substantial impact in the near future, given existing physical infrastructure. Policies to extend the school day to provide more time for mandatory participation in sports, dance, or other physical activities from kindergarten through high school would have a more immediate effect, as would incentives to employers to provide two 15-minute exercise breaks on the job directed by physical trainers. Some companies already provide incentives to encourage employees to stop smoking or lose weight. More would if encouraged by tax incentives.

Changing eating norms will require more aggressive strategies that start with children. It is time for Cookie Monster to retire from *Sesame Street*. Marketing any food product to children should be prohibited, whether it is done with television advertising or web-based games and promotions. School lunch programs need to be restructured to end policies that allow students to choose a soft drink, fries, and a piece of cake for lunch. Only meals that comply with USDA nutritional guidelines should be served as a way of educating students about healthy nutrition while satiating their hunger. Schools also should be prohibited from signing revenue-generating contracts that allow fast food businesses and vending machines on campus.

General strategies to change eating norms need to recognize that the demand for convenience foods is embedded in modern societies across all socioeconomic groups. The focus needs to be on creating healthier convenience foods, providing clear information about calorie content, and encouraging healthier consumption patterns. Most commercially processed foods and beverages already display nutritional information, but the calorie content is often obfuscated by unclear serving sizes. Policies need to require clear information about calories. Most importantly, the policy needs to be extended to require point-of-purchase menu labeling of the calorie content. The information would enhance consumers' ability to make healthier choices and influence the products offered by fast food and other restaurants.

Providing better nutritional information is a necessary, but insufficient, strategy. Growing income inequality in the United States is a public health problem that contributes to the obesity epidemic. Unhealthy fast food, snacks, and "treats" are less expensive, more convenient, more readily available, and more emotionally satisfying to consumers because they have been developed to taste good. This makes them particularly attractive to low-income Americans who lack the money, time, access, and alternative ways of indulging themselves. There is good reason to expect that fewer unhealthy food and beverage products would be consumed, if they were more expensive. The use of targeted taxes to raise the cost of tobacco has been a successful strategy for reducing use. Revenue from a "Twinkie" tax could be used to subsidize the cost of healthier foods and fund summer day camps for low-income children to promote increased physical activity. We must look upstream and think creatively and structurally. Unless interventions can be developed quickly and implemented, obesity will be the defining disease of the twenty-first century.

REFERENCES

Al-Nozha, M. M., Al-Mazrou, Y. Y., Al-Maatouq, M. A., Arafah, M. R., et al. (2005). Obesity in Saudi Arabia. *Saudi Medical Journal, 26*(5), 824–829.

American Society for Metabolic & Bariatric Surgery. (2008). Metabolic and bariatric surgery. Available at http://www.asbs.org/Newsite07/media/asbs_presskit.htm. Accessed on 13 November 2008.

Australian Bureau of Statistics. (2008). Overweight and obesity – Aboriginal and Torres Strait Islander people: A snapshot, 2004–05. Available at http://www.abs.gov.au/AUSSTATS/ abs@.nsf/mf/4722.0.55.006. Accessed on 10 November 2008.

Centers for Disease Control and Prevention. (2004). Trends in intake of energy and micronutrients – United States, 1971–2000. *Morbidity and Mortality Weekly Report*, *53*(4), 80–82.

Centers for Disease Control and Prevention. (2008). Preventing obesity and chronic diseases through good nutrition and physical activity. Available at http://www.cdc.gov/nccdphp/ publications/factsheets/Prevention/obesity.htm. Accessed on 13 November 2008.

Choudhary, T. (2006). *2005–2006 comprehensive economic development strategy of the Navajo Nation.* Window Rock, AZ: Division of Economic Development of the Navajo Nation.

Crossman, A., Sullivan, D. A., & Benin, M. (2006). The family environment and American adolescents' risk of obesity as young adults. *Social Science & Medicine*, *63*(06), 2255–2267.

Farley, R., & Haaga, J. (2005). *The American people: Census 2000.* New York: Russell Sage Foundation.

Flegal, K. M., Graubard, B. I., Williamson, D. F., & Gail, M. H. (2005). Excess deaths associated with underweight, overweight, and obesity. *JAMA*, *293*(15), 1861–1867.

Fontaine, K. R., Redden, D. T., Wang, C., et al. (2003). Years of life lost due to obesity. *JAMA*, *289*(2), 187–193.

Frohlich, F., & Potvin, L. (2008). Transcending the known in public health practice: The inequality paradox: The population approach and vulnerable populations. *American Journal of Public Health*, *98*(2), 216–221.

Glass, T. A., & McAtee, M. J. (2006). Behavioral science at the crossroads in public health: Extending horizons, envisioning the future. *Social Science & Medicine*, *62*(7), 1650–1671.

Institute of Medicine. (2005a). *Does the built environment influence physical activity? Examining the evidence.* Washington, DC: National Academies of Science.

Institute of Medicine. (2005b). *Preventing childhood obesity; health in the balance.* Washington, DC: National Academies of Science.

Institute of Medicine. (2007). *Progress in preventing childhood obesity how do we measure up?* Washington, DC: National Academies of Science.

Kaplan, G. A. (2004). What's wrong with social epidemiology and how can we make it better? *Epidemiology Review*, *26*, 124–135.

Katzmarzyk, P. T. (2008). Obesity and physical activity among aboriginal Canadians. *Obesity*, *16*, 184–190.

Loureiro, M. L., & Naygo, R. M. (2006). Obesity, weight loss, and physician's advice. *Social Science & Medicine*, *62*(10), 2458–2468.

Ludwig, D. S., & Nestle, M. (2008). Can the food industry play a constructive role in the obesity epidemic. *JAMA*, *300*(15), 1808–1811.

Marketdata Enterprises. (2007). *The U.S weight loss and diet control market* (9th ed.). Rockville, MD: Marketdata Enterprises Inc.

McDowell, I. (2008). From risk factors to explanation in pubic health. *Journal of Public Health*, *30*(3), 219–223.

McTigue, K., Larson, J. C., Valoski, A., Burke, G., et al. (2006). Mortality and cardiac and vascular outcomes in extremely obese women. *JAMA*, *296*(1), 79–86.

Mita, S. G., McCarthy, E. P., Phillips, R. S., & Wee, C. C. (2004). Obesity among US immigrant subgroups by duration of residence. *JAMA*, *292*(23), 2860–2867.

Must, A., Spadano, J., Coakley, E. H., & Field, A. E. (1999). The disease burden associated with overweight and obesity. *JAMA, 282*(16), 1523–1529.

National Center for Health Statistics. (2007a). *Health, United States, 2007*. Washington, DC: Government Printing Office.

National Center for Health Statistics. (2007b). *Summary health statistics for U.S. adults: National health interview Survey, 2006* (Series 10, No. 235). Washington, DC: Government Printing Office.

New Zealand Ministry of Health. (2008). Obesity in New Zealand. Available at http://www.moh.govt.nz/moh.nsf/indexmh/obesity-key-facts. Accessed on 10 November 2008.

OECD. (2009). OECD health data 2009 – Frequently requested data. Available at http://www.oecd.org/health/healthdata.

Office of Minority Health. (2008). Obesity data/statistics Available at http://www.omhrc.gov/templates/browse.aspx?lvl = 3&lvlid = 537. Accessed on 4 November 2008.

Ogden, C. L., Carroll, M. D., Curtin, L. R., McDowell, M. A., Tabak, C. J., & Flegal, K. M. (2006). Prevalence of overweight and obesity in the United States, 1999–2004. *JAMA, 295*(13), 1549–1555.

Ogden, C. L., Carroll, M. D., McDowell, M. A., & Flegal, F. M. (2007). Obesity among adults in the United States: No statistically significant change since 2003–2004. NCHS data brief. Available at www.cdc.gov/nchs/data/databriefs/db01.pdf. Accessed on 25 October 2008.

Pischon, T., Boeing, H., Hoffmann, K., et al. (2008). General and abdominal adiposity and risk of death in Europe. *New England Journal of Medicine, 359*(20), 2105–2120.

Popkin, G. M., & Udry, J. R. (1998). Adolescent obesity increases significantly in second and third generation U.S. immigrants: The National Longitudinal Study of Adolescent Health. *Journal of Nutrition, 128*(1), 701–707.

Rose, G. (1985). Sick individuals and sick populations. *International Journal of Epidemiology, 14*(1), 32–38.

Segal, D. R., & Segal, M. W. (2004). America's military population. *Population Bulletin, 59*(4), 20.

Simons-Morton, D. G., Obarzanek, E., & Cutler, J. A. (2006). Obesity research – Limitations of methods, measurements, and medications. *JAMA, 295*(7), 826–828.

Sturm, R. (2007). Increases in morbid obesity in the USA: 2000–2005. *Public Health, 121*(7), 492–496.

Sturm, R., & Wells, K. B. (2001). Does obesity contribute as much to morbidity as poverty or smoking? *Public Health, 115*(3), 229–235.

Surgeon General. (2001). *The Surgeon General's call to action to prevent and decrease overweight and obesity*. Rockville, MD: U.S. Department of Health and Human Services.

U.S. Bureau of Labor Statistics. (2007). Employment and earnings, January 2007. Available at www.bls.gov/cps/cpsaat11.pdf. Accessed on 12 November 2008.

U.S. Bureau of Labor Statistics. (2009a). Table 10, Employed persons by major occupation and sex, 1983 and 2002, annual averages. Available at www.bls.gov/cps/wlf-tables10.pdf. Accessed on 3 October 2009.

U.S. Bureau of Labor Statistics. (2009b). Women in the labor force: A databook. Table 1. Available at http://www.bls.gov/cps/wlf-databook2009.htm. Accessed on 3 October 2009.

U.S. Bureau of Labor Statistics. (2009c). The employment situation, September 2009. Available at www.bls.gov/news.release/pdf/empsit.pdf. Accessed on 4 October 2009.

U.S. Census Bureau. (2000). The changing shape of the nation's income distribution. Available at http://www.census.gov/hhes/www/income/incineq/p60204.html. Accessed on 3 October 2009.

U.S. Census Bureau. (2006). Asian/Pacific American heritage month, May 2006. Available at
    http://www.census.gov/Press-Release/www/releases/archives/facts_for_features_special_
    editions/006587.html. Accessed on 4 October 2009.
U.S. Census Bureau. (2008a). World population by age and sex. Available at http://
    www.census.gov/ipc/www/idb/worldpopinfo.html. Accessed on 29 October 2008.
U.S. Census Bureau. (2008b). Current Population Survey, 2004, Racial statistics. Tables 1
    and 8. Available at http://www.census.gov/population/www/socdemo/race/ppl-184.html.
    Accessed on 4 November 2008.
U.S. Department of Agriculture. (2008). Food CPI, prices and expenditures: food expenditures
    by families and individuals as a share of disposable personal income. Available at http://
    www.ers.usda.gov/briefing/CPIFoodandExpenditures/Data/table7.htm. Accessed on
    6 November 2008.
Wang, Y., & Beydoun, M. A. (2007). The obesity epidemic in the United States–gender, age,
    socioeconomic, racial/ethnic, and geographic characteristics: A systematic review and
    meta-regression analysis. *Epidemiologic Reviews, 29*, 6–8.
World Health Organization. (2004). *Obesity: Preventing and managing the global epidemic.*
    Geneva: World Health Organization.
World Health Organization. (2008). Obesity and overweight. Available at http://www.who.int/
    mediacentre/factsheets/fs311/en/index.html. Accessed on 29 October 2008.

WHO SAYS OBESITY IS AN EPIDEMIC? HOW EXCESS WEIGHT BECAME AN AMERICAN HEALTH CRISIS

Hanna Grol-Prokopczyk

ABSTRACT

Purpose – *To understand why obesity came to be considered an American epidemic, or even a global pandemic, in the mid-to-late 1990s. Why not decades earlier, given that by 1960 over 40% of Americans had body mass indexes (BMIs) above 25? Alternately, why at all, given the myriad ways in which obesity challenges standard definitions of an epidemic?*

Methodology/approach – *Four decades of American medical journal articles and best-selling diet books are reviewed for definitions, measures, prevalence estimates, and presumed causes of excess weight.*

Findings – *Developments paving the way for the "epidemicization" of American obesity include: (1) diffusion of the BMI as a standard measure of weight-for-height, and acceptance of increasingly low BMI cutoffs to define excess weight; (2) use of nationally representative surveys to estimate obesity prevalence; and, (3) the decline of psychoanalysis-driven prejudices predicating a wide gulf between a deviant obese minority and a nonobese majority.*

Understanding Emerging Epidemics: Social and Political Approaches
Advances in Medical Sociology, Volume 11, 343–358
Copyright © 2010 by Emerald Group Publishing Limited
All rights of reproduction in any form reserved
ISSN: 1057-6290/doi:10.1108/S1057-6290(2010)0000011022

Contribution to the field – *By showing how the obesity epidemic was able to transcend metaphor and become fact within the American medical community, this study demonstrates that health issues can come to the fore of public consciousness for a complex host of reasons. Better understanding of such reasons could help in evaluating, prioritizing, and ameliorating those health problems.*

INTRODUCTION

Why did obesity come to be considered an American epidemic, or even a global pandemic, in the mid-to-late 1990s? Why did such alarming designations come into widespread use at this particular moment in history? Indeed, why did the phrase "obesity epidemic" gain currency *at all*, given the many ways that obesity differs from historical or traditional epidemics? This chapter attempts to answer these questions from the perspective of the American medical community.

In Part I, I discuss the concept of "epidemic," and problematize obesity's inclusion in this category. In Part II, I review four decades of American medical journal articles to understand why the mid-to-late 1990s were a crucial turning point in the depiction of obesity as an epidemic. A central argument throughout is that changing definitions of and beliefs about excess weight were as important as changes in the actual American weight distribution in creating the idea of an obesity epidemic.[1]

BACKGROUND

Beginning in the mid-to-late 1990s, the American discourse about obesity changed strikingly, in both quantitative and qualitative terms. Quantitatively, the number of both professional and popular articles about obesity began to rise dramatically, as shown in Fig. 1.

Qualitatively, there was a change in the language and metaphors used to discuss excess weight. While by the mid-1960s public health professionals at times referred to obesity as "a major problem" (*New York Times*, 1966), only in the mid-1990s did obesity come to be spoken of as an "epidemic." Saguy and Riley (2005, p. 893) nicely track how an initially hesitant formulation in a 1994 *JAMA* editorial – "if this was about tuberculosis, it would be called an epidemic" – transformed over the year, as the trope spread from publication to publication, into more assertive statements that

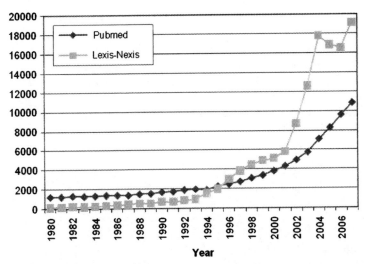

Fig. 1. Articles about Obesity in Medical Research and the Mass Media, 1980–2007. *Sources:* Lexis-Nexis and PubMed; adapted and updated from Saguy and Riley (2005, p. 876).

"obesity is an epidemic." Within a few years, "obesity epidemic" went from unknown concept to stock phrase.

Indeed, since the late 1990s, the depiction of obesity as an epidemic – or even a global pandemic – has become so common that it is nearly a cliché. And the observation that "[d]eclaring an epidemic" lends "a sense of urgency … like declaring war" (Saguy & Riley, 2005, p. 913) is borne out by the panic-inducing descriptions of obesity widespread in professional and lay publications [e.g., *JAMA*'s depiction of obesity as "a global calamity of biblical dimensions" (Roth, 2004)].

But how, and why, did obesity come to be considered an "epidemic" and a public health crisis in the United States? So common is the phrase "obesity epidemic" today that we may easily forget that, in fact, excess weight has none of the characteristics of a traditional epidemic; indeed, it is debatable whether obesity is even a disease. Even if we accept the designation as epidemic, we have a puzzle: the proportion of Americans with a body mass index (BMI) above 25 (and thus, by contemporary standards, overweight or obese[2]) has been well above 40% since at least 1960 (NCHS, 2002), a period when the health repercussions of excess weight were already acknowledged (e.g., Taller, 1961). Why, then, was it was only in the late 1990s that Americans' excess weight attained the status of an epidemic?

PART I: WHAT IS AN EPIDEMIC?

What is an epidemic? Medical and epidemiological definitions do not provide an unambiguous answer to this question. For example, Gordis's widely used epidemiology textbook (2004, p. 18) states,

> *Epidemic* is defined as the occurrence in a community or region of a group of illnesses of similar nature, clearly in excess of normal expectancy, and derived from a common or a propagated source.

But what is "clearly in excess of normal expectancy"? Disease prevalence that is always (and hence unsurprisingly) high is *endemic*, not epidemic. Acknowledging an element of subjectivity in distinguishing the normal from the excess, Gordis provides the following heuristic, accompanied by the graph below (Fig. 2): "With regard to excess, sometimes an 'interocular' test may be convincing: the difference is so clear that it hits you between the eyes" (p. 18).

Using data from all available waves of NHES and NHANES (NCHS, 2002), nationally representative surveys of the US adult population, I have created a graph of the percentage of Americans with BMIs above 25 (i.e., overweight or obese), from 1960 to 2000 (Fig. 3). Does this graph pass the "interocular test"?

The proportion of overweight/obese Americans rose from 45 to 64% in 40 years – not an unsubstantial change. But the slope of the graph does not resemble the dramatic peak in Gordis's image. The shape of any graph is, of

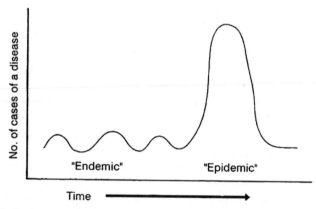

Fig. 2. Endemic versus Epidemic Disease. *Source:* Gordis (2004, P. 18). Reprinted with permission from Elsevier.

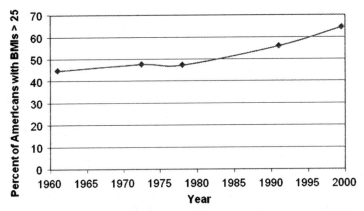

Fig. 3.   Rate of Overweight/Obesity, the United States. *Source:* NCHS (2002).

course, scale dependent. Still, the timeframe of the graph is not consistent with Slack's claim that epidemics take place over "days, months, or years" – but not decades (1992, p. 6); or Rosenberg's that a "true epidemic is an event, not a trend" (1992, p. 279).

Gordis specifies that an epidemic comes from "a common or a propagated source." But the causes of excess weight proposed today are extremely numerous and varied – and rarely literally contagious. Further-more, it is unclear if obesity even qualifies as a disease. Medical journals have at times proclaimed excess weight a disease (Jeffcoate, 1998), but more often the premise is asked rhetorically ["Is obesity a disease?" (Froguel, 2004)] or phrased hypothetically ["If obesity is a chronic disease ..." (Steelman, 2002)]; more often still, obesity is a condition or risk factor. And if obesity *is* now a disease (Glassman, 2004), it has the peculiar trait of having become one only *after* officially becoming an epidemic (WHO, 1998).

In short, obesity challenges standard definitions of "epidemic" in a number of ways. More generally, due to the imprecision and subjectiveness of such definitions – demonstrated here with the example of the "interocular test" – simple prevalence counts are often not sufficient to explain why something is or is not labeled "epidemic." The commonsense explanation that obesity came to be called an epidemic simply because it *is* an epidemic is, then, inadequate. To attempt a more nuanced explanation, I present a historical analysis of how American medical professionals came to see obesity as an epidemic.

PART II: MEDICAL JOURNALS AND DIET BOOKS ON OBESITY, 1960s–2000s

To assess how American doctors' understandings of excess weight have changed over the past four decades, I examined articles from *JAMA* and the *New England Journal of Medicine* (*NEJM*), the two best known and most widely circulating American medical journals. I identified articles containing one or more of the keywords "obesity," "overweight," "BMI," and "body mass," within the date range 1966–2004 for *JAMA*, and 1975–2004 for *NEJM*.[3] The search included not only research articles but also editorials and letters, to best observe professional debates and dialogues in progress. For a sense of lay beliefs about excess weight, I also reviewed American diet books that were top-five best sellers in the years from 1960 onwards, according to *Publisher's Weekly* (2004). I present my findings chronologically.

The 1960s and 1970s

By the 1960s, the health risks of excess weight were widely cited in the United States, in terms similar to those used today. The number one nonfiction best seller of 1962, the diet book *Calories Don't Count*, called "excess fat … a serious threat to health," and listed "heart disease, diabetes, hardening of the arteries, high blood pressure," and, with less certainty, cancer, as ailments "worsened or caused" by obesity (Taller, 1961, p. 46). Diet books throughout the 1970s mentioned similar health concerns, as did *JAMA* and *NEJM* articles (e.g., *JAMA*, 1970; Rivlin, 1975).

That excess weight entailed health risks was widely agreed upon, but a clear, generally accepted definition of "excess weight" did not yet exist in the 1960s and 1970s. Weight-for-height tables published by Metropolitan Life Insurance Company (henceforth MLIC), combined with their data on health outcomes, were the basis for a number of claims about excess weight's links to disease risks (*New York Times*, 1960), and were used as guides to "desirable" weights. But versions of the tables published in different years gave different goal weights, and were not consistent in their treatment of clothing weights, shoe heights, and "frame sizes" (Stearns, 1997; Kuczmarski & Flegal, 2000). The distinction between "average" and "desirable" weights was not always preserved, and the tables were assimilated into popular and medical writings in unstandardized ways.

Partially because of such inconsistencies, American diet books from the 1960s through the early 1980s presented a muddled sense of how much

Table 1.   Recommended Weight Ranges for a 5'4" Female.

Book (Publication Year)	Proposed Weight	Description of Weight Range	Source of Weight Range
Calories Don't Count (1961)	117–145 lbs	"Average"	MLIC
Dr. Atkins' Diet Revolution (1972)	108–138 lbs	"Desirable"	"Adapted" from MLIC
Weight Watchers Cookbook (1972)	127–144 lbs	"Goal weights"	"Recognized authorities"
Scarsdale Medical Diet (1978)	110–123 lbs	"Desired"	"Life insurance companies" (probably MLIC)
The Beverly Hills Diet (1981)	102 lbs	"Ideal"	Author's personal preference

Sources: Taller (1961, p. 43), Atkins (1972, p. 297), Nidetch (1972, p. 310), Tarnower and Baker (1978, p. 15), and Mazel (1981, p. 10).

people should weigh. Table 1 below shows the acceptable weight ranges given for a 5'4" female in the period's best-selling diet books (*Publisher's Weekly*, 2004). Strikingly, the last three weight ranges do not overlap at all. Had clear, standard definitions of excess weight already been firmly established and publicized by the medical community, such great variability of recommended weights would likely not have been possible.

If, in the 1960s and 1970s, Americans were not sure how much they should weigh, the US medical community was not well informed about how much Americans *did* weigh. MLIC height–weight tables were inadequate for generalizing about the United States as a whole, as MLIC policyholders were not a nationally representative sample. Furthermore, the tables excluded people with diseases such as heart disease and cancer, and applied only to people aged 25–59 (Kuczmarski & Flegal, 2000). Before the 1980s, I found only one estimate of total national prevalence of excess weight in the medical journals: a 1977 *NEJM* writer proclaimed that there were "40 to 50 million obese Americans" (roughly 20% of the US population), but gave no source for this figure (Mann, 1977).

Writers using MLIC data sometimes defined excess weight as 10 or 20% above the MLIC "ideal" or median (Nelson et al., 1973; Charney et al., 1976), but many other definitions were in circulation during this period. Letters to the *JAMA* editor expressed frustration at the lack of objective definitions of excess weight ("at times one believes that an obese patient becomes 'morbidly obese' only and as soon as he offends the esthetic sensitivity of the observer"), and argued for the "adoption of a precise quantitative measurement of obesity" (Boba, 1976). "[L]ively debate" (Charney et al., 1976) on this topic centered on the initially popular "ponderal index," a simple weight-to-height ratio, and a measure known as the Quetelet index or body mass index (BMI). The latter, argued to "correlate maximally with adiposity and minimally with height," was advocated by some writers as the "superior index," though no specific cutoffs between healthy and excess weights were yet proposed (Cork & Vaughan, 1979).

Medical articles from the 1960s and 1970s sometimes evinced great disdain for overweight people. For example, a *NEJM* author who hoped to find a "safe and comfortable way" for patients to lose weight continued immediately with the sarcastic and moralizing comment, "This process would, of course, require that the fat fellow be able to continue his sloth and gluttony even as the treatment works" (Mann, 1977; *cf.* Kirkpatrick, 1977).

One reason for such condescension may lie in the supposed causes of excess weight. In the 1960s and 1970s, excess weight was generally seen not as a result of sedentary lifestyles, genes, or sociobiological behavioral wirings, but of an underlying psychological defect. "What is crucial," wrote a *JAMA* contributor, "is the recognition that overeating per se is usually associated with a primary psychological problem" (Coodley, 1975). Doctors who studied obesity were often psychiatrists, and those eager to find "psychoneurotic complications" in their obese patients could easily so. In one study, obese patients were kept in a "metabolic ward" for 8 months of dieting, including 15 weeks at 600 calories a day. "Profound behavioral and psychological changes" were observed, including "anxiety, depression, hostility, concern over body-size changes, sexual psychopathology, and fantasies of food or eating." Rather than viewing most of these developments as an unsurprising result of long-term confinement and near-starvation, the author termed them a "severe manifestation of an inner conflict" (Vaisrub, 1974).

Possibly guided by such equating of large body size with psychological defect, the late 1970s and early 1980s saw a flurry of studies on the "psychosocial" effects of intestinal bypass surgeries, especially the surgeries' effects on patients' marriages. The syntactically ambiguous title of one *JAMA* article – "Surgery for Obesity and Marriage Quality" (Rand, Kuldau, & Robbins, 1982) – hints at the extent to which doctors' interest went beyond the biomedical to the interpersonal: Was this surgery to reduce obesity, or surgery to improve marriage quality?

As in the "metabolic ward" study, psychoanalytic preconceptions often shaped authors' findings in the bypass studies. Neill, Marshall, and yale (1978) interviewed 12 female patients who had undergone intestinal bypass.

After the surgery, when the women had lost weight and begun to spend more time outside the home, 3 (or 25%) of the "husbands became openly homosexual," another 25% "became impotent," and 3 of the couples eventually divorced or separated. The authors argued that the surgery, by allowing women to lose weight, disrupted the (perverse) balance of power between physically large, socially powerless, psychologically unhealthy women and their dependent, latent homosexual husbands. It is "suggested," the piece stated, "that these massively obese patients are neurotic," and "their spouses usually are noticeably psychopathologic" (p. 449). Such highly dubious findings were clearly informed by and served to reinforce prejudices about large women as incapable of healthy romantic relationships [a belief historian Peter Stearns interprets as a response to anxiety about women's growing enfranchisement, dating back to the 1920s (1997)].

As long as obesity was seen primarily as a moral failing or a psychiatric ailment, it was atypical, deviant, and, necessarily, relatively rare. Researchers who saw excess weight as a symptom of severe psychoneurosis would, quite likely, have resisted the notion that roughly 50% of Americans – themselves included – were subject to this disease. Medical attention was focused on the extremely or "morbidly" obese (though there was no clear definition of this term), and often only such patients were considered subject to the ill-health effects of excess weight (Van Itallie & Kral, 1981). From the point of view of the medical community of the time, the dangerously overweight American was the exception, not the norm; he was one of *them*, not one of us.

In summary, a number of factors made the American medical landscape of the 1960s and 1970s less than fertile ground for the development of an obesity epidemic. There were (1) no universally accepted measures of or definitions of excess weight; (2) no reliable, widely known estimates of the national weight distribution; and (3) a number of cultural prejudices, driven partially by psychoanalytic theories, predicating a wide gulf between a deviant obese minority and a nonobese majority. But this landscape changed considerably beginning in the 1980s.

The 1980s Through the Present

In the 1980s, the obsessive focus on "psychoneurotic" correlates of excess weight quietly disappeared from the medical radar. A 1982 response to the Neill et al. study – eschewing the latter's prurient details and psychoanalytic subtexts – used a larger sample size and a control group to argue that marriage quality could be enhanced by obesity surgery (Rand et al., 1982).

This article was the last of the studies on bypass surgery's effects on marriage. More broadly, it may have marked the end of obesity as a psychoneurotic or psychosocial problem. This no doubt reflected paradigmatic shifts in medicine as a whole: the heyday of psychoanalysis (the 1950s and 1960s) had passed, while the maturation of molecular biology led to the ascent of a genetic paradigm in the 1980s and 1990s (Conrad, 1997). Accordingly, in the 1980s obesity research moved its focus from the psychoanalytic to the genetic.

In early 1986, the psychiatrist A. J. Stunkard published "An Adoption Study of Human Obesity" in *NEJM*, followed by "A Twin Study of Human Obesity" in *JAMA* six months later. Finding that, in terms of body mass, children resembled biological parents more than adoptive ones, and that monozygotic twins had twice the BMI concordance rates of dizygotic twins, Stunkard concluded that "human fatness is under substantial genetic control" (Stunkard, Foch, & Hrubec, 1986), and even that "the family environment alone has no apparent effect" (Stunkard et al., 1986). An accompanying *NEJM* editorial was supportive (Van Itallie, 1986). The hunt for an obesity gene was officially on.

By 1995, the idea that (possibly psychopathological) "overeating causes obesity" was dismissed in the opening of a *NEJM* editorial as a flawed "folk belief" (Bennett, 1995). The author preferred an explanation involving a "set-point mechanism" (which "sets" an individual's weight to a level not easily deviated from), its effects on metabolic processes, and its response to the "*ob* protein" (the product of an "obesity gene"). Obesity had been medicalized – or, more precisely, biomedicalized, since it was no longer explained in terms of psychoneurotic ailments, but in terms of genes, hormones, and neurotransmitters.

The 1980s also saw a major change in the definition of excess weight. In the early 1980s, medical journal contributors still struggled to extract national overweight prevalence estimates from the unwieldy MLIC tables [though sometimes they more or less succeeded: Van Itallie & Kral in *JAMA* (1981) put the percentage of overweight Americans at 20%]. But in 1985, a NIH-sponsored "Consensus Development Conference on the Health Implications of Obesity," proclaimed that "overweight" (or obesity; the terms were not yet distinguished) would henceforth be defined as a BMI above 27.3 for women and 27.8 for men, since these BMIs roughly corresponded to weights 20% above the average, medium-frame, sex-specific MLIC weights (Kuczmarski & Flegal, 2000). The BMI metric, and the cutoff values proposed, were quickly assimilated by the medical community. *JAMA* published the recommendations in 1985 (*JAMA*, 1985), following soon with a diagram of BMI values for easy reference in clinical settings (Frankel, 1986).

Medical researchers and government agencies used the 27.3|27.8 cutoffs until the late 1990s.

Coupled with the National Center for Health Statistics' nationally representative surveys – NHES (1960-2), NHANES I (1971-4), and NHANES II (1976-80) – the BMI-based standards permitted, for the first time, a reliable estimate of the national prevalence of overweight. The fact that few studies before the 1980s used NCHS data to make such estimates could have reflected a lack of adequate computing technology, but the lack of a standard, easily calculable definition of excess weight was likely a factor as well.

The acceptance of the BMI-based definition of excess weight coincided almost exactly with diffusion of the news that, based on NHANES II data, 34 million Americans, or 15% of the population, were overweight. This figure (calculated with the 27.3|27.8 cutoffs) was cited repeatedly in medical journals in the mid to late 1980s (Frankel, 1986; *JAMA*, 1989). Furthermore, this figure was an increase over the 1971–1974 prevalence obtained from NHANES I data (Raymond, 1986). This was the first inkling doctors had that national rates of excess weight were rising.

In the 1980s–1990s, "lifestyle" factors were increasingly explored, often via large epidemiological studies, as possible causes of obesity. Again, this shift in approaches reflected more general disciplinary shifts, as enhanced computing power enabled a surge in epidemiological approaches to public health matters in the late 20th century (Rothman, Greenland, & Lash, 2008). Today the importance of lifestyle factors is taken for granted, but as late as 1993 "the health benefits of exercise" were called "controversial" in a *NEJM* editorial (Curfman, 1993), and provoked heated debate in letters to the editor (Livengood, Caspersen, Koplan, & Blair, 1993).

In 1994, initial NHANES III data put the prevalence of excess weight in the United States at 33.4% – more than double the figure presented a decade earlier (Kuczmarski, Flegal, Campbell, & Johnson, 1994). A media blitz followed. Commentators suggested various public health interventions that could help people maintain healthy weights. Excess weight was no longer seen as a plague of the deranged; it was a society-wide problem that, arguably, merited society-wide solutions.

In 1997, a group of international health experts met in Geneva to establish international definitions of excess weight, as the 1985 NIH Consensus Panel had done for the United States. But the "WHO Consultation on Obesity" proposed its own categorizations of weight: BMIs below 18.5 were "underweight"; between 18.5 and 24.9 were "normal"; above 25 were "overweight"; and above 30 were "obese." The Consultation's report on obesity (WHO, 1998) was preceded by a dramatic press release about the "escalating epidemic of overweight and obesity" (WHO, 1997). The WHO report was influential, and American agencies accepted the new weight categories almost instantly, as did medical journals: in mid-1998, *JAMA* declared that, by the new standards, 55% of Americans were overweight (*JAMA*, 1998). When NHANES IV data were released soon after 2002, the percentage of overweight/obese Americans was given as 64.5% (Hedley et al., 2004).

The now-common phrase "obesity epidemic" was nearly nonexistent in medical journals before the WHO's 1997 press release. An electronic search confirms this: *JAMA* shows no hits for "obesity epidemic" or "epidemic of obesity" before 1999, but 74 hits after; *NEJM* shows 3 mentions of either phrase before the press release (but just barely before – all are from 1996–1997), and 19 afterwards.

It is useful to present a graph of how doctors' conceptions of American excess weight have changed with time. Fig. 4 compares the percentage of Americans judged overweight by the current definition (BMI > 25) with the percent said to be overweight in *JAMA* articles, using the definitions *of the time.*[4]

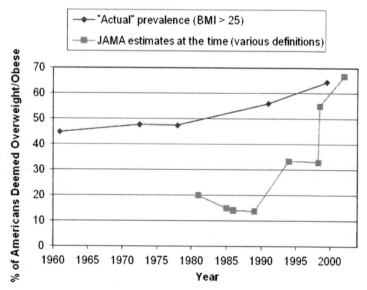

Fig. 4. Prevalence of Excess Weight (the United States): Contemporary vs. Historical Estimates. *Sources:* See footnote 4.

The top line in this graph is the same one as in Fig. 3, showing a relatively slow increase in the percentage of Americans with BMIs above 25. The lower line traces the story told in Part II: the first appearance of a national overweight prevalence estimate in *JAMA* (in 1981, using MLIC weight tables on NHANES II data), estimates using BMI cutoffs of 27.8 and 27.3 (in the mid-to-late 1980s), an estimate based on NHANES III data (1994), the switch to the 25|30 BMI cutoffs (1998), and finally, the release of NHANES IV data (in 2002). The nearly vertical rise in perceived overweight rates in mid-1998 had nothing to do with changes in the girth of the US population: it was the result of lowering BMI cutoffs to meet WHO recommendations. *JAMA* articles in March 1998, using the 27.8|27.3 cutoffs, estimated that 33% of Americans carried excess weight; articles published just 4 months later, using the 25|30 cutoffs, put overweight prevalence at 55%.

One reason American obesity has come to be widely seen as an epidemic is that public and medical awareness have followed the bottom line, not the top, in Fig. 4 above. For readers of *JAMA*, the proportion of overweight Americans jumped from 13.8% in 1989 to 66.7% just 13 years later – an astonishingly rapid change. The proportion of Americans with BMIs above 25, meanwhile, moved at a much less dramatic pace, from roughly 55% to 65%. The end point was (allowing for rounding) the same, but the former trajectory is much more likely than the latter to pass Gordis's "interocular test" – and to provoke a feeling of national panic.

DISCUSSION AND CONCLUSION

What has risen truly dramatically in recent decades, then, is not the weight distribution of Americans (though this has risen somewhat), but the proportion of Americans *considered* to have excess weight. This latter number depends as much on changing measures, definitions, data, and belief systems as it does on changing weight. Specifically, the "epidemicization" of obesity in the late 1990s was enabled by (1) the acceptance of the BMI, and of increasingly low BMI cutoffs (included those recommended by the WHO), to define excess weight; (2) the appearance of reliable, widely known estimates of obesity prevalence, based on nationally representative surveys; and (3) the decline of psychoanalysis-driven depictions of the obese as a deviant minority, supplanted by the notion of obesity as a biomedical or societal problem. These factors are not, of course, the whole story. But without the sense of rapid change in obesity rates enabled by the factors listed above, and the resulting sense of medical concern, or even panic, it is unlikely that the obesity epidemic would have been able to transcend metaphor and become fact within the American medical community.

To argue that the designation of obesity as an "epidemic" was historically contingent – and, indeed, that obesity does not qualify as a literal epidemic (unless the term is used in the broadest colloquial sense, to designate anything that is both undesirable and widespread) – is *not* to suggest that excess weight is not a risk factor for certain diseases, or that societal resources should not be directed toward improving population health via better nutrition and exercise. But it does demonstrate that public health issues come to the fore of the public consciousness for a complex host of reasons, not all of them directly related to the severity of the problem. Better understanding of such reasons could help us in evaluating, prioritizing, and ameliorating those health problems.

NOTES

1. For a more in-depth version of this paper, including a review of sociological literature on obesity and a discussion of obesity as a *global* epidemic, see Grol-Prokopczyk (2006).

2. The currently accepted measure of weight in relation to height is the BMI, calculated as weight-in-kilograms/(height-in-meters^2). US federal agencies currently define "overweight" as a BMI between 25 and 30, and "obese" as a BMI above 30. The "obesity epidemic" is often used to refer to the growing number of people with BMIs above 25, that is, it is also an "overweight epidemic."

3. JAMA allows full-text searches from 1998 on, abstract-only searches from 1975–1997, and table of contents searches from 1966–1974. NEJM allows full-text searches from 1993 on, and title/abstract searches from 1975–1992.

4. *Sources for Fig. 4:* Top line is from various waves of NHES and NHANES surveys of 20–74 year olds (NCHS, 2002), with the midpoint of the survey year range used as the *x*-axis value. Values are crude, that is, *not* age-adjusted. Bottom line is from the following *JAMA* articles: Van Itallie & Kral, 1981; Frankel, 1986; Raymond, 1986; JAMA, 1989; Kuczmarski et al., 1994; Andersen et al., 1998; JAMA, 1998; Weisberg, 2002; and Manson & Bassuk, 2003 (these last two presented as year 2002.5), and Hedley et al., 2004. For 1981, male and female prevalence are averaged to estimate overall prevalence. In 1986 and 1989, absolute numbers given are divided by Census Bureau population estimates of the given year to obtain a national percentage. Discrepancies between the two lines are due to lags in the release of survey data, rounding, and *JAMA*'s use of age-standardized, not crude, figures.

ACKNOWLEDGMENTS

I would like to thank Joan Fujimura, Doug Maynard, Jesse Norris, and Alberto Palloni for their helpful comments on an earlier version of this chapter.

REFERENCES

Andersen, R. E., Crespo, C. J., Bartlett, S. J., et al. (1998). Relationship of physical activity and television watching with body weight and level of fatness among children. *JAMA, 279*(12), 938–942.

Atkins, R. C. (1972). *Dr. Atkins' diet revolution* (pp. 297–298). New York: Bantam.

Bennett, W. I. (1995). Beyond overeating. *New England Journal of Medicine, 332*(10), 673–674.

Boba, A. (1976). Morbid obesity. *JAMA, 235*(23), 2476.

Charney, E., Goodman, H. C., McBride, M., et al. (1976). Childhood antecedents of adult obesity. *New England Journal of Medicine, 295*(1), 6–9.

Conrad, P. (1997). Public eyes and private genes: historical frames, news constructions, and social problems. *Social Problems, 44*(2), 139–154.

Coodley, A. (1975). Neurosis and obesity. *JAMA, 231*(6), 571.

Cork, R., & Vaughan, R. W. (1979). Indices of obesity. *JAMA, 242*(11), 1140.

Curfman, G. D. (1993). The health benefits of exercise – A critical reappraisal. *New England Journal of Medicine, 328*(8), 574–576.

Frankel, H. M. (1986). Determination of body mass index. *JAMA, 255*(10), 1292.

Froguel, P. (2004). Obesity: Mechanisms and clinical management. *New England Journal of Medicine, 350*, 1691–1692.

Glassman, M. (2004). Deletion opens Medicare to coverage for obesity. *New York Times*, July 16. Available at: http://www.nytimes.com/2004/07/16/politics/16obesity.html. Accessed on 17 July 2004.

Gordis, L. (2004). *Epidemiology* (3rd ed.). Philadelphia, PA: Elsevier Saunders.

Grol-Prokopczyk, H. (2006). *WHO says obesity is an epidemic? How excess weight became an American and global health crisis.* Master's thesis. University of Wisconsin-Madison, Madison, WI.

Hedley, A. A., Ogden, C. L., Johnson, C. L., et al. (2004). Prevalence of overweight and obesity among US children, adolescents, and adults, 1999–2002. *JAMA, 291*(23), 2847–2850.

JAMA. (1970). Obesity: A continuing enigma. *JAMA, 211*(3), 492.

JAMA. (1985). Consensus panel addresses obesity question. *JAMA, 254*(14), 1878.

JAMA. (1989). Prevalence of overweight – Behavioral risk factor surveillance system, 1987. *JAMA, 262*(4), 471 & 475.

JAMA. (1998). First federal obesity guidelines. *JAMA, 280*(4), 314.

Jeffcoate, W. (1998). Obesity is a disease: Food for thought. *Lancet, 351*, 903.

Kirkpatrick, R. A. (1977). A new problem from obesity. *JAMA, 237*(10), 961.

Kuczmarski, R. J., Flegal, K. M., Campbell, S. M., & Johnson, C. L. (1994). Increasing prevalence of overweight among US adults. *JAMA, 272*(3), 205–211.

Kuczmarski, R. J., & Flegal, K. M. (2000). Criteria for definition of overweight in transition. *American Journal of Clinical Nutrition, 72*, 1074–1081.

Livengood, J. R., Caspersen, C. J., Koplan, J. P., & Blair, S. N. (1993). The health benefits of exercise. *New England Journal of Medicine, 328*(25), 1852–1853.

Mann, G. V. (1977). Diet and obesity. *New England Journal of Medicine, 296*, 812.

Manson, J. E., & Bassuk, S. S. (2003). Obesity in the United States: A fresh look at its high toll. *JAMA, 289*(2), 229–230.

Mazel, J. (1981). *The Beverly Hills diet* (p. 10). New York: Macmillan Publishing.

NCHS (National Center for Health Statistics). (2002). *Health, United States, 2001. With chartbook on trends in the health of Americans.* Hyattsville, MD.

Neill, J. R., Marshall, J. R., & Yale, C. E. (1978). Marital changes after intestinal bypass surgery. *JAMA, 240*(5), 447–450.

Nelson, R. A., Anderson, L. F., Gastineau, C. F., et al. (1973). Physiology and natural history of obesity. *JAMA, 223*(6), 627–630.

New York Times. (1960). Public is advised to cut waistline. *New York Times*, February 2, p. 25.

New York Times. (1966). U.S. calls obesity a major problem. *New York Times*, November 1, p. 43.

Nidetch, J. (1972). *Weight Watchers program cookbook* (pp. 310–311). Great Neck, NY: Hearthside.

Publisher's Weekly. (2004). List of bestselling books for the entire [20th] century. *Publisher's Weekly*. Available at http://www.caderbooks.com/bestintro.html. Accessed on 19 Oct 2004.

Rand, C. S. W., Kuldau, J. M., & Robbins, L. (1982). Surgery for obesity and marriage quality. *JAMA, 247*(10), 1419–1422.

Raymond, C. A. (1986). Biology, culture, dietary changes conspire to increase incidence of obesity. *JAMA, 256*(26), 2157–2158.

Rivlin, R. S. (1975). Drug therapy: Therapy of obesity with hormones. *New England Journal of Medicine, 292*(1), 26.

Rosenberg, C. (1992). *Explaining epidemics and other studies in the history of medicine*. Cambridge: Cambridge University Press.

Roth, J. (2004). Spectre of Noah: 'Tell me a story!'. *JAMA, 292*(13), 1530.

Rothman, K. J., Greenland, S., & Lash, T. L. (2008). *Modern epidemiology* (p. 2). Philadelphia, PA: Lippincott Williams & Wilkins.

Saguy, A. C., & Riley, K. W. (2005). Weighing both sides: morality, mortality, and framing contests over obesity. *Journal of Health Politics, Policy, and Law, 30*(5), 869–923.

Slack, P. (1992). Introduction. In: T. Ranger & P. Slack (Eds), *Epidemics and ideas: Essays on the historical perception of pestilence*. Cambridge, UK: Cambridge University Press.

Stearns, P. N. (1997). *Fat history* (p. 111). New York: New York University Press.

Steelman, M. (2002). Pharmacotherapy for obesity. *New England Journal of Medicine, 346*, 2092–2093.

Stunkard, A. J., Foch, T. T., & Hrubec, Z. (1986). A twin study of obesity. *JAMA, 256*(1), 51–54.

Stunkard, A. J., Sorensen, T. I., Hanis, C., et al. (1986). An adoption study of obesity. *New England Journal of Medicine, 314*(4), 193–198.

Taller, H. (1961). *Calories don't count*. New York: Simon and Schuster.

Tarnower, H., & Baker, S. S. (1978). *The complete Scarsdale medical diet* (p. 15). New York: Rawson, Wade Publishers.

Vaisrub, S. (1974). Psychoneurosis and obesity – The hen and egg dilemma. *JAMA, 230*(4), 591.

Van Itallie, T. B. (1986). Bad news and good news about obesity. *New England Journal of Medicine, 314*(4), 239–240.

Van Itallie, T. B., & Kral, J. G. (1981). The dilemma of morbid obesity. *JAMA, 246*(9), 999–1003.

Weisberg, S. P. (2002). Societal change to prevent obesity. *JAMA, 288*(17), 2176.

WHO (World Health Organization). (1997). Press release for "WHO consultation on obesity, Geneva, 3–5 June 1997" (12 June). Available at http://www.who.int. Accessed on 7 Nov 2004.

WHO (World Health Organization). (1998). *Obesity: preventing and managing the global epidemic: Report of a WHO consultation on obesity*. Geneva, 3–5 June 1997. World Health Organization: Geneva.

"WHO ARE YOU CALLING 'FAT'?": THE SOCIAL CONSTRUCTION OF THE OBESITY EPIDEMIC

Alana J. Hermiston

ABSTRACT

Purpose – *In North America today, we are witnessing an unprecedented preoccupation with "excess" weight, with millions of people perceived to be part of the* epidemic *of obesity. While this chapter does not seek to contest medical evidence that average weights of North Americans have risen in recent years, nor deny the potential development of associated health problems, it offers a critique of the terminology invoked in these discussions and especially challenges the characterization of increased weight among the population as an "epidemic." This chapter suggests that what we are witnessing is more appropriately understood as a moral regulation project premised on ideas of risk, contagion, and neoliberal discourses of health.*

Methodology/approach – *In arguing that the concern about obesity may be understood as an example of moral regulation, this chapter employs the work of Alan Hunt, as well as Deborah Lupton's insights on governmentality and health.*

Findings – *In reviewing the scholarly literature on obesity as well as Canadian public health initiatives, a discourse of risk and contagion is*

Understanding Emerging Epidemics: Social and Political Approaches
Advances in Medical Sociology, Volume 11, 359–369
ISSN: 1057-6290/doi:10.1108/S1057-6290(2010)0000011023

evident. The overweight and obese (and these are commonly conflated) are presented as dangerous to themselves and others.

Contribution to the field – *In suggesting an alternative understanding of the obesity "epidemic" as a socially constructed and morally regulated phenomenon, this chapter aims to further discuss and reassess how those who are considered fat are understood and treated in North America.*

INTRODUCTION

Western ideals of body weight have shifted historically, from concerns about building strong bodies during the Depression and wartime eras, to admiration and condemnation of the "thin ideal" of the 1980s, to the current alarm generated by the "mass" of obese bodies identified in North America today. But where in previous eras particular populations (e.g., the working class, soldiers, and women) were the focus of corporeal concern, obesity is today seen as transcending categories, a risk to which literally *any body* may be susceptible, and against which all bodies must be protected.[1]

Over the last two decades, obesity has become a preoccupation for scientists, medical professionals, educators, social workers, and legislators. It has been defined as a significant public health issue, with both society and individuals being blamed for its dramatic increase. At the social level, factors identified as contributing to the increased body weights of North Americans include the proliferation of high-calorie "convenience" foods, a sedentary lifestyle, marketing strategies of the "fast-food" industry, and poor access to medical care. At the individual level, accusations of laziness, lack of motivation, and poor self-esteem are frequently levelled at those whose bodies are considered threatening.

While acknowledging that the average weights of adults and children in Canada and the United States have risen substantially, this chapter seeks to challenge the uncritical acceptance of the characterization of this phenomenon as an "epidemic." Is this really an appropriate description? Rather than an epidemic, I suggest that what we are witnessing is a moral regulation project related to neoliberal discourses of health. As Hunt (1999, pp. 6–7) explains, "moral regulation involves the deployment of distinctly moral discourses which construct a moralized subject and an object or target which is acted upon by means of moralizing practices." In contrast to the evangelistic discourse of earlier eras, modern moral regulation projects invoke the language of science, medicine, and social work (Valverde, 1994;

Hunt, 1999); the fat body is constructed as deviant and indeed, dangerous. The "risky" behaviours of the obese warrant intervention. In Canada, this is evident through the significant number of governmental initiatives introduced in recent years, such as the *Canadian Clinical Practice Guidelines on the Management and Prevention of Obesity in Adults and Children*, the Children's Fitness Tax Credit, and a more comprehensive revision of *Canada's Food Guide*, among others.

This chapter considers the strategic identification of obesity as an "epidemic," arguing that the terminology constructs increased weight as a risk to which we are all susceptible, and thus one which we must all take measures to avoid. Such a characterization supports the neoliberal call upon us to assume responsibility for ourselves, to take the necessary steps to ensure our emotional and physical health. And if being called "fat" does not encourage us to change our perceived behaviours, then perhaps being positioned within an "epidemic" will.

CONSTRUCTING AND DECONSTRUCTING THE OBESITY EPIDEMIC

Certainly the "obesity epidemic" is a popular tagline, with newspapers and medical journals alleging its rapid spread across the continent. Even respected international organizations such as the World Health Organization have embraced the terminology, arguing that it is in fact a global crisis, not limited to the slothful North American populace (1997, 2008). However, I submit the term "epidemic" is an inaccurate depiction, traditionally reserved for an infectious disease that spreads rapidly, resulting in sudden widespread death. As historian Slack (1992, p. 3) notes, epidemics have largely been understood as "being transmitted from person to person and as arising from particular, usually filthy, local conditions: notions of 'contagion' and 'miasma', of a more or less undefined kind, were combined." Medical historian Rosenberg suggests another "defining component of epidemics ... is their episodic quality. A true epidemic is an *event*, not a trend. It elicits immediate and widespread response" (1992, p. 279, emphasis added). Considered alongside these criteria, obesity does not seem to qualify.

Admittedly, there has been a shift in sensibility regarding epidemics (Slack, 1992), with the idea of contagion through poor hygiene practices and person-to-person contact being increasingly replaced with an understanding of contamination as "any event or agent that might subvert a health-maintaining configuration" (Rosenberg, 1992, p. 295). While this expanded definition may be rightfully lauded for moving us away from the "poor and infirm" blaming characteristic of the Victorian age (Valverde, 1991), it also serves to open up the possibilities of what may be considered "potentially epidemic" behaviour.

Consequently, the modern era is witnessing more than its share of "epidemics" – alcohol consumption, teenage sexual behaviour, obesity, and even apathy – that are presented as subverting the health of society. Rosenberg argues the term is intentionally used "to clothe certain undesirable yet blandly tolerated social phenomena in the emotional urgency associated with a 'real' epidemic" (1992, p. 279). Boero uses the term "post-modern epidemics" to describe this process "in which unevenly medicalized phenomena lacking a clear pathological basis get cast in the language and moral panic of 'traditional' epidemics" (2007, p. 41).

Indeed, critics of this strategic use of the term have argued that obesity does not even meet the criteria of a disease, let alone an epidemic. Gard and Wright (2005) and Oliver (2006) note the lack of objective standards for establishing "obesity" as a "condition," and question the association of weight and sickness. As Oliver (2006, p. 37) asks: "is someone who is only slightly overweight, only slightly diseased? Can someone catch or 'come down' with obesity?" Furthermore, the health problems commonly attributed to obesity are hardly exclusive to it. Ross (2005) points out that associated health problems such as mobility issues, high blood pressure, diabetes, or damaged joints are also commonly found among the non-obese population. Moreover, Ross argues that while excess weight may contribute to ill health, it does not itself constitute a specific state of ill health: "We would not classify car crashes as a disease yet they contribute significantly to ill health as does poverty and industrial pollution. In other words, obesity is not a diagnosable illness in its own right, meaning that if you are fat you are ill. Some fat people are well and some thin people are unwell" (2005, p. 95).[2]

It is not my intention to enter the debate surrounding the scientific and medical claims about the health risks of obesity. Rather, I am interested as to how obesity has itself become constructed as something "contagious" that poses a risk to all of us, and as such, is presented as a significant social problem.

Unlike earlier epidemics, where risk of contamination was commonly located within specific populations, everyone is perceived as being at risk of becoming obese.[3] When people are identified as being particularly susceptible, they are most often those for whom the larger society is expected to take responsibility (most notably children). Overwhelmingly, the obesity epidemic is presented as a predictable outcome of the North American "lifestyle," treating all of us as a homogeneous population. From an epidemiological standpoint, this is understood to facilitate the spread of contagion; from a sociological perspective, this might be considered "guilt by association." Parents, partners, or friends who "allow" their loved ones to become fat must share culpability.

But this is not a new issue. Concern with weight (among individuals and in terms of health demographics) has a lengthy history, and the evidence that, as a people, North Americans are getting fatter has been documented for over 20 years (Levenstein, 1993; Gard & Wright, 2005; Boero, 2007).[4] What *is* new is the intensity and scope of the attention being focused on this pattern of growth. There are many scholars, scientists, and health care professionals who argue that the availability of highly processed, calorie-laden foods and an increasingly sedentary lifestyle have created this epidemic, and thus express dire warnings of the ill health that will befall us unless we take immediate action to change our habits. In contrast, I suggest that the lack of popular concern and thus limited social and individual response to these "expert" predictions has led to the construction of the "obesity epidemic" as a strategic attempt to coerce North Americans into adopting a "healthier" way of life.

THE "RISK" OF BEING FAT

In his examination of the AIDS crisis, Rosenberg argues that for most people, the epidemic is a "media reality, both exaggerated and diminished as it is articulated in forms suitable for mass consumption. The great majority of Americans have been spectators, *in* but not *of* the epidemic" (1992, p. 290). I would suggest that until recently, a similar pattern has held true for obesity. Where many of us might carry "extra" pounds, we decline to see ourselves as "fat." Chubby perhaps, even "pleasantly plump," but not obese. The experts call this denial, but might it not in fact be considered a reasonable and healthy response, certainly healthier than being preoccupied with scales and pant sizes? The rejection of this description (or diagnosis) also makes sense when one considers the societal response to fat people in North America. Numerous studies have demonstrated strong prejudices against those considered fat, perceiving them to be morally suspect, lazy, and repulsive.[5] Who would want to identify with such a despised segment of the population?

But with ostensibly "objective" measurement criteria such as the body mass index and the increasingly popular tape measure test,[6] used in tandem with physiological, social, and psychological testing for "predisposition" towards obesity, it is increasingly difficult to avoid being placed in the ranks of the fat (or at least, the potentially fat). Following Rosenberg's description, North Americans are becoming *of* the epidemic.

Situated as such, citizens are expected to do something about it. If being obese is morally reprehensible, fighting obesity is morally commended. Identifying the trend towards heavier bodies as an "epidemic" serves to create fear among the population, not to mention further stigmatizing those who are (in many cases subjectively) determined to belong to the category of the "obese" of health. Hunt's work on moral regulation may be usefully employed to understand this process. As noted above, moral regulation involves a target that is acted upon: "Moral discourses seek to act on conduct that is deemed to be intrinsically bad or wrong" (Hunt, 1999, pp. 6–7). Furthermore, "moralizing discourses frequently invoke some utilitarian consideration linking the immoral practice to some form of harm" (Hunt, 1999, p. 7).

Hunt observes that the process of moral governance is not restricted to formalized relationships (such as that of patient–physician, or government–citizen), but can emerge from different social positions. He asserts that "moral regulation involves some people acting on other people and in so doing acting upon themselves" (Hunt, 1999, p. 19). Faced with an "epidemic," this is precisely what citizens are encouraged to do – monitor and regulate themselves and others, avoiding the "bad" behaviours which exacerbate the spread of contagion. In this, *risk* must be understood as a key component of moral regulation.

Again, I am not concerned here with the validity or probabilities of the "risks" of obesity, but rather, with the *problematization* of risk – that is, how the "obesity epidemic" has mobilized concepts of risk, and the motivations behind this strategy. While most sociocultural theorists concur that risk is a political concept, there is less agreement as to whether risk has some kind of objective tangibility, or is entirely a social construction. In popular usage, "risk" is less likely to be used to convey the odds of an event occurring, but rather, the phenomenon itself is presented as a risk. So, for example, obesity is portrayed as a risk in itself, something we may "catch." In the context of concerns about excess weight, Giddens' articulation of risk seems particularly relevant. He writes: "The notion of risk becomes central in a society which is taking leave of traditional ways of doing things, and which is opening itself up to a problematic future" (1991, p. 111). For Giddens, risk is a concept produced by a society preoccupied with controlling the unknown. Neoliberal discourses of health encourage (indeed *expect*) us to assume responsibility for our well-being; the literal growth of bodies creates concern and generates speculation about what *might* happen if left unchecked. Despite the conviction with which the obesity epidemic is reported upon, there is in fact little consensus as to what, exactly, the threat is (Gard & Wright, 2005; Oliver, 2006): "It is as if empirical confusion and uncertainty has created the perfect environment for rampant speculation" (Gard & Wright, 2005, p. 5). If eliminating, or at least minimizing, the risks of obesity is the goal, then people must first be educated as to their existence, and accept that they are harmful and to be avoided. While the risks may not yet be definitively articulated, the fear of fat is very real. As a society, we are uncomfortable with its symbolism of abundance, the suggestion of lack of self-discipline, and moral weakness (Sobal, 1995; Poulton, 1996; Gard & Wright, 2005; Oliver, 2006). This is a crucial element in enlisting the public in the moral regulation of obesity.

Leichter notes that "good health constitutes affirmation of a life lived virtuously" (1997, p. 359). Fat people are perceived to lack the willpower to resist "bad" foods and behaviours, as failing to adhere to the medical recommendations, and as such, as being disrespectful of the societal value of "healthy" (read: not fat) bodies. The overweight and the obese do not (to borrow a phrase from Foucault) practise "care of the self." Far from being a matter of individual choice and actions, care of the self is a "true social practice" (Foucault, 1986, p. 51). There is a sense of a communal goal (the fight against obesity) which may be met through individual discipline (adopting a healthy lifestyle). As Lupton (1995, p. 119) observes, those who fail to conform are seen as "not only socially unacceptable, but as selfishly endangering the health of all others around them."[7]

As noted above, obesity is not a new concern; the increase in body weights of North Americans has been tracked for many years, yet the pattern has continued. Through the use of an old strategy – that of moral regulation – the general public is being reminded of the common threat, and thus encouraged to share responsibility for the obesity "epidemic." Becoming the disciplined, healthy member of society, that is, the "good" subject requires action, diligence, and motivation: "This time is not empty; it is filled with exercises, practical tasks, various activities. Taking care of oneself is not a rest cure" (Foucault, 1986, p. 51). It seems to me quite straightforward that we strive to behave in accordance with the moral message because of the perceived risks associated with not doing so. Where being called "fat" is an insult, it is also a *diagnosis*, a warning of existing or impending health complications and reduced quality of life. And not just our own lives, but those of our fellow citizens: if the stigma of being fat were not enough, we now endure the stigma of allowing oneself or others to get fat, of not pursuing "healthy" choices, and of being a burden on the health care system.[8] Even ostensibly "scientific" discussions of obesity frame the trend in language that constructs the subjects in morally suspect ways. Fat people are routinely characterized as being too ignorant of nutritional recommendations and standards to eat properly and exercise regularly, or as lacking the discipline to do so.[9] In this, they help spread the "contagion." For instance, research now suggesting that fat is "catching" and that people who associate with the overweight are at greater risk of becoming fatter themselves[10] is a clear example of risk discourse being employed in an effort to modify people's behaviours.

Lupton (1999, p. 87) describes risk as "a governmental strategy of regulatory power by which populations and individuals are monitored and managed through the goals of neo-liberalism." Neoliberalism calls upon the individual to practise self-care, but this should not be confused with demedicalization; while viewed as a moral failure, obesity is still very much located within the realm of "illness."[11] Distinctions between "healthy" and "unhealthy" become blurred when everything is a potential source of risk (Petersen, 1997, p. 195). The expansion of health promotion and predetection results in the identification of more risks, and it is largely individuals who are expected to assume responsibility for risk avoidance. To avoid risk is to behave morally; failure to avoid risk, or moreover, voluntarily exposing oneself to risk represents a moral failing at the individual level, and a threat to the safety and well-being of the social body. Petersen (1997) describes the phenomenon of "healthism," in which those who do not live risk-free lives are seen as negligent in their duties to the self and others.[12] The undisciplined fat body is evidence of such negligence, and must be remedied.

CONCLUSION

As argued above, moral regulation projects invoke notions of risk and morality in order to gain support for the particular cause. As Hunt explains, they involve "a normative judgement that some conduct is intrinsically bad, wrong, or immoral" (1999, p. 7). Packaging obesity as an epidemic, a threat to all, is an effective means of motivating the population. But if the appeal to ideas of good citizenship, self-care, and stewardship of the larger society are not sufficiently persuasive, the obesity epidemic also relies heavily on the economic factor. Medical professionals and government legislators have issued dire warnings of the impact obesity will have on the already overburdened health care system. This line of argument is especially popular in Canada, where the projected costs of caring for an obese population are portrayed as the death knell for its highly valued system of universal health care.[13] In the United States, insurance providers are balking at covering anti-obesity treatments and therapies.[14] In more ways than one, fat people are seen as taking more than their share.

An assessment of the validity of the risks of excess weight is beyond the scope of this discussion, and indeed, not the point of it. In the face of conflicting scientific evidence and lack of consensus about the effects of extra pounds, experts caution the public not to rely on their own "feelings," but rather accept the idea that we are all at risk for obesity, and thus be vigilant against it (Gard & Wright, 2005; Oliver, 2006; Boero, 2007). The actual reality of the potential harm is less important than the moral arguments, as Hunt (2003, p. 167) explains: "[Moral and risk discourses] merge their characteristics into a distinctively new form. The most striking feature of the hybridization of morals and risks is the creation of an apparently benign form of moralization in which the boundary between objective hazards and normative judgments becomes blurred." Oliver agrees, noting "As with AIDS or even cancer, we attribute so much more to obesity than the reality of what is just a large amount of body fat" (2006, p. 57).

In this chapter, I have suggested that neither historical nor contemporary definitions of "epidemic" are appropriately applied to obesity. Instead, I have introduced the idea that the focus on obesity in North America may be more appropriately understood as a moral regulation project premised on ideas of risk, contagion, and neoliberal discourses of health. While the link of fatness and health problems is still contentious for some, the connection of fatness and immorality goes largely unchallenged in a society that values discipline and self-care. While fat bodies may have real, physical limitations, the idea that they present a threat to the larger society is overwhelmingly a social construction. Experts may warn that fat is "catching," but what is feared is a transfer of "bad" behaviours, and loss of self-control. And so, to return to the question that began this discussion – "Who are you calling 'fat'?" – the answer is: "potentially everyone." And it is the contagiousness of this *idea* that makes it an effective regulatory discourse.

NOTES

1. Admittedly, children have been identified as a group warranting particular concern, but there is considerable discussion of obesity addressing increased body weight among the general population.

2. There is also commonly a conflation of obesity and being overweight in regards to articulating potential health concerns.

3. Boero (2007) argues that there is a variation in degree of risk, and while I agree that is factually accurate, I would argue those differences are largely ignored in discussions of obesity, with the population being treated as a homogeneous entity.

4. In this, the trend towards being overweight fails to meet yet another of Rosenberg's criteria of the true epidemic, which he says "does not proceed with imperceptible effect until retrospectively 'discovered'" (1992, p. 279).

5. Oliver (2006) makes reference to a number of these. Similar findings are reported in Poulton (1996), Stearns (1997), and Gard and Wright (2005).

6. This test identifies health risks based on girth measurement alone.

7. Lupton uses the example of smokers in her analysis; I feel it can also be usefully applied to the overweight and obese.

8. This argument is particularly prominent in those nations with publicly funded health care systems, such as Canada.

9. Such responses may be found in both popular media (such as Internet blogs and columns) and more scholarly work.

10. According to the findings of Dr. N. Christakis and Dr. J. Fowler, as reported by the Canadian Press (2007a).

11. Although, as noted above, this is a contentious understanding.

12. Lupton (1995) uses the term "lifestyle risk discourse" to describe this process.

13. The Government of Canada report on "The Obesity Epidemic in Canada" (Starky, 2005) estimates the economic burden to be $4.3 billion annually including direct and indirect costs. In recent years there have been published reports of "obese" individuals being denied access to medical procedures due to their weight.

14. However, Oliver (2006) argues that the medicalization of obesity has been a financial windfall for many across the health care spectrum, including weight-loss doctors, researchers, and pharmaceutical companies. And in the province of Alberta, Canada, surgeons negotiated a 25 percent raise in their pay scale for surgeries on obese patients (Canadian Press, 2007b).

REFERENCES

Boero, N. (2007). All the news that's fat to print: the American "obesity epidemic" and the media. *Qualitative Sociology, 30*, 41–60.

Canadian Press. (2007a). Is obesity contagious? *Peterborough Examiner*, 26 July, p. A6.

Canadian Press. (2007b). Obesity pays more for doctors. *Peterborough Examiner*, 28 July, p. A5.

Foucault, M. (1986). *The care of the self.* New York: Vintage Books.

Gard, M., & Wright, J. (2005). *The obesity epidemic: Science, morality and ideology.* London: Routledge.

Giddens, A. (1991). *Modernity and self-identity: Self and society in the late modern age.* Stanford: Stanford University Press.

Hunt, A. (1999). *Governing morals: A social history of moral regulation.* Cambridge: Cambridge University Press.

Hunt, A. (2003). Risk and moralization in everyday life. In: R. Ericson & S. Doyle (Eds), *Risk and morality* (pp. 165–192). Toronto: University of Toronto Press.

Leichter, H. M. (1997). Lifestyle corrrectness and the new secular morality. In: A. M. Brandt & P. Rozin (Eds), *Morality and health* (pp. 359–378). London: Routledge.

Levenstein, H. (1993). *Paradox of plenty: A social history of eating in modern America.* New York: Oxford University Press.

Lupton, D. (1995). *The imperative of health: Public health and the regulated body.* London: Sage.

Lupton, D. (1999). *Risk.* London: Routledge.

Oliver, J. E. (2006). *Fat politics: The real story behind America's obesity epidemic.* New York: Oxford University Press.

Petersen, A. (1997). Risk, governance and the new public health. In: A. Petersen & R. Bunton (Eds), *Foucault, health and medicine* (pp. 189–206). London: Routledge.

Poulton, T. (1996). *No fat chicks: How women are brainwashed to hate their bodies and spend their money.* Toronto: Key Porter Books.

Rosenberg, C. E. (1992). *Explaining epidemics and other studies in the history of medicine.* Cambridge: Cambridge University Press.

Ross, B. (2005). Fat or fiction: Weighing the 'obesity epidemic'. In: M. Gard & J. Wright (Eds), *The obesity epidemic: Science, morality and ideology* (Ch.5). London: Routledge.

Slack, P. (1992). Introduction. In: T. Ranger & P. Slack (Eds), *Epidemics and ideas: Essays on the historical perception of pestilence* (pp. 1–20). Cambridge: Cambridge University Press.

Sobal, J. (1995). The medicalization and demedicalization of obesity. In: D. Maurer & J. Sobal (Eds), *Eating agendas: Food and nutrition as social problems* (pp. 67–90). New York: Aldine de Gruyter.

Starky, S. (2005). *The obesity epidemic in Canada* (PRB 05-11E). Ottawa: Library of Parliament.

Stearns, P. (1997). *Fat history: Bodies and beauty in the modern West.* New York: New York University Press.

Valverde, M. (1991). *The age of light, soap, and water: Moral reform in English Canada, 1885–1925.* Toronto: McClelland & Stewart.

Valverde, M. (1994). Moral capital. *Canadian Journal of Law and Society, 9*(1), 213–232.

World Health Organization. (1997). *Executive summary, preventing and managing the global epidemic – Report of a WHO consultation on obesity, 3–5 June.* WHO, Geneva. Available at http://www.who.int/nutrition/publications/obesity_executive_summary.pdf. Accessed on 1 November 2008.

World Health Organization. (2008). *Obesity and overweight.* Available at http://www.who.int/dietphysicalactivity/publications/facts/obesity/en/print.html. Accessed on 1 November 2008.